Praise for *The 30-Day Vegan C*

D0132070

"A beautiful and inspiring guide to the immense delight that can be yours
—John Robbins, author *Diet For A N*   ork

"With common sense, compassion, and crazy delicious recipes, Colleen Patrick-Goudreau takes you on a joyful journey that will heal your body, enrich your spirit, and nourish your mind (not to mention your belly). *The 30-Day Vegan Challenge* is a keepsake that will change your life for all its inspiration and information."
—Kris Carr, New York Times best selling author, *Crazy Sexy Kitchen*

"What a delicious way to get more energy, say good-bye to those stubborn pounds, and get healthy for good."
—Neal D. Barnard, MD, president, Physicians Committee for Responsible Medicine, and author of *21-Day Weight Loss Kickstart*

"In this beautiful and compelling book, Colleen Patrick-Goudreau becomes your personal mentor for a 30-day journey that will change your life, improve your health, and create a kinder world. The challenge takes a month; the gifts last a lifetime."
—Victoria Moran, author of *Main Street Vegan* and director, Main Street Vegan Academy

"A gorgeous, smart, insightful book to guide you through the ins and outs of eating a healthful vegan diet."
—Rip Esselstyn, bestselling author of *The Engine 2 Diet* and *My Beef with Meat*

"Whatever your motivation for making changes to your diet, *The 30-Day Vegan Challenge* is an extraordinary resource and guide by Colleen Patrick-Goudreau. She inspires, motivates, and informs - all while tantalizing your taste buds with delectable plant-based recipes. This is a book to treasure."
—Julieanna Hever, MS, RD, CPT, author of *The Complete Idiot's Guide to Plant-Based Nutrition* and host of *What Would Julieanna Do?*

"Colleen Patrick-Goudreau brings together in a beautifully produced book all the information anyone needs to make the transition to healthy, compassionate vegan living. And there's also much for vegans to learn!"
—Kim Stallwood, author, *Growl: Life Lessons, Hard Truths, and Bold Strategies from an Animal Advocate*

"I love everything about Colleen Patrick-Goudreau and the content she produces to help anyone go vegan. Colleen capably and gently guides readers on the basics by supporting, encouraging, and inspiring!"
—JL Fields, vegan cook, coach, and consultant, author of *Vegan Pressure Cooking*, and co-author of *Vegan for Her*

Books by Colleen

The Joy of Vegan Baking: The Compassionate
Cooks' Traditional Treats and Sinful Sweets
(Fair Winds, 2007)

The Vegan Table: 200 Unforgettable Recipes for
Entertaining Every Guest at Every Occasion
(Fair Winds, 2009)

Color Me Vegan: Maximize Your Nutrient Intake and
Optimize Your Health by Eating Antioxidant-Rich,
Fiber-Packed, Color-Intense Meals That Taste Great
(Fair Winds, 2010)

Vegan's Daily Companion: 365 Days of Inspiration for
Cooking, Eating, and Living Compassionately
(Quarry Press, 2011)

The 30-Day Vegan Challenge®: The Ultimate Guide to
Eating Cleaner, Getting Leaner, and Living Compassionately
(Ballantine Books, Original Edition 2011, OUT OF PRINT)

On Being Vegan: Reflections on a Compassionate Life
(Montali Press, 2013)

The 30-Day Vegan Challenge® Online Program

As a companion to the book you're holding in your hands, Colleen
Patrick-Goudreau also created The 30-Day Vegan Challenge® multi-
media online program, featuring outstanding written, audio, and video
content to give you everything you need to support you on your journey
towards optimal wellness and unconditional compassion. Sign up today
at 30dayveganchallenge.com for engaging videos, informative audio
messages, daily emails, and a community message board.

The 30-Day Vegan Challenge

The Ultimate Guide to Eating Healthfully and Living Compassionately

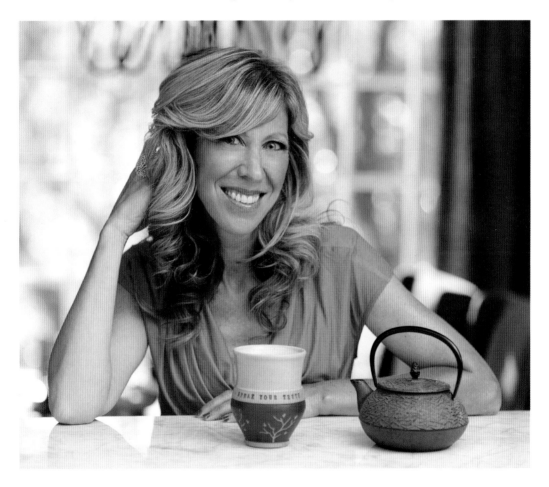

by Colleen Patrick–Goudreau

This Roundtree Press edition published in 2017.

First Compassionate Cooks, LLC, edition published in 2014.

Library of Congress Cataloging-in-Publication
Data available.

ISBN: 978-1-944903-14-5

Printed in China

10 9 8 7 6 5 4 3 2 1

Cover and interior design by Sarah Cadwell • sarahcadwell.com

Cover and interior photographs of Colleen, David, and cats
by Maria Villano Photography • mariavillano.com

Food photographs by Marie Laforêt • marielaforet.com

Photos of Colleen with Linus, Dawn, Lassen, and Waylon by Connie Pugh

Art direction by Colleen Patrick-Goudreau

Vegan Challenge is a trademark of Compassionate Cooks, LLC

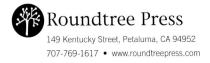

Roundtree Press

149 Kentucky Street, Petaluma, CA 94952
707-769-1617 • www.roundtreepress.com

Dedication

Michael, the Magnanimous.

Michael, the Mischievous.

Michael, the Magnificent.

You were here for the beginning but left before the end.

This renaissance is in memory of you, Michael Scribner.

In all likelihood, you have already made a spirited decision to accept the 30-Day Vegan Challenge and embark on a journey that may, at this moment, seem rather daunting. Fear not! You could not have chosen a wiser way to begin.

The 30-Day Vegan Challenge is no ordinary book; it is an extraordinary vehicle of change that is beautifully crafted to offer every morsel of support imaginable as you venture through unfamiliar territory. While your head may be spinning with questions, I can assure you that each and every one of those questions will be thoughtfully addressed in the pages that follow. Take a deep breath, and know that you are in very capable hands.

My personal experience is as a registered dietitian. When I first decided to become vegan in the late 1980s, I was employed as a public health nutritionist. I was not sure if there was another vegan dietitian on the planet. I thought that once the truth was uncovered, I might very well be ousted from the profession. I wondered how I could remain in a career that had at its very foundation 4 food groups, two of which were animal-based. The only reference to vegan diets made during my entire university training was a stern warning that such extreme regimes were downright dangerous. After considerable soul searching, I decided that I would stick with my chosen profession and make no apologies for my ethical choices. I decided that the balance of my career would be spent helping to ensure that those who had chosen a similar path would have the necessary nutrition information to succeed brilliantly.

With each passing year, the evidence in favor of plant-based diets grows stronger. Today, even the most conservative medical and dietetic organizations in the world acknowledge the safety, adequacy and health benefits associated with vegan diets. This shift is solidly reflected in the marketplace where mainstream manufacturers are increasingly using the word vegan on labels to sell their product. It is quite possible that these companies could find no single word that better captures the ideals consumers are seeking out: healthful, wholesome, responsible, ethical, and eco-friendly.

The evidence is quite clear that vegans have lower body mass indexes and are at reduced risk for most chronic diseases, including heart disease, hypertension, type 2 diabetes, and some forms of cancer. These are the very things that fill our doctor's offices, hospitals, and graveyards. We live in a food environment that is essentially toxic. The incontrovertible fact is that our food system is responsible for the vast majority of our health care expenditures. Well-planned vegan diets produce a dramatic shift in this paradigm. And while the personal health benefits of vegan diets are impressive, their consequences beyond personal health are perhaps even more compelling.

Adopting a vegan lifestyle is arguably the most powerful step any one individual can take towards the preservation of this planet. It takes about $\frac{1}{20}$th the resources to feed a vegan that it takes to feed a nonvegetarian.

But perhaps the most gripping argument of all is that of ethics. For many of us, the beautiful illustrations of family farms in children's story books stay indelibly etched in our minds. Unfortunately, for today's farm animals, their lives are about as far removed from these images as they could possibly be. A hundred years ago, over 40% of Americans lived on farms; today the figure is close to 2%. With the consumption of animal products rising, how is it possible to supply sufficient meat and milk for such a huge demographic? Every year in North America we slaughter over 10 billion land animals for food and over 90% of these animals are raised in concentrated animal feeding operations (CAFO's), otherwise known as factory farms. These facilities turn sociable, intelligent, feeling animals into production units. Their goal is simple - to produce the greatest amount of meat in the shortest possible time for the least amount of money. The consequences for animals are both unthinkable and unjustifiable. Although the average consumer is far removed from these establishments, efforts to invoke a sense of compassion in individuals are beginning to take hold. One can only hope that the words of Dr. Albert Schweitzer, one of the greatest humanitarians of all times, will soon ring true:

"...the time is coming when people will be amazed that the human race existed so long before it recognized that thoughtless injury to life is incompatible with real ethics. Ethics is in its unqualified form extended responsibility with regard to everything that has life."

Each and every one of us who dreams of a kinder, gentler world; who shares this vision of real ethics has the capacity to turn their thoughts into actions, and to bring us a little closer to this reality. By picking up this book, you have taken the first courageous step towards this end.

When I had the privilege of reading *The 30-Day Vegan Challenge* in its entirety, I was touched by the compassion woven through each and every word; I was awed by the painstaking attention to detail, and I was impressed by its reliability and readability. In a laudable effort to provide you with the most complete and practical guide possible, no stone was left unturned. Colleen Patrick-Goudreau is an outstanding writer and a remarkable human being. I cannot imagine finding a more capable and delightful partner in this journey. I am grateful that such a comprehensive resource exists and delighted that you have chosen to accept this challenge. May this journey be the journey of a lifetime. May it be a source of immeasurable rewards for you and for those with whom you are connected.

Get Ready!

Get Set!

Go!

CONTENTS

Get Ready!

CHAPTER 1

Welcome to Positive Change

Although our paths may look different, we are all facing the same direction. Perhaps you made your way to *The 30-Day Vegan Challenge* motivated by a need to get healthier or lose weight, by the desire to help decrease the use of the world's limited resources, or because, like me, you want to manifest your compassion for animals. Frankly, I think most people will tell you that although there was one single thing that sparked their desire to be vegan, they continue to remain so for a bevy of reasons. I think this is why this journey is so incredible: *you just don't know where it's going to take you.* I also think it's why this journey can be so scary for people: *you just don't know where it's going to take you.*

Fear not. I'm here to guide you every step of the way, and whatever your motivation, eliminating animal products from your diet—even for 30 days—will reap many benefits, some of which you may have never even considered before and some of which are very tangible and measurable.

Many of the changes people experience upon becoming vegan are immediate, and some are noticeable within 30 days, but all of them can be sorted into several categories of positive change, such as nutrient consumption, disease prevention and reversal, physical changes, palate sensitivity, and a sense of ethical congruency.

NUTRIENT CONSUMPTION

When people think about "being vegan," they often think about what you "give up" or—as I prefer, *let go of*. But being vegan is as much about what you take in as it is about what you eliminate.

What You Can Expect None Of

When you eliminate meat, dairy, and eggs from your diet, I can absolutely guarantee that you will be consuming *no* dietary cholesterol, no lactose, no animal protein, no animal hormones, no animal fat, and no aberrant proteins that cause "mad cow disease" (bovine spongiform encephalopathy)—all of which originate in animal products and not in plants. Not only are these things unnecessary, they can all be harmful to the human body.

What You Can Expect More Of

When you increase your consumption of plants, I can guarantee you will be eating more fiber, more antioxidants, more folate, and more phytochemicals because the source of these healthful substances is plants—not animals. You will also be taking in more essential vitamins and minerals because—as you will soon discover—the nutrients we need are *plant-based*.

What You Can Expect Significantly Less Of

Making whole foods the foundation of your diet means that you will significantly reduce your consumption of many other disease-causing substances, including:

- **Saturated Fat**—Though it exists mostly in animal flesh and fluids, saturated fat is also found in small amounts in plant foods, primarily coconuts. However, plant-based saturated fat is chemically different from animal-based saturated fat and does not seem to have the same negative affect on our bodies; in other words, a little virgin coconut oil, coconut butter, or coconut milk in your diet is fine—possibly even beneficial.

- **Heavy Metals**—Heavy metals such as mercury and other toxins settle in the fatty flesh of animals and are consumed by humans through their consumption of fish, dairy, and meat. The reason I didn't add them to the "Expect None" category is because even vegans consume low levels of heavy metals that end up on our food but in *significantly* less quantities.

- **Foodborne Illnesses**—Although there is still a risk of vegans consuming tainted fruits and vegetables that they buy in a store or restaurant, because they are not eating animals and animal products, the risk is much lower. When you keep a vegan kitchen, about the worst thing you might find is aphids in your kale and a borer worm in your corn.

- **Trans Fats**—By eating whole foods, you take in far fewer trans fats, which are prevalent in processed foods via partially hydrogenated oils and which are present also in animal meats.

DISEASE PREVENTION AND REVERSAL

Decades of peer-reviewed research have proven the many benefits of a plant-based diet in terms of disease prevention and reversal. If your goal is prevention, treatment, or reversal of cardiovascular disease (particularly the atherosclerosis that causes heart attacks and strokes), you couldn't make a better choice than switching to a plant-based diet based on whole foods. And even by the end of a short period such as 30 days, you will see changes in the markers for these diseases—especially if you had your blood work done before you begin.

Countless studies also point to the fact that a plant-based diet contributes to reduced risk of type 2 diabetes,[1] certain cancers—particularly prostate,[2] colon,[3] and breast[4]—macular degeneration,[5] cataracts,[6] arthritis,[7] and osteoporosis.[8]

PHYSICAL CHANGES

Typically, the physical changes people detect have to do with what they tend to lose, but there are gains to be made, as well.

What You Can Expect to Lose

People *tend* to lose weight when they remove fat- and calorie-dense meat, dairy, and eggs from their diet because fat-laden foods have more calories than protein- and carbohydrate-rich foods. Remember: there are 4 calories per one gram of protein and per one gram of carbohydrates; there are 9 calories per one gram of fat. So, when you cut out the most prevalent culprits of fat (animal products), you naturally reduce calorie intake—and thus potentially lose weight.

After a short time of eating no animal flesh or fluids (including eggs), people also tend to notice a decrease in the severity of their allergies;[9] and women tend to experience fewer PMS and menopausal symptoms.[10]

What You Can Expect to Gain

However, it's not just what you lose—it's what you gain, too! Many people who switch to a plant-based diet notice they have more energy, brighter skin with fewer blemishes, and an increase in the number of times they move their bowels, which is definitely beneficial for short- and long-term gastrointestinal health.

PALATE SENSITIVITY

Many people report that once their palate and body begin to know life without being coated by animal-derived fat and salt, cravings for these things are greatly reduced or completely eliminated. As a result, your palate may become more sensitive, you may taste flavors you never noticed before, and you may even have a more acute sense of smell.

ETHICAL CONGRUENCY

The harder-to-measure goals are those that relate to what it *feels* like to make choices that reflect our values. Prior to becoming vegan, I perceived myself as a conscious, compassionate, nonviolent person,

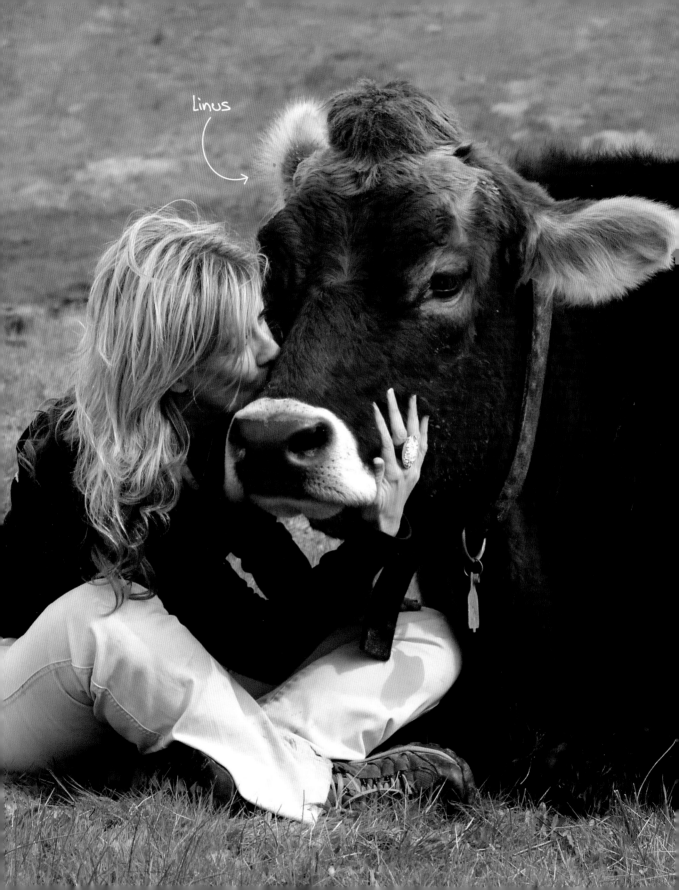

Linus

and yet I was funding what is no doubt the most violent industry in the world—one characterized by killing millions of individuals every day. I was paying people to be desensitized and to do what I would never do myself: hurt and kill animals. I still consider myself a conscious, compassionate, nonviolent person, but now those values are authentically reflected in my everyday behavior.

Since you're holding this book in your hands now, I'll assume that you know *why* you want to make some changes and that you're eager to reap one or more of the benefits I've already identified. Perhaps, though, you're unclear about *how* to make this transition—smoothly, joyfully, healthfully, and confidently.

Let me assure you that whatever compels you to become vegan, and however you identify yourself at this moment (carnivore, omnivore, pescetarian, flexitarian, plant-strong, or vegetarian), the transition process is the same for everyone: *it's a matter of undoing old habits and creating new ones.*

In my experience, when most people contemplate becoming vegan, they feel utterly overwhelmed because it seems so unfamiliar, and they don't know where to start. Many who try, but fail, mistakenly conclude that being vegan is an ideal that only a disciplined few can attain. They think being vegan requires willpower they don't have, so either they don't even try, or they give up after a short time. Filled with questions and misconceptions, what they need is a personal guide to hold their hand through the transition period, debunking myths and demystifying what it means to "be vegan."

Enter *The 30-Day Vegan Challenge*—your very own personal guide.

I take the approach that it is not the fault of "being vegan" that people revert back to eating meat and animal products or that they are unable to go even a month without eating them. Rather, I believe it's because core habits and perceptions remained unchanged, support during the transition process was nonexistent, and a dietary foundation was removed but not replaced with anything else to stand on. You won't have those issues. You will have my guidance and support the entire time.

Throughout the next 30 days, I will:

► Debunk myths using common sense so you will make informed decisions with confidence

► Get to the root of old perceptions and behaviors so that change is effortless

► Anticipate your challenges and provide validation and support

► Help you create a strong foundation of new habits

► Provide practical solutions for a variety of scenarios

You might choose to read only one chapter per day, or you may want to read well ahead. You may want to dive into the recipes dispersed throughout the book right away or wait until we've gone to the grocery store together. The content is broken up by each of the 30 days you're on this journey, but you don't *have* to read Day 4 before you read Day 5 or Day 16 before Day 17. There is a lot to take in during this 30-day period, and giving it to you day by day makes it easy to digest, but feel free to read ahead. Some people even read the book *all at once* before getting started and then use it as a resource guide during their transition.

> **CHALLENGE YOUR THINKING:**
> The more we keep telling people that it's too hard to change, the more they're going to believe it. But if we hold the bar high and have some expectations, we see amazing, life-altering changes take place in people—physically, emotionally, mentally, and spiritually.

You will notice, however, that there is a loose thematic structure to the book. Although the book's themes weave together throughout, the earliest chapters focus on *food:* shopping, cooking, prepping, and eating, which then lead into the chapters on *nutrition and health*, particularly the single nutrients with which we are so obsessed (protein, iron, calcium, and the like). Most of the remaining chapters address the *social aspects.* In other words, I think you will find that there is a linear journey to reading the chapters in order, but it is absolutely up to you.

Any way you choose to absorb the information, you can be sure that along the way, some old thought patterns will be challenged and some new behaviors will be created. And this I *guarantee:* if change is what you're looking for, then change is what you'll get, and I commend anyone who seeks it out. Change is often one of the most difficult things for humans to cope with—even when that change is positive. How many of us avoid making changes until we're absolutely forced to? How many of us engage in habits that make us sick, rather than simply change the way we eat? I've even heard doctors freely admit that they don't always give their patients the option of making significant diet changes—beyond advising them to switch from "red meat" to "white meat"—because they think people won't change.

You can call me crazy, but I have more faith in people than that. I know people change. I see it every single day. When the bar is raised, and people are given what they need to feel empowered, they *do* change. The problem is the more we keep telling people it's too hard to change, the more they just believe it.

The more we buy into the myth that there's something *radical* about eating vegetables, fruits, grains, legumes, mushrooms, nuts, seeds, herbs, and spices or that there's something *extreme* about *not* eating the mutilated bodies and secreted fluids of nonhuman animals, the less we'll expect of ourselves, and the less we'll expect of others. And nothing will change.

But when we hold the bar high and have some expectations of ourselves and one another, we see amazing, life-altering changes take place in people—physically, emotionally, mentally, and spiritually.

All I ask is that we remain open. Embrace the journey that encourages us to be humble, to learn new things, and to become better people. After all, that's what being human is all about: having the ability to make better decisions once we have new information.

By virtue of your picking up this book and being willing to take The 30-Day Vegan Challenge, you've raised the bar. I thank you for letting me be part of your journey, and may you find joy and abundance in the changes you make.

CHAPTER 2

Defining "Vegan"

Before we talk about all the exciting things you can expect in making this transition, I want to start out by defining "vegan." I also want to clear up some misunderstandings and misconceptions about what "vegan" means. In the most literal sense,

- To be "vegetarian" means to eat everything but the flesh of animals, whether they are from the land, air, or sea, so that includes fish.

- To be "vegan" means to eat everything but the flesh *and* fluids of animals (including their milk and eggs).

There is nothing new about people abstaining from meat, dairy, and eggs; only the terms have changed.

The sixth-century philosopher, Pythagoras, did not eat animals and advised his followers to do the same. All the way up to the 19th century, if you based your diet only on plants, you followed what was called a "Pythagorean diet," "vegetable diet," or a "vegetable regimen." The word "vegetarian" first appeared in print in *The Healthian* magazine in 1842, and it's clear from its context that the word would have been familiar to its audience by that time, which leads etymologists to surmise that it was in use by at least the 1830s. Then, in the middle of the 20th century, in reaction to the shifting definition of "vegetarian," a young British animal activist named Donald Watson conceived a new word to better convey the ethics behind the diet.

Watson was born in 1910 and died 95 years later in the northern region of England called Yorkshire. Intentional vegetarianism was not widespread in the rural, meat-eating community in which he grew up, but when asked about his journey to "becoming vegan," Watson would speak of his childhood memories of seeing and hearing animals slaughtered on neighboring small family farms or being dragged along alleyways to the local butcher. Repelled by violence and compelled by compassion, Watson became vegetarian (eventually vegan) and went on to co-found The Vegan Society (vegansociety.com), the first vegan organization in the United Kingdom, which is still active today.

Having been founded in 1847, a group called The Vegetarian Society was already in place. It was responsible for popularizing the word "vegetarian," which originally referred to a plant-based diet that excluded *all* animal products—meat, dairy, and eggs. Over time, however, diets called "vegetarian" began to include and embrace the consumption of eggs and animal's milk. Disheartened by this, Donald Watson set out to create a more precise word to describe ethical vegetarians who ate no animal products at all. In 1944, he—along with his wife, Dorothy—extracted the word "vegan" by taking the first three and last two letters of "vegetarian," because, as Watson explained, "veganism starts with vegetarianism and carries it through to its logical conclusion."

Watson emphasized its pronunciation (VEE-gun—not VAY-gun, VEE-jun, or VAY-jun) and wrote its definition,

> *a philosophy and way of living which seeks to exclude—as far as is possible and practical—all forms of exploitation of and cruelty to animals for food, clothing, or any other purpose.* [11]

The Oxford English Dictionary accepted the word, and there it remains—alive and increasing in recognition.

Aware that "veganism" is more than just a diet, many people—who eschew animal flesh and fluids strictly for health reasons—call themselves "plant-based." They may still wear leather and wool, go to the circus and aquatic animal shows, and not be concerned whether the products they use have been tested on animals.

Frankly, I don't care how people label themselves; anyone who eliminates animal products from their diet is making a positive contribution—to themselves, to the planet, and certainly to the animals. But I also know that when you begin this journey "only for health reasons," you become open to and aware of all the many other ways we exploit and hurt animals, and what was once a dietary choice often becomes an ideological one. The social aspects of eschewing meat, dairy, and eggs are the same—whether you're "plant-based" or "vegan." All of those issues are covered in this book.

Still, many people have a problem with the word "vegan," but I don't think it's because there's anything wrong with the word itself. I think it's because of the many misconceptions surrounding its meaning.

A MEANS TO AN END

The word has certainly gained traction in the public consciousness, especially in recent years, but misunderstandings still prevail about what it actually means. There is a misconception that the goal of being vegan is to be perfect or pure, as if there is such a thing as a certified vegan. Watson himself anticipated this when he clarified that all we can do is make the most compassionate choices "as far as is possible and practical."

I think one of the reasons people tend to equate veganism with perfection is that they're operating under the mistaken idea that being vegan is an *end* in itself, and so you find nonvegans trying to *catch* vegans in all the ways they're imperfect—stepping on insects while walking, driving a car whose tires contain animal products, wearing leather shoes left over from their pre-vegan days. And you have vegans, too, beating themselves up for accidentally eating something that contains eggs or for not being able to afford to replace the leather couch they bought just before becoming vegan. All of this entirely misses the point about what it means to "be vegan." Being vegan is not an *end* in itself; it's a *means* to an end. And for me, that end is unconditional compassion: doing everything we can to make choices that cause the least amount of harm—both to ourselves and others.

Being vegan is a powerful and effective means towards attaining that end, but it is not the end itself.

Because veganism is often characterized as a "diet," it is often associated with sacrifice, deprivation, or any number of negative words that characterize diets: temperance, cheating, abstaining, suppressing, portion-controlling, losing, and failing. Sometimes it's called "difficult," "temporary," or "extreme."

I think the problem is the perception that being vegan is about saying "no"—about refusing things that are offered to us. It *appears* that being vegan is about restriction and sacrifice, and that's the problem—the *perception* of what it means to live vegan. If people are on the outside looking in, they tend to see what vegans *don't* choose. They don't see what we *are* choosing. Perhaps in public settings, people see vegans rejecting things far more than they see them embracing things.

Another misconception about veganism is that there are *rules* about what vegans "can" and "cannot" eat, of what we're "allowed" or "forbidden" to eat. Let's be clear: vegans can eat whatever we want. There's nothing we *can't* have. But, there are some things we simply *don't want*. Choosing to avoid putting in our mouths or on our bodies the flesh and fluids that came off of or out of an animal is just that: a *choice*. We're "allowed" to eat whatever we want. Nobody is *preventing* us. We aren't adhering to rigid dietary *laws*. We aren't *forbidden* to eat animals. We don't *want* to eat animals.

Being vegan is not about rules or doctrine. It's not about restriction or self-denial. And though being vegan does involve saying "no" to some things—such as unhealthy foods, destructive environmental practices, cruelty, and violence—at its core, being vegan is about saying "yes."

It's about saying "yes" to our values. What's the use in having values if they don't manifest themselves in our behavior? And how many of us actually translate our values into action? It's nice to say that we are kind, caring, trustworthy, and helpful people. It's nice to say that we're in favor of eating healthfully or that we're against violence and cruelty. Most of us are. But how many of us actually take these abstract values and put them into concrete action? For me, being vegan, which extends to every area of my life, is an opportunity to do just that: to put my abstract values into concrete action.

By choosing to eat life-giving rather than life-taking foods, we're saying "yes" to our values of wellness and health, of peace and nonviolence, of kindness and compassion.

By choosing to *look* at what we do to other animals—human and nonhuman—on our behalf and for our convenience, we're saying "yes" to our values of accountability, of responsibility, of commitment to truth and knowledge.

By standing up for our beliefs and speaking up on behalf of those who have no voice, we're saying "yes" to our values of justice, courage, unity, and service to others.

Being vegan is about saying "yes" to the bounty of plant-based food available to us.

Being vegan is about embracing abundance—whether you *call* yourself vegan or not.

CHAPTER 3

Why 30 Days?

Most behavioral experts agree that it takes three weeks to change a habit and that to do so successfully, the key is to replace old behaviors with new ones. *The 30-Day Vegan Challenge* is all about creating new habits and new perceptions, and I provide an extra week just to make sure I cover all of your questions and needs. I also like the roundness of a 30-day cycle: giving your body enough time to respond in such a way that will enable you to *measure* improvement. (The best way to chart physical changes is to get a blood panel done. See Chapter 4: Know Your Numbers.)

Most people find it remarkable that the body can change and heal so quickly—with food and not pharmaceuticals, although it's been demonstrated again and again. We know this simply on an anecdotal level—feeling energized and clean after eating a healthful nutrient-dense meal, or heavy and sick after a rich fat-laden meal—and this is validated on a clinical level by taking blood before and after a meal, noting differences in blood cholesterol, blood pressure, blood glucose, and the like. With our ability to measure such specifics, we know that after *one meal*, our body chemistry changes negatively or positively depending on what we eat.

AFTER *ONE* MEAL!

To be sure, the body is a complex organism, but in many ways, its needs are simple. In fact, if we whittled it down, we can say that a healthy body is all about blood flow—keeping that blood flowing through our arteries to get to all the places it needs to go, easily and without hindrance.

Each time we eat, we have the choice to consume substances that hinder this blood flow or help it. After decades of research in the field of food and health, one thing is certain: animal products (meat, dairy, and eggs) hinder blood flow; plant foods increase blood flow.[12]

This is why people see significant, tangible, measurable changes in their blood within 30 days of eating vegan. Like water that runs through an unblocked hose, the blood is able to run easily through the arteries—both because of the improved consistency of the blood and because of the openness of the arteries themselves.

To experience these changes, however, requires a little openness. It requires surrendering to some old notions and being willing to have a new understanding. I've heard every excuse in the book for not letting go of meat, dairy, and eggs, and I know how attached people are to these products—and habits.

Some people are skeptical. Having been utterly disempowered by the modern medical system and persuaded by the industries that have the most to gain, many people believe that their genes have already determined their fate. Rather than believe they have a part to play in their health, they have made scapegoats of their ancestors and thrown up their hands. To them I say, try it for 30 days. You have nothing to lose.

Some people say they "don't eat a lot of meat and dairy" and thus conclude that they wouldn't benefit very much from taking this stuff out of their diets completely. In the many years I've been doing this work, I haven't met one person who doesn't have this perception of themselves. But I have to ask: Compared to what? Compared to how much you *could* eat? Compared to how much humans ate 100 years ago? What barometer are we using when we say that? Part of the problem is that our perception of our habits and ourselves isn't always aligned with reality. The truth is you don't know how much of this stuff you're eating until you stop! That's one of the benefits of The 30-Day Vegan Challenge. Your dietary habits become crystal clear.

So to those who don't think you eat "that much meat, dairy, and eggs," I say *great*. It just means it will be that much easier for you to stop completely for 30 days!

Some people think they're too old to make changes. Resigning themselves to the "inevitable" diseases and medications associated with "getting old," these folks insist you can't teach an old dog new tricks. I disagree. It doesn't matter how old we are when we decide to make changes. Our food habits were ingrained in us by the time we were about five years old, and we carry these habits with us into adulthood. It doesn't matter if you're 30 years old or 40 years old, 18 or 80. *A habit is a habit is a habit.*

> **CHALLENGE YOUR THINKING:**
> You don't know how much meat, dairy, and eggs you eat until you stop.
>
> **CHANGE YOUR BEHAVIOR:**
> Recognize (and change) your habits by not eating meat, dairy, and eggs for 30 days.

The behaviorists who say that it takes three weeks to change a habit don't make qualifications based on age. They don't say it takes three weeks to change a habit if you're 25 years old but three months to change a habit if you're 70. It's the same no matter how old you are. You just have to be willing to cast off some familiar behaviors and perceptions and try on some new ones.

Although they are deep-seated, our habits do not reflect who we really are. By definition, a habit is just a behavioral pattern we've created over time. In fact, the word "habit" originally referred to something that was worn (and is still used to refer to the garb of some religious persons, such as nuns), which means it can just as easily be put on as taken off.

This may seem like cold comfort, because we all know how hard it is to change a habit, but truly, we're all capable of learning new habits, and 30 days gives you plenty of time to take off the old and don the new. Some habits you never thought you'd be able to let go of will fall away effortlessly and some habits you'd never thought you'd form will become second nature.

But you don't have to take my word for it. You will experience it for yourself.

Get Set!

CHAPTER 4

Know Your Numbers

By the time you complete The 30-Day Vegan Challenge, you will no doubt experience changes. Some will be impossible to measure—changes in your outlook, energy level, perspective, and overall well-being. Some you will be able to track and measure, such as physiological and biochemical changes. It may surprise you to know that many of these changes will be detectable within 30 days.

Because some readers will want to see these tangible differences in black and white, I recommend you visit your health professional before you begin the Challenge to get a complete health check as well as a full blood and urine panel. The results of these laboratory tests will be helpful tools for evaluating your health status. Many people get their blood and urine work done during their annual physical exam, but they tend to trust what their doctor says without ever really looking at, or understanding, the laboratory results themselves. This section will help you understand what the numbers mean so you can compare yours to the optimal numbers in each category.

Common laboratory tests span a wide spectrum, so I'm including only a few main ones here. Your health professional can help you interpret others not listed below.

BODY WEIGHT

When it comes to evaluating weight and its impact on your health, it's not just a matter of what the scale says. You need to consider your percentage of body fat, waist circumference, and body mass index (BMI).

In the last several decades, a number of different tables have been devised to help people determine their "ideal weight." The ones that were most widely used were those created by Metropolitan Life Insurance Company in 1942 and subsequently updated over the years.[13]

These height/weight tables provide very little information about an individual's health risk, though they may be helpful when used in conjunction with other measurements to indicate whether you are within a healthy weight range.

BODY MASS INDEX (BMI)

One of the most accurate ways of assessing whether you are overweight or obese is to determine what percentage of your body weight is fat. However, getting accurate body fat measurements can be expensive and difficult, so the National Institutes of Health (NIH) created the Body Mass Index (BMI) in 1998. This guide has essentially replaced the old life insurance tables as a method to gauge healthy weight, and it helps doctors, researchers, dietitians, and government agencies get on the same page regarding weight recommendations. The same scale is used for men and for women.

BMI is a measure of body weight relative to height. According to NIH standards, you are overweight if you have a BMI between 25 to 29.9, and obese if you have a BMI of 30 or higher. A healthy weight provides a BMI of 18.5-24.9. See the BMI table below.

BODY MASS INDEX (BMI)

WEIGHT

HEIGHT in/cm (lbs)	100	105	110	115	120	125	130	135	140	145	150	155	160	165	170	175	180	185	190	195	200	205	210	215
(kgs)	45.5	47.7	50.0	52.3	54.5	56.8	59.1	61.4	63.6	65.9	68.2	70.5	72.7	75.0	77.3	79.5	81.8	84.1	86.4	88.6	90.9	93.2	95.5	97.7
5'0" – 152.4	19	20	21	22	23	24	25	26	27	28	29	30	31	32	33	34	35	36	37	38	39	40	41	42
5'1" – 154.9	18	19	20	21	22	23	24	25	26	27	28	29	30	31	32	33	34	35	36	36	37	38	39	40
5'2" – 157.4	18	19	20	21	22	22	23	24	25	26	27	28	29	30	31	32	33	33	34	35	36	37	38	39
5'3" – 160.0	17	18	19	20	21	22	23	24	24	25	26	27	28	29	30	31	32	32	33	34	35	36	37	38
5'4" – 162.5	17	18	18	19	20	21	22	23	24	24	25	26	27	28	29	30	31	31	32	33	34	35	36	37
5'5" – 165.1	16	17	18	19	20	20	21	22	23	24	25	25	26	27	28	29	30	30	31	32	33	34	35	35
5'6" – 167.6	16	17	17	18	19	20	21	21	22	23	24	25	25	26	27	28	29	29	30	31	32	33	34	34
5'7" – 170.1	15	16	17	18	18	19	20	21	22	22	23	24	25	25	26	27	28	29	29	30	31	32	33	33
5'8" – 172.7	15	15	16	17	18	19	19	20	21	22	22	23	24	25	25	26	27	28	28	29	30	31	32	32
5'9" – 175.2	14	15	16	17	17	18	19	20	20	21	22	23	24	24	25	25	26	27	28	28	29	30	31	31
5'10" – 177.8	14	14	15	16	17	18	18	19	20	20	21	22	23	23	24	25	25	26	27	28	28	29	30	30
5'11" – 180.3	14	14	15	16	16	17	18	18	19	20	21	21	22	23	23	24	25	25	26	27	28	28	29	30
6'0" – 182.8	13	13	14	15	16	17	17	18	19	20	20	21	21	22	23	23	24	25	25	26	27	27	28	29
6'1" – 185.4	13	13	14	15	15	16	17	17	18	19	19	20	21	21	22	23	23	24	25	25	26	27	27	28
6'2" – 187.9	12	13	14	14	15	16	16	17	18	18	19	19	20	21	21	22	23	23	24	25	25	26	27	27
6'3" – 190.5	12	12	13	14	15	15	16	16	17	18	18	19	20	20	21	21	22	23	23	24	25	25	26	26
6'4" – 193.0	12	12	13	14	14	15	15	16	17	17	18	18	19	20	20	21	22	22	23	23	24	25	25	26

Legend: Underweight | Healthy | Overweight | Obese | Extremely Obese

WAIST CIRCUMFERENCE

One of the main problems with using the Body Mass Index *alone* is that it doesn't consider muscle mass, so people such as body builders can have a high BMI but low actual body fat. Thus, it's useful to factor in waist circumference.

Waist circumference is a helpful measurement because your health is affected not only by excess body fat but also by *where that fat is located.* Some people gain weight in the abdominal area (the so-called "apple shape"), while others store it around their hips and buttocks ("pear-shaped" bodies).[14] People with the former are at higher risk for heart disease and type 2 diabetes.

According to the National Institutes of Health, a waist circumference greater than 40 inches for men and 35 inches for women is linked to a higher risk of type 2 diabetes, high blood pressure, high cholesterol levels, and heart disease.[15]

To measure your waist properly, place a tape measure around your middle, just above your hipbones but below your rib cage. Breathe out, and measure.

PERCENTAGE OF BODY FAT

You can determine your body fat by using one of those little devices called calipers, often available at your local gym or doctor's office. This is a skinfold test to determine the thickness of the subcutaneous fat layer at three or seven sites on the body, which is then converted to estimate fat percentage. According to the American Council on Exercise[16], a body fat level greater than 25% in men and 32% in women indicates one is obese.

BLOOD PRESSURE

Blood pressure is a measure of how hard blood is pressing against artery walls, like water running through a hose. Ideally, you want the systolic (top number) to be under 120 and the diastolic (bottom number) under 80. The risk for strokes and heart attacks starts progressively climbing above 115/75 mmHg.[17] You can measure your blood pressure using machines available in many pharmacies and doctor's offices, or buy a device to check at home.

BLOOD GLUCOSE

According to the Centers for Disease Control and Prevention, as of 2012, an estimated 21.0 million people (children and adults) in the United States have been diagnosed with diabetes, another 8.1 million are undiagnosed, and 86 million are prediabetic.[18]

Doctors use one to three different glucose tests to make a diagnosis.

- The first test checks the amount of glucose in your blood at any given time during the day, regardless of the last meal eaten. A glucose value of 200 mg/dl (plus diabetes symptoms) is a good indicator of diabetes.

- The second test is a fasting blood glucose, which is done after you have fasted for a minimum of eight hours. Fasting glucose should be in the range of 70 to 100 mg/dl; a fasting glucose level of 126 mg/dl or more indicates diabetes.[19]

- The third test is an oral glucose tolerance test to see how well your body deals with sugar. Normally, blood sugar rises after you eat and then returns to normal levels (70 to 110 mg/dl) within an hour or two. Higher values mean your body has trouble moving glucose out of the blood and into the cells.

The 86 million people with "prediabetes" means their fasting blood glucose level is 100 to 125 and post-meal level is 140 to 200 mg/dl—not high enough for a diagnosis of diabetes but higher than what is considered normal.[20]

CHOLESTEROL

When it comes to talking about cholesterol, we throw around labels such as "good" and "bad," though many of us don't even know what cholesterol is or what it does. Made in the liver of animals, cholesterol is a fat-like substance we consume in our diets via meat, dairy, and eggs (there is no dietary cholesterol in plant foods). Though our bodies also produce cholesterol (we are, after all, animals), we have no requirement to *consume* dietary cholesterol. The cholesterol made by our bodies travels through the bloodstream in little packages called *lipoproteins:*

- Low-density lipoproteins (LDL or "bad" cholesterol) deliver cholesterol TO the body.

- High-density lipoproteins (HDL or "good" cholesterol) take cholesterol OUT of the bloodstream.

When there is too much cholesterol in the bloodstream, it's a major risk factor for heart and blood vessel disease. To determine cardiovascular disease risk, doctors look at total cholesterol, LDL, HDL, and the ratio of the latter two.

Total Cholesterol: Because the average cholesterol level in the United States is so high (around 200), recommendations from organizations such as the American Heart Association are that levels must be reduced to "below 200." Although people with a level of 200 are at lower risk than those at 235, they are still at significantly high risk, according to the Framingham Heart Study. In fact, "about 35% of those who have heart attacks have cholesterol levels between 150 and 200."[21]

According to such longtime landmark studies as the Framingham Heart Study and the China Diet Study, the optimal level for total cholesterol is below 150.

LDL ("Bad") Cholesterol: Less than 100 is the optimal number.

HDL ("Good") Cholesterol: Between 40 and 60 is optimal.[22]

Important Note: A nutrient-dense plant-based diet makes the HDL portion of cholesterol *lower* because *all* portions of the *total cholesterol* are reduced.[23] That is to say, it is not necessarily an indication that something is wrong when your HDL level falls. On the other hand, a very *high* HDL level (60 or above) is not always a good sign either.[24] It means the HDL is working harder to get cholesterol out of the bloodstream. The more cholesterol, the more work it has to do. However, *always* check with your doctor to understand what your numbers mean.

TRIGLYCERIDES

Triglycerides are fatty substances that—like cholesterol—are made in the liver and circulate in the bloodstream. High levels indicate a risk of cardiovascular disease and are associated with pancreatitis.

Although medical establishments consider triglyceride levels of 100 to 150 mg/dL "normal" or "good," many experts feel that optimal fasting blood triglyceride levels should be 50 to 150 milligrams mg/dL. Levels of 200 to 500 mg/dL are considered high and very high, respectively.[25]

HOMOCYSTEINE

Homocysteine is an amino acid that is normally found in small amounts in the blood. Higher levels are associated with increased risk of cardiovascular disease, venous thrombosis, dementia, and Alzheimer's disease.

The optimal range is between 6 and 8 μmol/L.

Helpful Note: Keeping homocysteine at levels associated with lower rates of disease requires adequate intake of vitamin B_{12} (through supplements or fortified foods) and folate (through green leafy vegetables) or folic acid (the synthetic version of folate found as single supplements or in multivitamins).

VITAMINS

Because there are some vitamin deficiencies in the typical American diet, it is also worth looking at the following:

- **Vitamin D:** Americans are deficient in vitamin D more any other vitamin. Opinions vary between shooting for 40 to 70 ng/mL with 50 to 60 ng/mL as the optimal range with the most expert agreement.[26]

- **B_{12}:** >400 pg/mL is optimal. (In the case of getting an accurate B_{12} level checked, it's recommended that you request a urine MMA test or order it online.)

CHAPTER 5

Create Your Intentions and Goals

Because our motivations tend to determine our experience, I think it's important to be clear about why you want to take The 30-Day Vegan Challenge and what you hope to get out of it. Therefore, I highly recommend taking a few minutes to write down some intentions and goals. Seeing your goals and intentions in black and white makes them more concrete and more satisfying to look at when the 30 days are over. At the end of the 30 days, you'll want to revisit the answers to these questions and take stock.

You'll notice I recommend thinking about both your *intentions* and *goals*, and there is a difference between the two. Goals tend to be tangible and measurable; intentions are more about having a particular mindset.

For example, your intentions for the Challenge might be

- to remain open-minded
- to be willing to confront information or images that may be difficult or painful
- to be joyful and enthusiastic
- to not let fear (of the unknown, of something new, of something painful) guide me

Your goals might be

- to learn three new recipes
- to lose five pounds
- to lower my cholesterol
- to get a better understanding of nutrition
- to know a little more about the ethical component

Intentions create a framework of awareness, a motivation for *why* and *how* you want to approach something. They're more about the *process* than the *end result*.

Goals, on the other hand, are about results, and there's nothing more satisfying than returning to a list of goals and crossing off the accomplishments you set out to do.

As important as it is to create goals, I do encourage you to keep them realistic. The benefits of living vegan are numerous, but as we transition, it's important to have reasonable expectations so we're not surprised or disappointed. While it is perfectly reasonable to set a goal to lose some weight, you will want to be realistic about your expectations. For example, to lose weight safely and consistently, experts recommend losing no more than 2 pounds a week. Although some people may lose more than 8 pounds in 30 days, depending on what their starting weight is, I *do not recommend* making your goal "lose 30 pounds in 30 days." If you want to keep it less specific, just make "lose weight" be a goal; even if you lose one pound by the end of the 30 days, you'll have accomplished your goal!

This goes for any number you may be measuring, including how many points your cholesterol and blood pressure drop. The idea is to create goals that are realistic so that you can feel proud of yourself by the end of 30 days. Perhaps just going 30 days without meat, dairy, and eggs is enough of an accomplishment for you; if that's the case, make *that* your goal and then be pleasantly surprised by anything you may experience.

I also recommend writing your intentions and goals down on paper (or type them on a document on your computer and print them out). Seeing them in black and white makes them more concrete and more satisfying to look at when the 30 days is over.

Take a few minutes to answer the following questions. Take as much time and space, as you need. At the end of the 30 days, I'll ask you to refer to them again.

How do I feel now—before I begin The 30-Day Vegan Challenge?

Physically?

Emotionally?

Spiritually?

What are my intentions for doing The 30-Day Vegan Challenge?

What goals do I want to attain by the end of the 30 days?

What am I most afraid of or anxious about?

What am I anticipating being the most challenging aspects of these 30 days?

What am I anticipating being the most exciting aspects of these 30 days?

CHAPTER 6

Complete Your 3-Day Diary

Though many people protest that they "don't eat a lot of meat, dairy, and eggs," the truth is you have no idea how much you're eating until you stop and examine your daily food choices more closely. For this reason, I recommend keeping a food log for three days prior to starting the Challenge to help you see in black and white what your diet is like before you begin. Try to include at least one weekend day since we tend to eat differently and more decadently on Saturdays and Sundays.

For three days before beginning (perhaps while you're waiting for your blood test results), simply write down everything you eat and drink (except water). Be sure to include every morsel: condiments, what you put in your coffee, the soda you order at lunch, a candy bar you get from the vending machine at work, and even the cheese you sprinkle on your pasta.

Carry a small notebook around with you to make it easier, and be as thorough as possible. This kind of food tracking will not be necessary once you begin the Challenge. It's simply to enable you to accurately assess your current diet as compared to how you'll be eating once The 30-Day Vegan Challenge begins.

CHAPTER 7

Find a Buddy

Whether you're taking The 30-Day Vegan Challenge on a whim, as a bet, or because you want to make long-lasting changes in your life, the process will be a lot more enjoyable if you involve someone else in the journey—perhaps a family member, friend, or co-worker. Together you can exchange ideas, compare notes, provide support, and cook with and for each other.

In addition, I encourage you to ask your family members or anyone with whom you live to join you in the Challenge. Because you share meals and values together, it will make the process less stressful when everyone is on the same page and eating the same foods at home.

Change is hard, and the more support you can get from your loved ones, the more successful you will be. However, the changes we make may affect the people closest to us, and this can create waves—sometimes tidal waves—in our relationships, especially when food is involved. I hear from so many people whose otherwise loving and supportive family members become irate at the idea that their spouse or sibling or child has become vegan. Because they have not experienced the same desire to eschew animal products, they don't understand why their loved one has, and they may feel threatened by any change in their normal routine. Even if you've said nothing to make them feel this way, they might feel judged or guilty for wanting to continue to eat meat, dairy, and eggs.

Taking The 30-Day Vegan Challenge together can lessen the tension that mixed households experience, particularly in the first few weeks when everyone is struggling with new habits, new routines, and new ways of seeing the world.

If they protest, remind them that it's only for 30 days!

Also, if you do find resistance or hostility as you continue on this path, please take comfort in the fact that given time, that initial reaction usually subsides. Over and over, I've seen loved ones come around after they've had time to adjust to the changes. But whether you choose to do it on your own or with someone else, please know that I'm here with you every step of the way, and I promise you're in good hands.

A Note about the Recipes and Meal Ideas

Between *The Joy of Vegan Baking, The Vegan Table, Color Me Vegan,* and *Vegan's Daily Companion*, I've created and published well over 600 recipes. It's such a pleasure to know that my recipes are part of people's regular repertoire; it's such an honor to know that people cook from my books in their own kitchens and share the dishes with their loved ones.

RECIPE INDEX

The 30-Day Vegan Challenge is not a cookbook, but collectively, there are over 100 recipes and meal ideas within this book to guide you on your journey. Aware of the vast spectrum of cooking skills of the people picking up this book, each recipe was chosen carefully and created solely for this Challenge. They run the gamut of breakfast dishes, lunch options, dinner mains and sides, and desserts; and many of them can be used for special occasions and holidays.

Reluctant to simply stick them in one section at the back of the book, I've purposefully placed them within the various chapters so you can recognize them within the context that made sense for each one. Certainly, you can mix and match them. Don't hesitate to use a recipe I included in the Packing Lunches chapter as a recipe for dinner or a holiday. To make it easy for you to find the recipes and create your own menus, I've created a Recipe Index (on page 316) in addition to the regular index. It's organized by alphabet and by type of recipe.

ADDITIONAL RECIPES

Whether for my previously published cookbooks or for this new edition of *The 30-Day Vegan Challenge*, I'm meticulous about which recipes to include. My hope is that the recipes within will give you what you need to embark upon (or continue on) a healthful and compassionate way of living—whether or not you have experience with or an affinity for cooking. If you would like more recipes, of course I can highly recommend those in my earlier titles. Occasionally, when relevant to the content in a particular chapter, I might refer to recipes in *The Joy of Vegan Baking, The Vegan Table, Color Me Vegan,* or *Vegan's Daily Companion*. Copyright laws prevent me from simply reprinting the recipes from those books, but I mention a few throughout this book so you know they exist should you want them.

PLEASING EVERYONE

Always striving to create a balance between providing easy-to-prepare meals and encouraging people to get into the kitchen to cook, I create recipes that are meant to be accessible, familiar, healthful, and delicious. But, as they say, "You can't please all of the people all of the time." No one knows this better than someone who creates recipes. Some readers will want more salt. Some readers will say there is too much salt. Some will complain I use oil. Some will complain I include soy, gluten, wheat, sugar, or peanuts.

Although I don't subscribe to one particular type of diet, I'm aware that there are people who do, which is why I indicate whether or not each recipe is gluten-, wheat-, soy-, or oil-free. Most recipes can be adjusted to suit your desire. I believe once my recipes are in the hands of my readers, they're not mine anymore. And so, short of adding animal products, please feel free to modify the recipes within to customize them to your palate or preferences.

For instance,

► If the baked goods are too sweet, add less sugar.

► If you want more salt in any of the recipes, then add a little more.

► If you want less salt in any of the recipes, then reduce the salt.

► If you want to reduce (the little) oil I recommend, then use water to sauté vegetables instead.

► If you prefer your food spicier, just increase the heat.

► If your oven temperature is different from mine and requires that something cook a little longer than I've indicated, then follow your oven and not my instructions.

NUTRITIONAL INFO

As for the nutritional information, we did our best to indicate the size of the serving when it was possible to do so ("2 tablespoons," "$\frac{1}{2}$ cup," or "1 cookie"), but that wasn't always possible, and so please note that when the yield for a finished recipe is a range (such as "serves 6 to 8"), the nutritional information "per serving" was calculated using the larger number. Also, we defaulted to soy milk for the nutritional information when I offered a choice of "plant-based milks."

DEDICATION

You'll notice that some recipes have a dedication. The production of this book was funded by individuals who believed in its value and importance, and so in order to honor certain people for their generosity, I offered the opportunity to dedicate a recipe to a loved one, and it was a joy to implement this reward.

FLEXIBILITY

Finally, I very purposefully did not include daily menus or "what to eat today" directives for each of the 30 days. There is nothing *prescriptive* or *programmatic* about this book or this Challenge. It is a *manual*, a *guide*, and a *resource* for you wherever you are on this path. I'm also aware of the fact that we eat differently depending on the day of the week, so recommending something that feels too complicated before leaving for work may not work for you.

However you consume this book and the recipes, may you enjoy the process of sensitizing your palate to the myriad of flavors in the plant kingdom.

Go!

"Vegan" is Not a Separate Food Group: Demystifying Plant Foods

In the many years I've been doing this work, it's become clear to me that people want to make healthful choices, but they also want these choices to be convenient and familiar, and they assume being vegan is neither.

This assumption has more to do with our perception than reality.

We've all been taught to consider animal-based meat, dairy, and eggs as "normal" or "regular" food and "vegan food" as "alternative" or "different," as if the latter were a category unto itself. The fact of the matter is "vegan food" is food we're all familiar with; it's vegetables, fruits, grains, legumes, lentils, mushrooms, nuts, seeds, herbs, and spices. In the case of baked goods, it's flour, sugar, cocoa, chocolate, vanilla, spices, baking soda, baking powder, cornstarch, and yeast.

> **CHALLENGE YOUR THINKING:**
> Recognize that "vegan food" is "normal food" you're already familiar with: fruits, vegetables, beans, legumes, lentils, mushrooms, grains, nuts, seeds, herbs, and spices.

When you get down to it, "vegan food" is food we already cook with and already love. You just might not call it "vegan." But if you've had an apple, you've had "vegan food." It's just *regular* food; you don't call it a "vegan apple." If you've ever eaten spaghetti with marinara sauce, you've had "vegan food." If you've had pretzels, peanuts, and popcorn at a baseball game, you've had "vegan food."

When we take it out of the box called "vegan," we recognize that it's not so unfamiliar after all.

It's no surprise we have these misconceptions about veganism. We're taught early on in our culture that meat, dairy, and eggs is "normal food" for regular folks and that "vegan food" is unsubstantial and lacking, reserved for counter-culture types, "health freaks," or the allergy-prone.

These misperceptions also lead people to believe that many familiar favorite foods are not vegan. And so on your first day of The 30-Day Vegan Challenge, let's set the record straight here and now.

Bread is vegan. Some brands and types of commercial loaves of sliced breads have animal's milk added to them—but not all. Good bread—real bread—is naturally vegan. Just think of the definition of bread according to French law, "it can contain nothing more than flour, salt, water, and yeast."

Pasta is vegan. Although some types of pasta have chicken's eggs added to them—namely *egg* noodles—by definition, pasta is really just made from flour and water. In fact, the word originally meant "pastry dough sprinkled with salt."

Chocolate is vegan. Some people mistakenly believe that if you're vegan, you have to forego chocolate, having to settle only for carob! *Au contraire.* By definition, chocolate is vegan; it comes from the cacao tree. Cocoa powder, cocoa butter, bittersweet chocolate, semisweet chocolate, dark chocolate, even white chocolate, are all vegan by nature.

Cocoa *butter* is vegan. We tend to associate the word *butter* with dairy, but it really has more to do with *fat* than cow's milk. Peanut butter, cocoa butter, coconut butter, almond butter, and shea butter—are all plant-based fats. Cocoa butter is simply the fat in the cacao bean, so just because a label says "butter" it doesn't mean it's an animal product. I think we need to take back the word "butter," which is why you'll find me often referring to "nondairy butter" or "plant-based butter"—not margarine and certainly not "fake butter."

Vegans eat yeast. Considering the fact that yeasts are microorganisms classified as fungi—not animals, of course vegans eat yeast, which means, as I said, "Bread is vegan."

Now this doesn't mean that there aren't some new foods and ingredients you'll be learning about throughout your transition, but that's all part of growing, evolving, and experiencing new perceptions.

Eggplant

Artichoke

Tempeh

Tofu

Seitan

Nutritional Yeast

Trying New Foods

Before we go to the grocery store, I want to invite you to look through a new lens. One of the most common assertions I hear nonvegans make is, "I don't eat a lot of meat, dairy, or eggs." I haven't met one person who hasn't said this. Everyone seems to have this perception of themselves, and yet 45 billion land and sea animals are killed every year in the United States for human consumption.[27] Someone is eating the animals!

The truth is you really don't know how much meat, dairy, and eggs you're eating until you stop. When you stop—when you participate in something like The 30-Day Vegan Challenge—you become conscious of how many times you automatically reach for things that contain animal products. You become acutely more aware of your habits once you make an effort to change them.

If you've been looking in one direction your whole life, choosing the same foods over and over and not crossing any comfort zones, you're most likely stuck in habits and routines that compel you to make snap judgments against "vegan food." You place it in an ugly box marked "other," allowing yourself to remain unchanged.

Think about the process of going from eating Italian cuisine your whole life to learning how to prepare Indian cuisine. You're intuitively aware that you need to learn some new techniques and explore some new ingredients, but you don't judge Indian cuisine for being *inferior* to Italian cuisine. You just recognize that it's *different* and *unfamiliar* to *you*.

CHALLENGE YOUR THINKING: If you've been cooking Italian food your whole life and decide to master Indian cuisine, you realize there are things you don't know and need to learn. You don't judge Indian cuisine for being *inferior* to Italian cuisine; you recognize that it's *different* and *unfamiliar* to *you*.

CHANGE YOUR BEHAVIOR: Embrace new "vegan foods" you discover on your journey, resisting the temptation to judge them as *inferior* to the animal-based foods with which you're familiar.

When you become vegan—when you stop long enough to recognize your ingrained habits—you become aware of the fact that you have more food choices than ever before. It's not that those choices weren't available to you when you were eating meat, dairy, and eggs; it's just that you weren't looking outside of your comfort zone. When you shift your gaze from one direction to another, an entire world opens up—of new cuisines, new flavors, new textures, new aromas, and new experiences. And how exciting is that?

KEEPING IT FAMILIAR

We'll get to some of those new foods in a moment, but first, let's talk about what is already familiar to you. When people contemplate making the vegan transition, they often think it means having to create an entirely new repertoire of foods. You don't have to do this unless you want to, but I'm guessing, if you're like most people—vegan or not—you're most likely rotating the same dishes again and again. You make the same favorite meals, go to the same restaurants, and order the same items each time. We're such creatures of habit that experts estimate that we rotate the same seven foods every week.[28] This is one of the reasons I find it so ironic that people say vegans don't eat a variety of foods; it's really quite the opposite.

So, how do you keep things familiar while removing such staples as meat, dairy, and eggs from your daily diet? First, consult the 3-Day Food Diary you created before you started the Challenge. Grab a piece of paper, and do the following:

1. **Write down what you already eat that's vegan.** Common examples include:
   a) pasta with marinara sauce
   b) pasta primavera
   c) peanut butter and jelly sandwiches
   d) tortilla chips and salsa
   e) corn or flour tortillas with rice, beans, and guacamole
   f) vegetable stir-fry
   g) tossed green salad
   h) raw veggies
   i) bean chili (canned or homemade)
   j) minestrone / vegetable soup (canned or homemade)
   k) hummus (homemade or store-bought)

You'll most likely find that at least three dishes in your current repertoire are already vegan. Highlight or circle those.

2. **Next, look at your diary and pick out three of your favorite meat-, dairy-, or egg-based dishes. Now think of ways to easily "veganize" them."** For instance, you can:
   a) use vegetable stock in place of chicken stock in your favorite soup.
   b) add a few drops of liquid smoke, a chopped chipotle pepper, or chipotle chili powder to your favorite Split Pea Soup (instead of ham) to get that smoky, salty flavor.

c) toast some pine nuts or walnuts, crush them or pulse them in a food processor with a little salt (and even some nutritional yeast), and sprinkle on your favorite pasta dish instead of Parmesan cheese. Fat, salt, familiarity, texture, and flavor—we'll talk more about this on Day 12: The Power of "Cravings."

d) replace dairy-based sour cream with nondairy sour cream or guacamole. (See brands in Day 3: Stocking a Healthful Kitchen.)

e) replace egg-based mayonnaise with eggless mayo. (See brands in next chapter.)

f) add vegan meat crumbles or crumbled thawed tofu to marinara sauce and serve over pasta. (See brands or commercial vegan meats in next chapter; see my method for freezing and thawing tofu in Day 17: Demystifying Tofu: It's Just a Bean!)

g) use mushrooms, tofu, or tempeh in place of meat in a stir-fry.

h) grill portobello mushrooms for a hearty sandwich or main dish.

i) make pesto without the Parmesan cheese, enjoying the rich flavors of the pine nuts, basil, garlic, and olive oil—with a little salt.

Now you have *six* vegan recipes—and they're all familiar favorites!

3. **Next, learn three new recipes.** Consult the recipes throughout this book for breakfast, lunch, dinner, dessert, and snack ideas. Choose three to make part of your repertoire.

EXPANDING YOUR HORIZONS

Without making much effort, you've just discovered *nine* vegan recipes for your rotation, and only three of them are entirely new. This enables you to still enjoy your favorites while discovering new dishes. One of the most common comments I hear from people is that in becoming vegan they find a love of cooking. They find themselves excited to try new recipes and cuisines, and they gain a confidence in the kitchen they never had before. Even if you don't wind up *loving* cooking, just being willing to try new foods is improvement.

As time goes on, I encourage you to continue to rotate these nine dishes, as well as add new ones. I'm always struck by people who say they tried being vegan but became "bored" eating the same foods over and over again. The fact that we get stuck in ruts is not the fault of—and certainly not unique to—"being vegan." It's because we become lazy and don't rotate or expand our repertoire. Rotating the same meals is fine—for a while—but be sure to explore the thousands of plant foods and flavors out there to keep things exciting and new.

For all intents and purposes, plant-based foods are available to everyone—vegans and nonvegans, but some plant foods have become so identified with vegan eating that it's worth taking a few moments to

CHALLENGE YOUR THINKING: The fact that we get stuck in cooking and eating ruts isn't the fault of "being vegan." It's because we become lazy and don't rotate or expand our repertoire.

CHANGE YOUR BEHAVIOR: Periodically rotate your favorite dishes; even changing one meal every couple of months keeps things dynamic rather than static.

elaborate on them. Besides, a few may be completely new to you. On Day 12: The Power of "Cravings," I discuss the role each of these foods plays in satisfying our "cravings" for meat, dairy, or eggs, but let's talk about them briefly here in the context of including them in your new repertoire.

Mushrooms

I was a mushroom-hater for years; unless they were totally puréed in something like raviolis or gravies, I just hated the texture. Little by little, I came around, and now I'm a mushroom-junkie. My gateway mushroom was the shitake, and I regularly kick myself for not trying them sooner. There is a wonderful world of mushrooms out there, and I encourage you to learn from my silliness and just try them. Check out brown mushrooms (also called cremini or baby portobello), shitake, maitake, oyster, and many more. You can incorporate them into your dishes in a variety of ways.

- ▶ Sautéed brown and shitake mushrooms pair beautifully with pasta.

- ▶ Add mushrooms to your favorite vegetable- miso-, or lentil-based soups.

- ▶ Roast or grill them.

- ▶ Make the Creamy Leek Polenta on page 95 and top with sautéed mushrooms.

- ▶ Sauté mushrooms, then use them as a pizza topping.

- ▶ See page 117 for Tofu, Mushroom, and Sausage Scramble.

- ▶ Check out many more recipes for a variety of mushrooms in *The Vegan Table* and *Color Me Vegan*.

Seitan

Originating in China by vegetarian Buddhist monks looking for chewy plant-based alternatives to animal-based meat, seitan (pronounced SAY-tan) is simply a wheat-based food made much like bread. The difference is that you use just vital wheat gluten (gluten is the protein in wheat) as your flour, which produces a very chewy texture. It's plain-tasting on its own—just like any meat—and relies on herbs, spices, and other seasonings to flavor it. You can make it from scratch very easily (see recipe for Homemade Seitan on page 50) or find it in the refrigerated case of grocery stores where the tofu tends to be; it will be sold as "seitan," "wheat gluten," or "wheat meat." Seitan is a protein-rich food that can be stir-fried, sautéed, grilled, baked, barbecued, or fried. It can also be chopped up as a base for a "no-chicken salad" or my Waldorf Salad on page 51.

Tempeh

Made from whole soybeans, tempeh (pronounced TEM-pay) has a delicious nutty flavor and hearty texture. A staple in Indonesian cuisine, it has made its way west, where it's enjoying its time in the spotlight.

Cremini Mushrooms

Shitake Mushrooms

Portabello Mushrooms

Oyster Mushrooms

Both the flavor and texture are different from tofu, and because it's fermented, some people complain that it is slightly bitter. For that reason, I always recommend steaming it first. Just slice or dice it up, place it in a steamer basket in a 3-quart saucepan over medium heat for 10 minutes, then do anything you want to it, such as adding it to a stir-fry, sautéing it, grilling it, or tossing it with BBQ sauce and baking it. You can also visit my videos on my website, joyfulvegan.com, where you'll see me demonstrate how to cook with tempeh.

Tofu

An entire day is devoted to this food based on the versatile and protein-rich soybean, so jump ahead to Day 17: Demystifying Tofu: It's Just a Bean!, if you like. Some people automatically assume that if you're vegan, you eat tofu, but here's a secret: tofu is for everyone. *And* you don't have to eat tofu if you *are* vegan. (That's two secrets for the price of one!) I *adore* tofu, and you'll find recipes for it throughout my books, including a couple in this one. Check out page 215 for Tofu Cacciatore and page 117 for Tofu, Mushroom, and Sausage Scramble.

Eggplant

Admittedly, I started appreciating eggplant late in life and always surprised people who couldn't believe that someone could be vegetarian *and* not eat eggplant. (I was vegetarian for years before becoming vegan.) Interestingly, just as it was the Japanese shitake that sparked my love of mushrooms, it was also Asian cuisine that turned me on to eggplant. It's one of my go-to dishes in Thai and Vietnamese restaurants. When I do cook with it at home, I tend to steam it before doing anything else with it—to moisten it up and ensure that it's cooked thoroughly first. Grilled eggplant makes a great main dish, and stuffed eggplant makes a pretty focal point. It melts in your mouth rather than offer a chewy mouthfeel, so if you're looking for something "meaty," I'd stick with mushrooms, tempeh, seitan, or tofu (especially frozen/thawed tofu, which you can read all about in the tofu chapter on Day 17: Demystifying Tofu: It's Just a Bean!).

Nutritional Yeast

Don't judge this food by its name! It's flaky, yellow, cheesy, and delicious and is probably one of those foods you aren't really aware of until you become vegan. Nutritional yeast is used to make cheese sauces, add a pretty color and cheesy flavor to dishes like tofu scramble, and is a favorite in the Patrick-Goudreau household for sprinkling on popcorn and on our cats' food (they love it!). You can also sprinkle it on pasta upon serving, though I think it doesn't have the appeal that Parmesan has unless you mix it with some fat and salt. (See Day 12: The Power of "Cravings": Fat and Salt Taste Good.)

The idea is to be open to trying foods that are unfamiliar to you. Of course, you can do this whether you're vegan or not, but this 30-Day Vegan Challenge is the perfect opportunity to expand your horizons a bit.

You may find what so many others do: that being vegan is actually more expansive than anything you've experienced before. You think it's going to be restrictive because you've been looking in one direction your whole life. Yet, when you look a little more closely, you see how expansive your choices now are, you realize how limited you made your options before: choosing the same foods again and again, going to the same restaurants over and over, picking the same menu items in those same restaurants *ad nauseam*. There's nothing wrong with finding comfort with what is familiar, but when it hinders us from trying something new, it can be restrictive.

REVOLUTIONIZING OUR RHETORIC

I often put "vegan food" in quotation marks, because what falls into that category is food we already eat but don't call "vegan:" vegetables, fruits, nuts, seeds, mushrooms, grains, legumes, herbs, and spices. We don't say "vegan banana" because we know that a banana is "vegan" by virtue of being a fruit. When we understand that "vegan food" is just food, we're more inclined to embrace it.

On that same note, some of the words we use elevate meat, dairy, and eggs to such a degree that they make "vegan food" seem inferior, words such as "alternative," "substitute," "imitation," "replacement," "faux," "fake," "mock," and "analog." The use of these words in this context denigrates plant foods and exiles them from the realm of the "normal" to the realm of the weird or inedible. After all, who wants to eat something that is "fake"? When we use words that make plant-based foods sound unappetizing or unreal, we perpetuate the perception that these foods are just that, and we make it seem as if animal-based products are the barometers by which we should measure everything else.

We see this when we talk about animal-derived milk, referring to it as "regular milk," "normal milk," or "real milk" and to plant-based milk as "imitation milk" or "milk substitute." Sometimes—much to my chagrin—I even see it spelled "*mylk*." I address this in detail on Day 16: Plant-Based Milks, but in short: we don't drink "milk *substitutes*." The only imposter in our diets is animal milk, which is, quite literally, a replacement for our own species' milk: the only mammalian milk we have a physiological need to consume until we're weaned.

I suggest we call animal-based milks what they are: "cow's milk," "goat's milk," "buffalo milk," "rat's milk"—or whatever animal's milk people are being sold these days—and that we call plant-based milks what they are: "plant-based milk," "soy milk," "almond milk," "rice milk," "oat milk," "coconut milk," "hazelnut milk," and so on. I might say "dairy-based milk and butter" to distinguish them from "nondairy milk and butter," but I never say "fake butter." Nondairy butter is not fake. It is simply butter made from plant fats rather than animal fat.

When it comes to cheese, I also say "dairy-based cheese" and "non-dairy cheese," or I name it based on what it's made from, such as "cow's milk cheese," "goat's milk cheese," "nut-based cheese," "cashew-based cheese," "soybean-based cheese," "almond cheese," and so on.

> **CHALLENGE YOUR THINKING:**
> When we recognize that "vegan food" is just food, we're more inclined to embrace it.

I even advocate for reclaiming the word "meat." As I explain in my fourth book, *Vegan's Daily Companion,* "The word meat comes from the Old English word *mete* and originally referred to something that was *eaten* to distinguish it from something that was *drunk*."[29] It referred to solid food rather than a beverage, and we still say it today when we say "coconut meat" and "the meat of a nut." In the same spirit, I recommend that we use such phrases as "vegan meat," "plant-based meat," "grain meat," "nut meat," and "wheat meat" to distinguish them from "animal-based meat." Seitan, burgers, sausages, deli slices made from these plant foods are not *fake;* they're made from *real*, authentic ingredients.

It may take us a moment longer to say these words and phrases, but that's a small price to pay for normalizing our consumption of plant foods.

RE-PLATING OUR FOOD

Some of our blocks and misperceptions about a diet centered on plant foods aren't simply about the food itself but also about *how we plate our food.* In our meat-centric culture, we're accustomed to having a piece of animal-based meat at the center of our plate surrounded by some token vegetables (most likely covered in dairy-based butter and cream sauces). Many people perceive a "vegan meal" as lacking because they imagine that piece of meat being removed—leaving the plate full of "only side dishes." This is one of the reasons people think vegans eat "only sides" or "only salads." They can't see past the familiar-looking plate with meat as the star and a few side dishes playing runner-up.

> **CHALLENGE YOUR THINKING:**
> The way we plate our food is purely cultural—what we were taught in our families and society.
>
> **CHANGE YOUR BEHAVIOR:**
> Rethink what a plate of food "should" look like, using cuisines from around the world as inspiration. Give yourself permission to create a plate based on what we typically call "side dishes."

The way we plate our food is purely cultural—what we've been taught in our families and in our society. If you think about how the food is plated in various cuisines around the world, you'll notice that it looks very different from a Western meal. Think of Indian, Mexican, Japanese, Chinese, Thai, Vietnamese, Italian, or Ethiopian cuisines. The plates are made up of what we would somewhat derisively call "side dishes," and yet they're comprised of the most healthful and flavorful foods: vegetables, grains, lentils, beans, and greens. So, on the one hand, we need to rethink what a plate of food "should" actually look like, *and* we need to embrace the notion of centering our meals around what we were taught should only be "on the side": grains, greens, legumes, mushrooms, and colorful vegetables.

Moreover, aside from simply being familiar to us or being characterized as "the protein" on the plate, the lifeless slab of animal meat plays another role: it creates a focal point: the center around which everything else is built. Therefore, the idea is to use *plant foods* to the same—and much *prettier*—effect. There are so many ways to create a focal point on the plate using plant-based foods, starting with the vegetables themselves.

► Hollow out any of the following and fill with a flavorful stuffing made of grains, veggies, spices, and herbs: squash (acorn, butternut, delicata, or zucchini), bell peppers, mushrooms (portobello or cremini), potatoes (yellow or sweet), eggplant (globe or the long purple Asian version), tomatoes (any variety), cornhusks, artichokes, cabbage, olives, or pea pods!

► You don't necessarily have to use the vegetables themselves as the "container." Fill small, colorful individual bowls, custard cups, or ramekins with a filling—or even use them as the "mold." Overturn your filled bowl (assuming the filling is compact enough to keep its form when overturned), onto the plate, and you have a mound o' beauty atop which you can garnish with fresh herbs or edible flowers.

► Some foods, such as polenta, ravioli, socca (see page 92), and tortillas are ideal for cutting into simple geometric shapes—or for using a cookie cutter to do so. Top with filling or garnish for a pretty main dish.

► Some plant foods are hearty enough to play the role of the main dish, such as tempeh, tofu, seitan, and portobello mushrooms.

Homemade Seitan

YIELD 3 pounds or 6 seitan cutlets

INGREDIENTS *BROTH*

8 cups (2 liters) vegetable broth
  (or 8 cups water + 2 vegetable
  bouillon cubes)

2 tablespoons tamari soy sauce

INGREDIENTS *DOUGH*

1 cup (120 g) vital wheat gluten

2 tablespoons nutritional
  yeast flakes

1 teaspoon garlic powder

½ cup (120 ml) vegetable broth
(room temperature or cold)

3 tablespoons tamari soy sauce

1 tablespoon olive oil

PER SERVING (1 CUTLET):
Calories: 126, **Protein:** 17 g, **Fat:** 2.7 g,
Carbohydrates: 8.6 g, **Fiber:** 0.5 g,
Cholesterol: 0 mg

FOR YOUR
MODIFICATION

There are as many variations for
this dough as your imagination
could conjure. You can add a few
teaspoons of dried herbs (any
variety), ⅛ teaspoon of fine black
pepper, or a little cayenne pepper
for a slight kick.

The exact derivation of the word "seitan" is unknown, though the meaning is quite clear: it refers to the wheat-based meat made from gluten. Gluten is the protein in wheat and is what gives this meat its chewy texture. This recipe can be made in no time and can be used as the base for countless recipes for which you want a meaty texture. The trick to attaining the perfect texture is to simmer the gluten slowly and not overcook.

DIRECTIONS

⊙ Fill a large soup pot with the eight cups of vegetable broth and the two tablespoons of tamari. Cover, and bring to a boil over medium heat.

⊙ Meanwhile, stir together the flour, nutritional yeast, and garlic powder. Next, add the vegetable broth, tamari, and olive oil.

⊙ Stir the wet ingredients into the dry, and combine with a wooden spoon until the wet and dry are combined. Use your hands to finish combining, kneading at the same time for about one minute. The resulting texture will be an elastic dough.

⊙ Using a sharp knife, divide this dough into three or four pieces and briefly knead and stretch those pieces in your hand.

⊙ Once the broth has come to a full boil, carefully drop the dough into the broth, lower the heat to low-simmer, and place the lid on only partially.

⊙ Allow to simmer for 45 to 60 minutes, turning occasionally. Remove from the heat, remove the lid, and let sit for 15 minutes.

⊙ At this point, you can either transfer the dough and broth to a container, let cool, and store in the fridge for up to a week. Alternatively, if you'd like to use it right away, remove the dough from the broth, and place it in a strainer or colander until it is cool enough to handle.

⊙ From here, you can use the seitan however you'd like. Slice it and serve on a sandwich, sauté it, marinate it, or add it to the Waldorf Salad on page 51.

Waldorf Salad

YIELD Makes 4 servings

INGREDIENTS

Homemade Seitan (use about
⅔ of the finished recipe on
page 50), sliced

1 cup (150 g) seedless red
grapes, halved

1 medium crisp apple (Fuji,
Granny Smith, Gala), cored
and chopped

½ cup (62 g) chopped walnuts,
raw or toasted

¼ cup (40 g) chopped red onion

⅓ cup (75 g) eggless mayonnaise
(Wildwood, Just Mayo,
Vegenaise)

2 teaspoons lemon juice

Salt and pepper, to taste

PER SERVING:
Calories: 338, **Protein:** 21.1 g, **Fat:** 19 g,
Carbohydrates: 23.5 g, **Fiber:** 3.1 g,
Cholesterol: 0 mg

Our 30-Day version retains all the elements of the classic Waldorf salad—apples, celery, grapes, and walnuts dressed in mayonnaise—but with a compassionate twist: eggless mayonnaise and seitan instead of chicken. You can also use tofu or steamed tempeh.

Note: *You can absolutely use store-bought seitan for this recipe, although I recommend using our homemade version. If you do use the latter, since you have to prepare it first, you will want to factor that in to your total prep time for this salad.*

DIRECTIONS

◉ Add the seitan, grapes, chopped apple, walnuts, mayonnaise, and lemon juice to a large bowl, and thoroughly combine all of the ingredients. Taste, and add salt and pepper to your liking.

FOR YOUR
MODIFICATION

❧ The Homemade Seitan, especially once it's been chilled in the refrigerator, is perfect as it is for this recipe, but you can also fry it up in a little oil, if you prefer.

❧ Dried cranberries, raisins, a chopped pear, or chopped plums or pluots also add sweetness if you don't have grapes and apples.

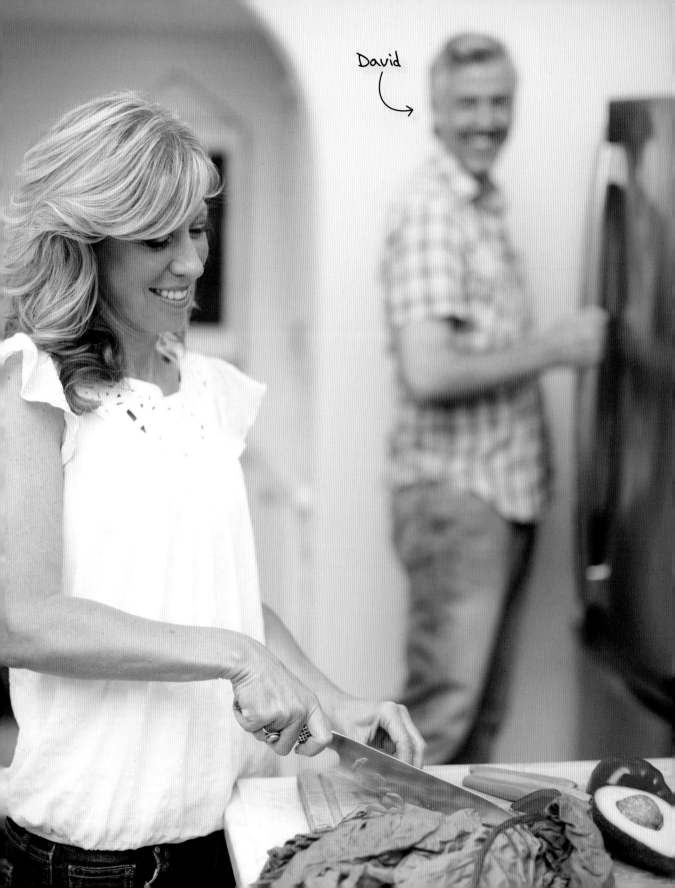
David

Stocking a Healthful Kitchen

Before I send you to the grocery store, I encourage you to look in your cupboards, refrigerator, and freezer and note what you already have that is "vegan." You will most likely find pasta, marinara sauce, peanut butter, jelly, jam, preserves, rice, canned beans, and frozen and fresh vegetables and fruits.

Just as when you wrote your 3-day food diary and noticed how many animal-based foods you may have been eating prior to starting the Challenge, so too may you notice all the nonvegan food in your kitchen, whether they are such obvious things as the meat in your freezer; animal-based milk, dairy-based cheeses, and eggs in the fridge; or the processed and packaged foods with animal-derived ingredients in your cabinets, such as boxed macaroni & cheese and Jell-O.

Having familiar animal products in the kitchen makes it too convenient to reach for them when you're ravenous or in a rush. It is best to make a clean break. Some people will discard all the animal products immediately, some will decide to eat them up, and still others may decide to donate them to a local animal shelter/wildlife center or feed it to their cats or dogs.

However, one mistake people make when getting rid of what is undesirable and unhealthful is not replacing them with healthful—and in our case, vegan—versions. Having a variety of nutritious ingredients on hand—particularly fresh fruits and veggies—is key to ensuring that you can whip up delicious, healthful, compassionate meals anytime. Though a lot of junk food is technically vegan (Cocoa Puffs, Oreo Cookies, and Skittles), my intention is to guide you toward *healthful* plant-based foods, and I'm always walking the line of making suggestions that allow for fast, easy cooking, while recommending foods that are as whole as possible.

There are many vegan-friendly brands in addition to the ones I name below; once you know what to look for on the label (see Day 5), you'll find options everywhere you look.

> **TIP:** *As you look over these categories, you may want to begin writing out your shopping list in preparation for going to the grocery store.*

CANNED GOODS

☞ **Canned Beans:** Some people mistakenly believe that canned beans are lower in nutrition than beans made from scratch; it's not true. In fact, many people digest canned beans much better than they do beans made from scratch because canned beans have been extensively soaked and cooked to remove the sugars (called oligosaccharides) that give people the discomfort, bloating, and gas. The only thing you sacrifice with canned beans is money, because you pay extra for convenience. You can decide which means more to you.

TIP: Always rinse and drain canned beans to get rid of the liquid they've been sitting in. This also rinses away some excess sodium.

Varieties to Stock: adzuki, chickpeas (garbanzo beans), kidney, black, cannellini, navy, Great northern, black-eyed peas, pinto, soybeans, and vegetarian refried.

Favorite Brands: Eden Foods, Whole Foods 365, Westbrae, Trader Joe's

☞ **Canned Lentils:** I recommend dried lentils below, but canned lentils can speed up things even more! The same brands that sell canned beans also sell canned lentils.

☞ **Canned Tomatoes:** When fresh tomatoes are out of season, canned tomatoes save the day.

Varieties to Stock: To have a variety for different dishes, buy cans of diced, whole peeled, stewed, crushed, and fire-roasted tomatoes. Also, stock up on tomato paste, since it adds so much depth of flavor to sauces, stews, stir-fries, pasta, and chili.

Favorite Brands: Muir Glen, Eden Foods, Whole Foods 365, Trader Joe's Progresso, Hunt's, and Red Pack (Note that Muir Glen, Eden Foods, and Trader Joe's don't have BPA in their linings)

☞ **Canned Soups:** Though it's infinitely less expensive (and yummier) to make your own soups from scratch, canned soups are great when you're in a pinch.

TIP: Many brands carry fat-free, low-fat, and low-sodium versions of their soups, and many are also organic. Some come in a jar, some come in a can, and some come in an aseptic, vacuum-sealed, cardboard box.

Varieties to Stock: Split pea, lentil, minestrone, carrot, tomato, bean, and chili are typical choices across all brands. (Look for the more "natural" brands to ensure that the soup is made with vegetable stock rather than animal-based stock.)

Vegan-Friendly Brands: Amy's, Health Valley Foods, Muir Glen, Simply Organic, Trader Joe's, Walnut Acres, Whole Foods 365, Westbrae. Instant soups, such as Dr. McDougall's, are also available, and some soups are packaged in aseptic (cardboard) boxes that don't need to be refrigerated until opened, such as Imagine Foods and Pacific Foods of Oregon.

SAUCES AND DRESSINGS

Pasta, Marinara, and Pizza Sauces: Choose sauces that have the fewest and most recognizable ingredients. Some brands add cheese or chicken broth, so check the label, and sometimes you'll see sugar in the list of ingredients. (Homemade pasta sauce often calls for a little sugar.) Better brands will use *sugar* and *not* corn syrup. Flavors that are typically vegan include arrabbiata, marinara, spicy red pepper, and tomato & basil.

> **Vegan-Friendly Brands:** Muir Glen, Whole Foods 365, Newman's Own, Amy's, Five Brothers, Classico, Walnut Acres, Barilla, Rao's, Prego, Trader Joe's

Salad Dressings: Some commercial dressings are made with eggs, honey, cow's milk, or cow's milk derivatives; just check the labels and look for more healthful brands, which also tend to be free of corn syrup and hydrogenated oil. Common flavors that tend to be vegan include Asian sesame, balsamic vinaigrette, French, goddess (tahini), green garlic, Italian, mango, miso ginger, raspberry vinaigrette, and shitake & sesame. Some brands are now even selling a commercial bottled "Caesar" dressing.

> **Vegan-Friendly Brands:** Annie's Naturals, Whole Foods 365, Spectrum Organics, Newman's Own, Organicville, Trader Joe's, Follow Your Heart, Briannas

Curry Pastes: Having curry pastes on hand allows you to whip up fast, flavorful meals by simply combining them with coconut milk and adding to sautéed vegetables. The best stuff can be found in Asian markets or large natural food stores, but wherever you're shopping, look for versions without fish sauce or fish paste. Green, red, yellow, Massaman, Panang, and Prik Khing are common varieties.

> **Vegan-Friendly Brands:** Thai Kitchen, Mae Anong, Maesri, A Taste of Thai, Cock, Jyoti

Stir-Fry Sauces: Although you can always opt for making your own stir-fry sauce, bottled varieties provide convenience. Many are vegan and can be added while vegetables are sautéing for instant flavor.

Salsa and Hummus: Kept in the fridge, these are two essential foods that add instant flavor and nutrients to many dishes. Choose fresh salsa in the refrigerated section over salsa in jars.

CONDIMENTS

If you take a closer look at all your condiments, you'll realize that most of them are naturally vegan. In fact, most of the things we flavor meat with are plant-based, as illustrated by all the condiments listed below and by the ones you most likely have in your pantry already, such as ketchup, mustard, relish, and chili sauce.

Other vegan-by-default cupboard essentials that may be less familiar to you depending on where you live are hoisin sauce, Marmite, Vegemite, and miso paste.

- **Tamari Soy Sauce:** Brewed longer than Chinese soy sauce, Japanese tamari is much fuller bodied and just tastes better. Try Shoyu or Bragg's Liquid Amino Acids for a similar flavor.

- **Tahini:** Essentially sesame butter (similar to peanut butter but grinding sesame seeds instead of peanuts), tahini is used to make hummus, salad dressings, and sauces.

- **Eggless Mayonnaise:** Vegan mayo just relies on the fat from plant oils rather than fat from eggs. The best vegan brands are Vegenaise by Follow Your Heart, Garlic Aioli by Wildwood, Just Mayo by Hampton Creek Foods, and Mindful Mayo by Earth Balance, although Spectrum Organics and Trader Joe's have eggless versions, too.

- **Barbecue Sauce:** Many people have half-consumed bottles of BBQ sauce in their fridge. Now's the time for a fresh start! Look for flavors and brands without honey.

- **Worcestershire Sauce:** Considered essential for Bloody Mary cocktails, vegan Worcestershire sauce contains no anchovies, reflected in such brands as Annie's Naturals, Edward & Sons, and The Wizard's.

SPREADS AND SYRUPS

Most jams, jellies, relishes, nut butters, and syrups are naturally vegan, but while you're in clean-out mode, look at the labels and get rid of those spreads and syrups that contain unhealthful corn syrup and hydrogenated oils.

- **Liquid Sweeteners:** Agave nectar, maple syrup, and brown rice syrup can generally be used interchangeably. Vegan-friendly brands include Karo, Lundberg, Eden Organic, Madhava, and Wholesome Sweetners.

- **Jams, Jellies, Preserves:** Look for those sweetened with fruit concentrate.

- **Nut and Seed Butters:** Almond, peanut, cashew, macadamia, sunflower seed, hemp seed, and coconut butters are all fabulous.

VINEGARS

I have an entire cupboard shelf dedicated to vinegars, since they lend so much flavor and depth to a variety of dishes and dressings. Now is the opportunity to experiment with new tastes and infusions.

- **Seasoned Rice:** "Seasoned" means a little sugar is added, taking the edge off the vinegar and making it a little sweeter. If you can't find seasoned, just buy plain rice vinegar and add a little of your own sugar.

- **Balsamic:** Use the cheap stuff for cooking and the good stuff for dressings. (Hint: if the label says "Modena," it's on the cheaper side.) Try different varieties, such as Balsamic Cherry Vinegar or White Balsamic Vinegar. Each is as special as the next and makes a great base for salad dressings.

- **Apple Cider:** Great for making for salad dressings and baked goods.

OILS

All cooking oils are vegan, but not all are created equal. Choose olive, sesame, canola, grapeseed, and coconut for cooking and baking (the latter three are best for baking), and avoid those high in polyunsaturated fats, such as vegetable, corn, safflower, and sunflower. My favorite instant-flavor oil is truffle. I use it sparingly and mostly at the end of recipes (like a lentil soup) to add flavor and richness; just a small amount packs a lot of flavor. Regardless, I recommend that you use oils sparingly just for a little added flavor or to keep food from sticking to pots and pans.

> **TIP:** *Buy an oil mister at a kitchen supply store, which enables you to use very little oil but still enough to coat pans to prevent food from sticking.*

HERBS, SPICES, AND VEGETABLE STOCKS

- **Dried Herbs and Spices:** Because herbs and spices tend to overwhelm or intimidate people, they sit on the spice rack for years until they're stale and flavorless. Learn to use them!

- **Vegetable Stock:** A wonderful ingredient that adds depth to so many dishes, vegetable stock is an easy switcheroo from chicken or beef stock. Prepared broths and stocks (also in low-sodium versions), such as No-Chicken, No-Beef, Vegetable, and Mushroom, are available in aseptic boxes, but I prefer veggie bouillon cubes for their convenience.

  Vegan-Friendly Brands (Prepared): Imagine Foods, Health Valley, Pacific Foods of Oregon **(Bouillon Cubes/Powder):** Massel, Rapunzel, Edward & Sons, Better Than Bouillon, Herb-Ox

- **Nutritional Yeast Flakes:** Although it suffers from what I think is a terribly unappetizing name, nutritional yeast is found in the bulk bins of natural food stores and adds cheesy flavor to sauces, pasta dishes, and popcorn. (And, I know from experience that cats and dogs also love it sprinkled on their food!)

BAKING ITEMS

Along with various flours (all-purpose, whole-wheat, pastry, and bread), you most likely already keep yeast packets (for making leavened breads), baking soda, baking powder, vanilla extract, and unsweetened cocoa powder in your pantry. Great. You might want to have muffin, scone, and cake mixes on hand in your kitchen as well. They're more expensive than when you bake from scratch, but sometimes the convenience is worth that extra expense. If the mix you buy calls for eggs or dairy-based milk, just follow the guidelines in Day 14: Baking Without Eggs (It's Better!), to make them vegan.

Other essential items you may want to add to your baking cupboard are whole flaxseeds (once you grind them, you should keep them in the refrigerator), commercial egg replacer (see Day 14: Baking Without Eggs), kudzu, arrowroot, agar agar, molasses, cornmeal, and chocolate chips. You may also want to keep some marshmallows on hand for classic hot cocoa, and yes, a number of vegan brands are available, including Dandies (made by Chicago Vegan Foods, chicagoveganfoods.com) and Sweet & Sara (sweetandsara.com).

> **Favorite Brands of Prepared Cake/Muffin Mixes:** Simply Organic, Oetker Organics, Bob's Red Mill, Arrowhead Mills, Hodgson Mills.

> ❦ **Premade Pie Crust:** All types of store-bought pie crusts are available these days, whether you're looking for Whole Wheat, Corn, Gluten-Free, or Graham Cracker

> **Vegan-Friendly Brands of Pie Crust:** Whole Foods 365, Wholly Wholesome, Trader Joe's, Vicolo, Oronoque Orchard's, and Keebler

> ❦ **Chocolate:** Chocolate is essential in baking (at least in my house, it is). Some companies (such as Hershey's and Nestle) play with definitions by adding cow's milk to what they call semi-sweet and dark chocolate bars and chips. Just take a quick peek at the ingredients to make sure there is no added "milk fat," "milk powder," or "casein." Check out foodispower.org for a list of the most ethically sourced cocoa beans.

DRIED BEANS AND LENTILS

Cooking beans from scratch is a breeze; lentils are even easier, since they don't have to be soaked first. Keep red lentils, brown/green lentils, Puy (French), Umbrian, and yellow or green split peas on hand for quick soups, stews, salads, pates, and loaves.

WHOLE GRAINS

Acting as a base or complement to many of the dishes you'll be preparing, whole grains are also simply delicious. Stock up on a variety—from Amaranth to Quinoa—so that you have options aplenty. Most whole grains have cooking instructions on the packaging, but in general, the ratio is 1 cup of grain to 2 or 3 cups of liquid.

PASTA AND NOODLES

Most commercial pastas (penne, angel hair, spaghetti, fettuccine, and linguine) and noodles (soba, udon, and rice) are vegan, made with semolina, buckwheat, or rice flour, water, and salt. (Gluten-free pastas are also available.) A few brands may add eggs, so just check the label.

NONDAIRY FOODS

Nondairy versions of familiar foods abound in the dairy section of the supermarket. No deprivation here!

- **Yogurt:** Cultured with all the "good bacteria" such as L. Acidophilus and B. Bifidum that people look for in dairy-based yogurts, there are soy milk-based (Silk, Wildwood, Trader Joe's, Whole Soy & Co.), coconut milk-based (Turtle Mountain/So Delicious), almond milk-based (Turtle Mountain/So Delicious and Almond Dream), and rice milk-based (Ricera) yogurts available.

- **Butter:** Earth Balance is my favorite; free of hydrogenated oils and trans fats, it's made from nongenetically modified ingredients, and comes in soy-free, organic, whipped, and stick versions. My preference is the organic version.

- **Milk:** Most plant-based milks come in aseptic boxes you can keep in the cupboard until they're ready to open. (Then they get stored in the fridge.) Soy, rice, oat, almond, hemp, hazelnut, and coconut are available in a number of brands and flavors.

    Vegan-Friendly Brands: Trader Joe's, Whole Foods, Wildwood, So Delicious/Turtle Mountain, Earth Balance, Silk, Soy Dream Vitasoy, Blue Diamond, Pacific, Almond Dream, Tempt Living Harvest, Hemp Bliss, Eden Soy

- **Cheese (Shredded, Sliced, and Spreadable):** You can find vegan cheeses in all shapes and sizes these days, and more will continue to flood the market. Larger health-oriented grocery stores will have the largest selection, but vegan stores online and off will most definitely carry them. (See Day 13 for more.)

    Vegan-Friendly Brands: Dr. Cow's Tree Nut Cheese, Kite Hill, Sheese, Sunergia Soy Foods, Parma in the Raw, Galaxy Nutritional Foods, Daiya, Teese

- **Sour Cream:** Make your own sour cream by puréeing silken tofu or cashews with lemon juice and salt, or check out the many commercial varieties, such as those made by Tofutti, Wayfare, Vegan Gourmet, and Galaxy Foods.

- **Cream Cheese:** The commercial versions are very good for spreading on bagels or for making cheesecake! Brands include Daiya, Tofutti, Vegan Gourmet, and Galaxy Foods.

VEGAN MEATS

Many vegan meats provide the salt, fat, texture, and familiarity that you crave in animal-based versions. Though they're certainly healthier than the animal-based versions, some of these lil' buggers are definitely highly processed and should be treated as convenience or transition foods—not daily health food.

> *TIP: Even within the category of vegan meats, there is a spectrum of how processed they are. Tofu and wheat gluten meats are less processed than soy isolate protein and soy protein concentrate meats. (See Day 17: Demystifying Tofu for more on this topic.)*

- **Deli Slices:** Soy-based Yves and Tofurky brands carry vegan turkey, ham, bologna, salami, and pepperoni, and wheat-based (soy-free) Field Roast's deli slices come in Lentil Sage, Wild Mushroom, and Smoked Tomato flavors.

- **Cutlets and Strips:** Field Roast makes delicious wheat-based (soy-free) nut-breaded cutlets, and Gardein and Beyond Meat specialize in soy-based versions.

- **Meatless Meatballs, Ground Veggie Meat, and Meatloaf:** Nate's, Trader Joe's, Match Meat, Gardein, and Yves are all vegan-friendly brands. Field Roast makes a fantastic meatloaf.

- **Sausages:** My favorite brands are Field Roast (wheat-based and soy-free) and Tofurky (tofu-based) for dinner-type sausages; Lightlife makes a gluten-based version called "Gimme Lean" that is ideal as a breakfast sausage. Sol Cuisine makes a wheat- and gluten-free breakfast sausage, and Field Roast makes delicious breakfast links called Apple Maple Sausage.

- **Veggie Dogs:** Field Roast "Frankfurters" (my favorite), Yves ("Tofu Dogs" and "Veggie Dogs"), and Lightlife ("Smart Dogs" and "Tofu Pups") will be in the refrigerated section; Loma Linda's "Little Links" are sold in a can.

- **Chicken-Free Nuggets:** A great transition food for kids because of their crispy coating, just pop them in the oven, and serve with ketchup or BBQ sauce.

  Vegan-Friendly Brands: Gardein, Trader Joe's, Health is Wealth, Lightlife, Boca—found in both the refrigerated and freezer sections.

- **Bacon:** Lightlife makes "Smart Bacon"; Turtle Island makes "Smoky Maple Bacon Marinated Tempeh."

- **Veggie Burgers:** Whether you're looking for tofu-based, veggie-based, or wheat-based, meatless burgers abound. Some are more processed than others are, some are vegetarian (not vegan) and contain chicken's eggs, so check the label.

Vegan-Friendly Brands: Dr. Praeger's, Amy's Kitchen, Trader Joe's, Sol Garden, and Gardenburger are found in the freezer section. Wildwood Foods, Soy Deli, and Trader Joe's all make tofu burgers found in the refrigerated—not frozen—section.

FREEZER ITEMS

Many healthful foods are found in the freezer section.

~ **Fruit:** Keep a combination of frozen fruit on hand for delicious smoothies.

   TIP: *When bananas are at their ripest, peel them, break the bananas into chunks, place in freezer bag, and store in freezer for instant, thick smoothies any time of the day. Check out the recipe for my Green Machine Smoothie on page 111.*

~ **Bread:** Some brands of sliced whole grain sandwich breads contain honey; others contain cow's milk derivatives, such as whey or casein. However, pita bread, lavash, sandwich rolls, fresh bread, French baguettes, and nice Italian rolls in the bakery section are more often vegan than the sliced breads meant to have a long shelf life.

   Vegan-Friendly Brands (Sliced Bread): Ezekiel (often in the freezer case), Rudi's Organic Bakery, Arnold's, Alvarado Street Bakery, Garden of Eatin'; **(Hot Dog and Hamburger Buns)** Alvarado Street Bakery, Rudi's Organic Bakery; **(English Muffins)** Rudi's Organic Bakery

~ **Frozen Pizza:** Varying in the type of crust and nondairy cheese they use, the most popular brands are Tofutti, Amy's Organic Kitchen, and Tofurky.

   TIP: *Prepared pizza crust, cornmeal crust, and phyllo dough found in the freezer are typically vegan.*

~ **Frozen Waffles:** Although you can make your own from scratch (see *The Joy of Vegan Baking!*), there are several brands that make vegan frozen waffles, including Van's and Nature's Path.

ICE CREAM AND SORBET

I grew up with a father who owned ice cream stores, so I'm a staunch critic. Once you get dairy out of your palate, though, you stop comparing what you *knew* with what's *new*. There are more options in grocery stores than I name here. Check the freezer section.

   Vegan-Friendly Brands: Turtle Mountain/So Delicious, Whole Soy, Temptation, Soy Dream, and Tofutti are popular soy milk ice creams with lots of flavors and frozen treats;

Coconut Bliss is a delicious coconut milk ice cream; Rice Dream is made from rice milk, and Almond Dream is made from almond milk.

TIP: Though sherbet and frozen yogurt are dairy-based, sorbet is vegan by definition. Choose brands that use cane sugar as a sweetener—not corn syrup.

SNACKS

- **Energy Bars:** Great for a quick refuel, many—if not most—energy bars are vegan. 22 Days Nutrition, Clif Bar, Luna, Lara, Organic Food, ProBar, Kind Bar, Raw Revolution, 18 Rabbits, and Vega bars are some of the brands to look for.

- **Chocolate Bars:** Good brands that carry vegan chocolate bars include 365 (Whole Foods), Divine, Endangered Species, Equal Exchange, Sjaak's, TCHO, and many more. (See foodispower.org for list of ethically sourced vegan chocolate.)

- **Dried Fruit Crisps:** More and more companies are making very simple, incredibly healthful snacks made simply from dried fruit. Check health food stores for the widest variety.

- **Bagged Crisps/Chips:** Not as healthful as fruit and veggies, but not as greasy as potato chips: pretzels, tortilla chips, crackers, Veggie Booty (aka Pirate Booty: Veggie) and Tings by Robert's American Gourmet are great treats for the lunch box.

- **Bottled Smoothies:** When you don't have time to make your own, try one of the many dairy-free smoothies in the refrigerated section of most grocery stores: Odwalla, Naked Juice, Bolthouse Farms, and Sambazon.

That should be enough to get you started. Many more brands and products are mentioned throughout the book in various sections.

My Favorite Kitchen Tools

I've seen it time and again: people think they don't need to invest in the proper kitchen tools (and gadgets) because they aren't cooking a lot, but what they don't realize is that they'd probably cook more—and more quickly and with lots of pleasure—if they invested in a few good tools. If you find it difficult, uncomfortable, or even dangerous to prepare food, then you're going to be less inclined to do so. Here are ten essentials I think every kitchen should have.

- **Knife**—One 8- or 9-inch chef's knife and a serrated knife for bread are really all you need.

- **Cutting Board**—In a vegan kitchen, you don't have to obsess about using separate cutting boards for meat and vegetables, so one sturdy wood or bamboo cutting board is all you need. Make sure the cutting board is at least 12 inches—preferably 18 inches wide.

- **Food Processor**—Most food processors have one single bowl with one blade, but the KitchenAid offers a large bowl and large blade and a small bowl with small blade you just insert into the large one.

- **Blender**—Do you need a blender *and* a food processor? I think so. There are some things that one can do, but the other can't. For instance, you cannot make a fruit smoothie in a food processor, and you wouldn't chop an onion in a blender. Get the highest-power blender you can afford and enjoy it for decades (many have lifetime guarantees).

- **Toaster Oven**—Perhaps I'm old-school, but I *love* my toaster oven! It uses a lot less energy than an oven, and you can cook and bake a lot of things besides toast without turning on your range.

- **Sturdy Pots and Pans**—Stainless steel has made a comeback; nonstick pans are now being made without Teflon, and people still swear by their beloved cast-iron pots. You decide what works best for you.

- **Coffee Grinder**—I use this little gadget to grind flaxseeds, which, once ground, must be kept in the refrigerator or freezer to avoid going rancid. (See Day 14: Baking Without Eggs)

- **Microplane**—Fantastic for grating ginger root, hard chocolate, fresh nutmeg, and for zesting lemons.

- **Electric Handheld Mixer**—I've had the same one since 1985; I use it regularly for both mixing cake batter and whipping potatoes.

- **Unbleached Parchment Paper**—*Not* wax paper (which burns when used in the oven). Parchment is perfect for creating a nonstick surface without oil.

- **Pizza Stone and Peel**—Find a simple pizza kit at any kitchen store. Foolproof pizza dough recipes can be found in my book *The Vegan Table*.

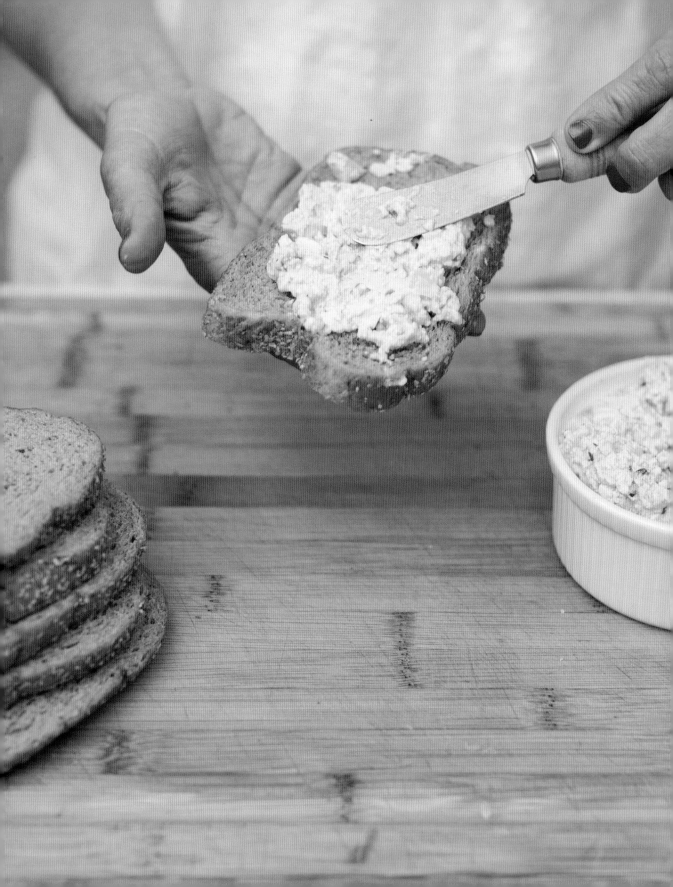

Eating Healthfully Affordably

The economic situation for many people today has made eating affordably a major topic of discussion around the dinner table and in the media. People are looking for ways to cut back on expenses, reduce the grocery bill, and pinch pennies just to get food on the table for their families. And whenever I hear this discussion, I just want to shout, "Eat a plant-based diet based on whole foods!"

When people make the transition to a whole foods plant-based diet, one of the things they notice is how much less money they spend on food. I've seen it time and again. Now, I realize you may be saying, "But wait! I'm about to go to the store to spend a lot of money restocking my kitchen!" I understand you may have to replace some animal-based products with plant-based ingredients, but I imagine we're talking mainly about condiments and the like. Because these items will last you a long time, keep in mind that you won't be buying these staples week after week. I think once you get beyond the initial 30 days, you'll be better able to more accurately calculate what you're spending on your weekly groceries, and unless you're relying on prepackaged, premade, convenience foods, I would wager that your grocery bill will decrease.

My hope here is to debunk the myth that "eating vegan" is more expensive than eating an animal-based diet and guide you to eating healthfully affordably. Looking through this lens will help you as you plan your trip to the grocery store.

CHALLENGE YOUR THINKING: Convenience foods—vegan or nonvegan—simply cost more than whole foods.

CHANGE YOUR BEHAVIOR: To make the most healthful and affordable choices, make whole plant foods the foundation of your diet.

CHALLENGE YOUR THINKING: The problem isn't that organic, locally grown, ethically produced foods are expensive; the problem is that unhealthful, ethically questionable products—such as meat, dairy, and eggs—are subsidized and thus artificially cheap.

COST COMPARISON

Even with the government subsidies that the meat, dairy, and egg industries enjoy, animal proteins are still more expensive than plant proteins. The cheapest cuts of beef, such as ground meat, average $3.00 per pound in the U.S; boneless chicken breasts average $3.40 a pound; and canned tuna fish is about $2.00 per pound. Contrast that with dried beans and lentils at less than $1.00 a pound and rice well below $1.00 per pound. Tofu is also usually under $2.00 a pound. The cost of nuts and seeds vary, and although pine nuts tend to be expensive, you can always choose sunflower seeds, which contain nearly the same amount of protein at a fraction of the price.

If you price out vegan meats, such as veggie dogs, they do tend to cost about $5 a pound, so this is just another reason I emphasize basing your diet on whole foods. If you want to indulge in these convenience foods once in a while, that's fine, but keep in mind that even when you buy *nonvegan* convenience foods, you're paying more than if you bought whole foods. Ultimately, in terms of the most healthful and most affordable food, whole plant foods win every time—over processed foods *and* over animal products.

COSTS BEYOND DOLLARS

Notice I'm using the word "affordable"—not the word "cheap." There's a big difference between eating affordably and eating cheaply. I'm not talking about eating cheap food, which is what we've all become accustomed to primarily due to government subsidies and buy-backs for meat, dairy, and eggs. Because of these artificially cheap products, we tend to complain when we have to pay the true cost of whole, organic, nonsubsidized foods. The problem isn't that these foods are expensive; the problem is that animal products are priced artificially low.

Aside from changing our buying habits, we need to change our *thinking* when it comes to the money we spend on what we eat. Traditionally, people have praised "cheap" animal products that allow more people to buy what are—in fact—very expensive things to produce, but they are ignoring the full costs beyond the actual dollars we spend—costs to our health, our planet, the people who produce our food, and the animals.

The people who live in North Carolina, the heart of the pig-meat industry, have a lot to say about the high cost of cheap hot dogs, ham slices, and bacon strips. 10 million pigs are confined on North Carolina "hog farms," and there are serious, serious public health and environmental concerns as a result (not to mention concerns about the animals).

One of the biggest problems stems from the fact that pigs excrete four times as much waste as humans do, and that pours into huge open-air waste lagoons, often as big as several football fields. These lagoons are prone to leaks and spills, and there have been several instances of lagoons bursting and spilling millions of gallons of pig waste into nearby rivers, killing fish, destroying wetlands, contaminating water supplies, sickening people, and destroying anything that lives.

The animal waste consumes the oxygen in the water and destroys everything and everyone in that water. Where there is no oxygen, there is no life. Hence, there is the "dead zone" in the Gulf of Mexico, the size of which fluctuates each year, but it is about 7,000 to 8,000 square miles large.[30] Luckily, our choices are not limited to "cheap animal-based hot dogs" or "expensive veggie hot dogs." That's a false dichotomy. The options for affordable, healthful plant-based foods are endless.

HEALTH CARE COSTS

Anyone who claims those cheap animal products are good for the consumer hasn't considered another way we pay for them: our health care costs, which are much lower for vegans than they are for nonvegans and nonvegetarians.[31] Vegans have less chronic disease, better heart health, and a lower risk of certain cancers. In fact, health insurance agencies are promoting lifestyle changes to try to offset the costs associated with heart disease, and yet there are still no discounts available for those who follow a vegan diet. I am, however, optimistic that this is on the horizon.

Coronary bypass surgery, stents, cholesterol-lowering drugs, diabetes drugs, and dialysis—all correlated with animal-based diets—are incredibly expensive; a bypass surgery or angioplasty procedure can cost about $40,000.[32] Some 16,000,000 people (8,700,000 men and 7,300,000 women[33]) are living with some form of coronary heart disease. An estimated 1,065,000 people suffer a (new or recurrent) coronary attack every year.[34] As a result, in 2010, there were 397,000 coronary artery bypass graft surgeries performed in the United States each year, making them two of the most commonly performed major operations.[35]

And people complain that an organic apple costs more than a nonorganic one.

What's more: how many people undergoing these expensive treatments have no insurance? How many of them are the working poor or the elderly? How many of them are not told by their physicians that they have options other than getting their chests cut open and going through a risky procedure only to have a temporary band-aid applied.

In the vast majority of cases, an unhealthy cardiovascular system is the result of lifestyle, namely a poor diet. A 2003 study published in the Journal of the American Medical Association concluded that a vegan diet is as effective as statin drugs in lowering LDL cholesterol levels—without the side effects.[36]

Every time we don't choose a healthful plant food, we're making a decision about how we want to feel in the short term as well as in the long term. And, we're making these decisions for our children, too. Research indicates that the food habits instilled in us as children dictate how we eat as adults. Research also indicates that the food choices we make as children are strong predictors of disease later in life. In other words, what children eat during their formative years has a profound impact on their future health, and since American children eat so few whole plant foods, there is much room for improvement.

MONETARY COSTS

I admit I tend to romanticize the stories my father tells me about how his family lived during the Depression. They had very little money and literally counted every penny. He tells me how exciting it was for him and his siblings when they had enough money to buy a half a loaf of bread for dinner one night or a lollipop for each as a treat. I'm certainly not trivializing the difficulties he and his family experienced, but rather, I appreciate the simplicity of how they lived and the gratitude they felt when they were able to afford something "extravagant," such as a lollipop or an extra piece of bread. We all know how much we appreciate something we have to fight for. And, in our days of plenty, we don't have to fight for much, and so I think we tend to appreciate less.

I'm actually overwhelmed when I go into a grocery store, because the choices we have are frankly ridiculous—almost embarrassing. Although I'm grateful for the privilege of having so many options, it actually just makes me more inclined toward simplicity—the simplicity we're often forced into when we're in a recession, or when income is low, or when we need to get a better handle on our budget. This simplicity that has so many benefits, including

- ► appreciating what we have

- ► saving up for what we really want

- ► using up what we have in our cupboards before going shopping

- ► choosing healthful whole foods rather than expensive packaged products

- ► cooking simple meals that rely on just a few ingredients

Here are some ways I recommend choosing simplicity and thus experiencing a myriad of benefits.

EAT AT HOME

Cooking at home is one of the best and easiest ways to eat affordably. Today, Americans are spending over 43% of the food budget eating out,[37] and fast food accounts for over 50% of the 11 billion meals eaten outside the home in the UK.[38] Eating out that much takes a toll on our wallets, on our bodies, and even on our taste buds. Restaurant chefs are trained to maximize the use of fat and salt, so their calorie-dense dishes not only contribute to weight gain and health problems but also to our palates lacking sensitivity, coated as they are with fat and salt. Eating out should be an occasional treat, not a daily rite.

I say this aware that people working in offices are often bound by lunchtime meetings and that people who travel extensively for work have little choice but to eat in restaurants. What I'm suggesting is that *when we are able*, we choose home-cooked meals over restaurant fare. This may not always be as possible for the lunchtime meal (although you can pack sandwiches and salads—see Day 10: Packing Lunches for School and Work), but I do recommend that you at least strive to eat breakfast and dinner at home. You will notice a huge difference in how you feel and in how much less money you spend.

BUY IN BULK

When I suggest buying in bulk, I'm not necessarily referring to buying 50 packages of paper towels. I'm talking about shopping in the bulk section of grocery stores and natural food stores, where you can buy dried foods, such as pasta, grains, flour, oatmeal, lentils, beans, and even herbs and spices from bins, choosing exactly how much you want and paying for the weight of that food rather than for the brand name or packaging. Buying in bulk is not only less expensive; it is also much more Earth-friendly, especially if you bring your own bags and containers to the store.

COOK FROM SCRATCH

Of course, there are times you want to just call the pizza guy (and yes, most regular pizza restaurants and pizza delivery places will happily leave the cheese off of the pizza upon request), and when you do, you pay more in money than you do in time. Sometimes, that's the choice we make, and that's fine, but in the end, cooking from scratch is always healthier and more affordable than eating out or buying premade, convenience foods, including when it comes to baking. It's true there are vegan cake, brownie, and biscuit mixes out there (See Day 3), as well as fantastic vegan bakeries (and nonvegan bakeries that make vegan baked goods), but if you're looking to save money, those are unnecessary expenses. When you parse out the ingredients for any of the recipes for baked goods in this book (or any other), you'll find that it costs a couple dollars to make them from scratch, even using organic, fair trade ingredients.

CHOOSING NUTRIENT-DENSE FOODS

We provide a car with high-quality fluids for it to run well, and *we* need high-quality fuel for our own bodies to run well. If we fill our car or bodies with junk, they may still run, but not optimally, and optimal health should be our goal. We want to get the best *caloric* bang for our buck (eating enough food to have the energy to function well), but ideally, we want to get the most *nutritional* bang for our buck, as well.

Physiologically, we need calories for energy, but we also need other nutrients to function properly. The best food choices provide calories with lots of nutrients. This is the principle behind avoiding eating "empty calories." They may fill you up, but they don't provide you with the nutrients you need to function well. It's like filling up a gas tank with water. The tank might be full, but it's not filled with a

CHALLENGE YOUR THINKING: Highly processed and refined foods as well as animal products may fill you up, but they don't provide much nutrient value in return.

CHANGE YOUR BEHAVIOR: Get the most nutritional bang for your caloric buck: choose nutrient-dense foods.

substance that enables it to run, and soon the car will break down. Processed and refined foods are mostly "empty calories"; although they have the same energy content per calorie, they lack vitamins, minerals, antioxidants, phytochemicals, and fiber that are vital to health. The same can be said of meat, dairy, and eggs: they provide many calories but very little nutrient value in return. No fiber. No antioxidants. No phytochemicals.

In other words: in order to make the *most* of the calories we eat, we want to choose nutrient-dense calories. Think of how much money we spend in the form of empty calories—including beverages, such as sodas, juices, and fancy coffee drinks. Many calories are consumed with very little return in terms of nutrition.

Based on their nutrient-per-calorie density, the winners are:

- 1st Place: dark leafy green vegetables such as kale, collard greens, chard, mustard greens, and turnip greens

- 2nd place: other green vegetables: brussels sprouts, broccoli, artichokes, asparagus, celery, cucumbers, peas, green peppers, snow peas, snap peas, string beans, and zucchini squash

- 3rd place (but still complete winners): non-green veggies like beets, tomatoes, carrots, squash, bell peppers, and cauliflower and fresh fruits

BECOME A SAVVY SHOPPER

Don't fall into the traps of overspending and making unhealthful food choices at the grocery store. To avoid this:

▶ **Make a list.** Having a list and sticking to it is vital to saving money. This is where planning your meals ahead comes in handy (See Day 7: Making the Time to Cook). Knowing what you want to eat for the week enables you to look through your recipes carefully enough to create your shopping list and prevents you from running out to the store for one item, which always winds up turning into several by the time you leave the store. Commit to buying only what you need and resist temptations along the way. Keep a chalkboard or eraser board in the kitchen to note items you're low on or out of.

▶ **Look down.** Items on the lower shelves of the grocery store tend to be less flashy, less processed, less intensively packaged—and thus less expensive.

▶ **Eat before you shop.** It may be obvious, but it's helpful advice nonetheless. We never make the best choices when we're ravenously hungry. Eat first.

▶ **Choose local.** Because most supermarket produce travels thousands of miles before arriving, it's bred for having a long shelf life—not for optimum flavor. To experience maximum flavor and freshness—while supporting your own local farms—choose locally grown fruits and veggies as much as possible either by buying them at farmer's markets or by shopping in grocery stores that adhere to the law that requires them to notify customers the source of where certain foods are grown.

► **Know when to choose organic.** Because organic produce is priced according to its true cost, it feels more expensive than subsidized, artificially priced conventionally grown produce. To help make the best decisions about when to buy organic, check out the Environmental Working Group's "Shopper's Guide to Pesticides in Produce" at ewg.org.

At a glance, "The Dirty Dozen" is the category of fruits and veggies that tend to be so highly sprayed with harmful chemicals that they should be eaten only when labeled organic: apples, strawberries, grapes, celery, peaches, spinach, sweet bell peppers, imported nectarines, cucumbers, cherry tomatoes, imported snap peas, and potatoes.[39] Those least-sprayed are called the "Clean 15" and include avocados, sweet corn, pineapples, cabbage, frozen sweet peas, onions, asparagus, mangoes, papayas, kiwis, eggplant, grapefruit, cantaloupe, cauliflower, and sweet potatoes.[40]

► **Don't browse.** Think of the different grocery departments as separate stores within the supermarket. Just as you wouldn't shop at every store at the mall, think of the grocery store this way. Walk down only the aisles that house the products on your list. Skip the others.

► **Put off going to the grocery store.** When you "haven't a thing to eat," take a long hard look at your newly veganized cupboards, freezer, and refrigerator. Most likely, you have enough to make a few more meals before heading to the store. Make a stew with those canned beans; make a pilaf with that brown rice. Spoiled as we are, we think we have to run to the store every time we're low in the staples. Be creative, and stretch out your visits a little longer. You'll save a little money and perhaps enjoy seeing what you can come up with.

Applying these principles, you'll save loads of money and make huge strides in preventing costly and life-threatening diseases.

Reading Labels

With a good idea of what to fill your cupboards with and in preparation for going to the grocery store to stock up *and* save money, let's look at how to read labels so you can identify the most prevalent animal products that appear in various items.

Contrary to what some people think, vegans do not spend all their time deciphering labels. Once you know what to look for, one quick glance at the label will tell you whether something has an animal product in it. Having said that, if you have to weed through a long list of ingredients to determine if it's vegan or not, you probably shouldn't be eating that product anyway. Why would you want to eat something that resembles a chemistry experiment rather than real food? You shouldn't feel like you're in science class when you read a label.

The best way to avoid labels altogether is to eat whole foods as much as possible. The more you eat whole foods, the less you have to worry about animal products or unnecessary and potentially harmful ingredients in your food.

However, there are plenty of commercial foods available to us that are perfectly healthful to consume; some may come in a box, some in a jar, some in a can, some in a bag, and all of them—by law—have to have ingredients listed on their labels. Although making whole foods the foundation of our diet is optimal, it's helpful to know what to look for when we're buying perfectly healthful things such as canned beans, canned soups, packaged tortillas, jarred tomato sauce, condiments, and the like.

When reading labels, I recommend looking for:

► foods with the fewest ingredients possible (making exceptions, of course, when something includes a long list of spices and herbs)

► ingredients with recognizable names

► ingredients that are animal-free

Some people argue that once you eliminate the most obvious animal products from your diet (meat, animal's milk, and eggs), you can relax a bit when it comes to the animal products hidden in commercial foods. Although I agree that being vegan is not about obsessing over being perfect, I simply don't want to consume the blood, bones, or fat of animals—even when they're hidden among other ingredients. I would never buy any of these things if they were sold individually, and I don't want to eat them shoved into my food as filler or fat. In fact, many of these animal products are given names other than what they really are because even the manufacturers know that people wouldn't buy them if they knew exactly what they were.

Look out for the following:

Gelatin: Made by boiling the skin, bones, and connective tissues of slaughtered animals—most often cattle, pigs, horses, and fishes—gelatin is the by-product of the meat and leather industries. If it says "gelatin" on the label, it is from an animal. Though there are vegetable-derived "gelatins" available, particularly in the form of agar, guar gum, carrageenan, and pectin, they are NOT the source if a label simply says "gelatin."

Products most associated with gelatin are Jell-O, marshmallows, vitamin capsules, gummy bears, and ice cream. Vegan versions of all are available.

ETHICAL CONSIDERATION: Though gelatin is made from the "byproducts" of slaughterhouse waste, it is misguided to think that using the remains of the animals is a noble use of what would "go to waste," as many people assert. We unnecessarily kill 10 billion land animals and countless marine animals every year, and the industries that profit off these animals have come up with sundry ways to make even more money by selling their byproducts. These very profitable byproduct industries simply wouldn't exist if we didn't systematically kill animals in the first place. By purchasing animal byproducts, we are supporting the primary industries we ethically oppose.

Whey and casein: Both are both derived from animal's milk. When you curdle dairy-based milk (to make cheese), you are essentially separating the milk solids (casein) from the milk liquid (whey). If the label says "casein," "caseinate," "milk protein," "sodium caseinate," or "whey," these ingredients are most definitely animal-derived. Some soy- and rice-based cheeses contain casein.

Products most associated with casein and whey: Some—but not all—brands of protein powders, boxed cereals, cereal bars, processed sandwich breads, prepared breadcrumbs, and crackers contain these cow's milk derivatives. Vegan versions of these foods are definitely available, so just check the label.

HEALTH CONSIDERATION: When you separate the curds from the whey to make cheese, you're tangling up all the milk proteins (the casein) into solid masses or "curds." What remains contains only whey proteins. In cow's milk, 80%-87% of the proteins are caseins, which is not a good thing. According to renowned researcher and Professor Emeritus of Nutritional Biochemistry at Cornell University, T. Colin Campbell, casein is the "number one carcinogen (i.e. cancer-causing substance) that people come in contact with on a daily basis."[41] In dairy-based cheeses, the casein is even more concentrated, and in low-fat dairy-based milks, there tends to be more casein to make up for the fat that has been removed.

Lactose: The sugar in all mammalian milk (including human's), lactose appears on labels as such. However, "lactate" or "lactic acid" is not animal-derived.

HEALTH CONSIDERATION: There seems to be a misunderstanding about the components that make up mammalian milk, since I often hear people mistakenly assert that they're "allergic to milk" and thus drink lactose-free cow's milk. Casein is the milk *protein* to which people can become allergic; lactose is the milk *sugar* that gives many people gas, bloating, and cramps. Since so many people are suffering from "lactose intolerance," which is our body's natural revulsion to a sugar we're not equipped to digest after we're weaned, the dairy industry came up with a profitable solution: lactose-free milk. Though the milk may not contain lactose, it still contains saturated fat, dietary cholesterol, and casein. If you want truly lactose-free milk, drink those derived from plants.

Lanolin: A fat derived from sheep's wool, lanolin is a by-product of the wool industry, and it is most commonly found in cosmetics, lotions, moisturizers, and lip balms. The Procter & Gamble product "Oil of Olay" comes from the word "lanolin," which is a primary ingredient. (When contacted, the company confirmed that now only their body washes do not contain lanolin.) Plenty of beauty products are made without lanolin.

Stearate or Stearic Acid: A fat derived from either plant or animal sources, it's used for making candles, soaps, and plastics; it's sometimes used in chewing gum and candy. The best way to know its source is to read the label. If it's plant-derived, it will most likely say so.

Carmine or Cochineal: Both of these terms refer to the ground-up bodies of beetles that are then used as a coloring in red-color juices, dairy-based yogurt and ice cream, and cosmetics. The word carmine is derived from a word that means "crimson," so essentially you'll find it in products that are some shade of red, pink, or purple. It also appears on labels as "carminic acid."

Bonito are dried fish flakes frequently seen in Japanese foods.

Lard is the fat taken from pigs' stomachs. Many Mexican restaurants make their refried beans without lard and use vegetable-based oils, instead. If they use lard for their refried beans, order the whole beans!

Lipoids or Lipids are the fat and fat-like substances found in both animals and plants. When they're from plants, the label usually says so.

Rennet or Rennin is an enzyme taken from the fourth stomach of young ruminants (e.g. cattle, goats, bison, buffalo, deer) to make dairy-based cheese. (Read more about this on Day 17: Demystifying Tofu: It's Just a Bean!) Each ruminant produces the special kind of rennet needed to digest his or her mother's milk. There's kid-goat rennet especially for goat's milk cheese, lamb-rennet for sheep's milk cheese, and calf rennet for cow's milk cheese. Most of the stomachs are from the discarded males of the dairy industry who are sold to the veal industry.

Aside from learning to recognize these animal products, another way to tell if a product (food, clothing, personal care item) is vegan is to look for the trademarked "Certified Vegan" symbol, managed by an organization called Vegan Action (vegan.org).

WARNING LABELS

These days, we also see many warnings on labels that say the food was manufactured in plants and on equipment that have also been used for cow's milk and other allergens. This is mainly about liability protection. The Food Allergy Labeling and Consumer Protection Act now requires labeling of any food that contains or was in contact with machinery that saw one or more of the following allergens: peanuts, soybeans, cow's milk, eggs, fish, crustacean shellfish, tree nuts, and wheat.

People have asked me if I—from a vegan perspective—buy or eat products processed using machinery that also processes nonvegan products. My answer is: yes, I do. That kind of low-level concern about purity is not why I'm vegan, and it doesn't mean I'm less vegan if I eat chocolate chips that were processed on machinery that may also process nonvegan chips.

Being vegan is about doing the best we can in an imperfect world. It's not about being perfect or pure. If we lose sight of that, if we treat veganism as the *end* rather than the *means*, then we'll not only drive ourselves crazy, we'll also forget what being vegan is all about. There are some things we have no control over, and I think it makes more sense to focus on what we *can* do rather than on what we *can't*.

And, there's *so* much we *can* do.

> **CHALLENGE YOUR THINKING:**
> Being vegan is not about obsessing over being perfect, but if we wouldn't buy the blood, bones, and fat of animals sold separately, why would we want to eat them hidden among other ingredients?

> **CHALLENGE YOUR THINKING:**
> If we treat veganism as the end rather than the means, then we'll not only drive ourselves crazy, we'll also forget what being vegan is all about.
>
> **CHANGE YOUR BEHAVIOR:**
> Focus on what you *can* to do manifest your values of compassion and wellness—not on what you *can't* do.

Getting to Know the Grocery Store

I took the first five days of the Challenge to prepare you for today. After all, the goal of *The 30-Day Vegan Challenge* isn't simply to help you make a better shopping list; it's to provide a new foundation for you to stand on and a new lens for you to look through. So now that you have cleaned out your cupboards, made your shopping list, learned some tips for eating affordably, and learned how to identify animal-based ingredients at a glance, it's time to go shopping!

Habituated to choosing the same items again and again, we're not even aware of how unconscious we are when we shop: hypnotically choosing the same brands over and over, never venturing down certain aisles, avoiding looking at foods that might be unfamiliar to us, or making impulse purchases precisely because product-placement makes it incredibly easy for us to do so. Make no mistake about it; though it appears you're exercising personal choice and freedom when you choose one product over another, massive efforts and huge amounts of money go into influencing—i.e. manipulating—your decisions. Careers are built on the study of consumer behavior such that each item sold in the grocery store—and the average supermarket sells 40,000 edible products—is methodically shelved, priced, and advertised based on the results of these studies.

At a time when cardiovascular disease, diabetes, and obesity are at an all-time high, food companies famously shirk responsibility and deny their own influence, claiming that individuals have the freedom to make their own personal choices and are clearly choosing the foods that they want.

You often hear this type of reasoning in the attempt to justify people's consumption of meat, dairy, and eggs, "If people didn't want these

CHALLENGE YOUR THINKING:
Though it appears you're exercising personal choice and freedom when you choose one product over another, massive efforts and huge amounts of money go into influencing—i.e. manipulating—your decisions.

CHANGE YOUR BEHAVIOR:
Make informed food choices by becoming a conscious, informed, savvy shopper.

things, they wouldn't buy them. The animal products industries are just filling a consumer demand." Never mind that the demand is created and shaped by the very companies who have the most to gain. Every day, every moment—whether it's through radio and television commercials; magazine, newspaper, and Internet advertisements; supermarket product placement; billboards; or celebrity endorsements, *we are told what to eat,* especially when it comes to animal products. We're told, "Real men eat meat," that humans are *supposed to* consume another animal's milk, and that chickens' eggs are "nature's perfect food." Unless you live in a hovel in the ground, no one is immune to these messages, which are so powerful, so prevalent, and so effective that any recommendations *against* consuming meat, dairy, and eggs are called *biased.*

This plays out in the number of times I've I heard people declare that vegans have an *agenda.* "It's fine if they want to eat that way, but they shouldn't tell other people how to eat. They shouldn't impose their opinions on others." Yet, the companies who have the most to gain are telling us how to eat *all the time.* We've been conditioned to believe that to consume meat, dairy, and eggs is to take a neutral position, but to be vegan is to have an "agenda." Just one critically minded walk through a typical grocery store is enough to demonstrate that we choose—almost hypnotically—what the food companies *want* us to choose—primarily in the form of unhealthful animal products and highly processed junk.

So how do you take this inevitable weekly or bi-weekly trek through the supermarket and make the most healthful, conscious, compassionate choices possible?

- ▶ **Learn the layout.** When you seek it, you'll find "vegan food" all over the place, everywhere you look. Here are some tips for finding "vegan" items that may be new to you. Placement may vary from store to store, but in general:

  - » Nondairy milks are next to dairy-based milks in the refrigerated section; however, the aseptically packaged/cardboard-boxed milks are often on the shelves near similarly packaged juice boxes.

  - » Nondairy butters, yogurts, and cheeses are next to dairy-based butters, yogurts, and cheeses.

  - » Tofu and vegan meats tend to be shelved together in the refrigerated produce or dairy section. Silken tofu, however, sold in cardboard aseptic boxes, tends to be shelved either with baking ingredients or in the aisle where Asian products are shelved.

  - » Some brands of eggless mayonnaise are in the condiment section, but most are in the refrigerator case with nonvegan mayo.

  - » Commercial egg replacer powder tends to be with baking ingredients. Don't be lead astray by a grocery clerk who brings you to the refrigerated section to show you the "egg beaters" in the little carton. They're still eggs—they're just egg *whites.*

  - » Nondairy ice creams are in the freezer with dairy-based ice creams.

» Veggie burgers and other vegan convenience foods are often in the frozen section, though tofu-based burgers tend to be in the refrigerated section—next to the tofu. Burger *mixes* would most likely be in the aisle with similar types of prepared boxed foods that just call for adding hot water.

► **Pick up a new food.** The most familiar "vegan" foods will be vegetables, fruits, legumes, grains, mushrooms, nuts, seeds, herbs, and spices. But just because you know what a vegetable or grain is doesn't mean you've tried them all. Pick up a new plant-based food today in any of the aforementioned categories, and try it.

► **Go international.** Check out the shelves reserved for Asian, Middle Eastern, Mexican, and Indian food items. You'll find sauces, condiments, prepared meals, spices—most of which happen to be vegan.

► **Spice it up.** Most people have spices and dried herbs in their kitchen, and most people have dust collecting on those cute little jars. The shelf life of dried herbs and spices is about 6 and 12 months, respectively. If yours are past their prime (or if you can't remember when you bought them), replace them with fresh herbs and spices. Over the course of this Challenge, you'll gain more confidence using fresh herbs and spices in your cooking.

► **Ask for what you want.** If your store doesn't carry an item you're seeking, ask them to stock it. If their distributors carry it, they will probably be happy to sell it—especially if they know at least one person will buy it. (Most likely, more people will buy it once it's stocked, and the store will continue selling it.)

► **Shop on the perimeter.** The outside aisles are where you'll find the fresh, whole foods, such as produce and bulk items such as grains and nuts. More processed products are in the center aisles.

► **Shop by color.** This is easy to do when you're centering your diet on whole foods (not colorfully packaged items). When in the produce section, fill your cart with as much color variety as possible. (See my cookbook, *Color Me Vegan* for everything you need to know about the advantages of eating according to color, as well as dozens and dozens of recipes.)

In addition to health food stores and online vegan grocery stores (see Sidebar), don't forget to check out those little neighborhood markets that cater to specific cuisines. You can find an array of tantalizing plant-based condiments, spices, and herbs in Indian, Middle Eastern, Asian, or Mexican markets.

Vegan Grocery Stores

Although you can find almost any of the vegan food items I recommend in large or small natural food stores, online and offline vegan grocery stores are popping up all over the world. These vegan-owned companies specialize in food but also carry an array of compassionate products such as clothing, shoes, and toiletries.

- **Food Fight Vegan Grocery** in Portland, Oregon
  Online and retail store · foodfightgrocery.com

- **Nooch Vegan Market** in Denver, Colorado
  Shop in person · noochveganmarket.com

- **Park + Vine** in Cincinnati, Ohio
  Retail storefront · parkandvine.com

- **Republic of V** in Oakland, California
  Retail storefront · republicofvegan.com

- **Vegan Haven** in Seattle, Washington
  Shop online or in person · veganhaven.org

- **Vegan Essentials** in Wisconsin
  Online shopping; no in-person shopping, but they welcome you to pick up orders that are placed online or visit to try on footwear · veganessentials.com

- **Vegan Store** in Rockville, Maryland
  Online store and open for walk-in customers during select hours · veganstore.com

- **Viva La Vegan** in Rancho Cucamonga, California
  Online store and open for walk-in customers · vivalavegangrocery.com

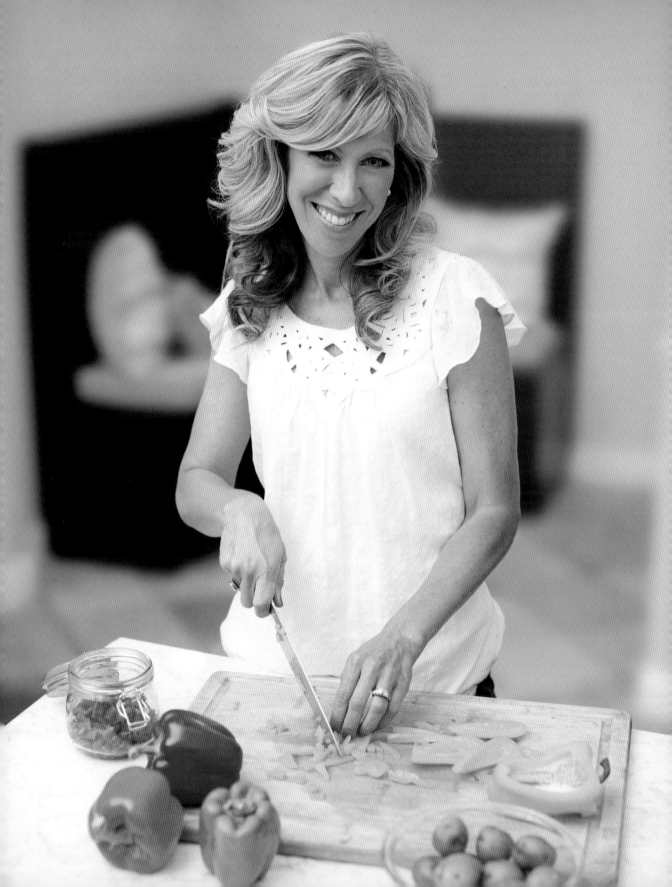

Making the Time to Cook

Let's assess things thus far. You've been to the grocery store, learned to recognize animal-derived ingredients on labels, restocked your kitchen with healthful foods, and realized that many of the things you were already eating were "vegan." Now it's time to demystify *cooking*. Although I expect (and hope!) that you will have prepared some meals before today, this chapter is about helping you lay a strong foundation that will empower you to feel confident in the kitchen all your live-long days. It's also an opportunity to start trying some of the recipes featured throughout this book.

One of the most common excuses for not eating a healthful, plant-based diet is, "I just don't have time to cook."

We've become so dependent on processed, packaged, frozen, and fast food that our barometer for how much time we should spend on preparing our meals has become completely skewed. Our idea of how long we should spend on cooking (and eating!) has become completely distorted. Our threshold for chopping vegetables tends to be about "zero."

We need a new measuring stick. It's true that cooking requires a little extra time, but compared to what? Compared to throwing a package of processed food-like substances into the microwave? Sure, I'll concede. Cooking requires more time than that, but is that really the measuring stick we want to use?

Even if you think you're eating well but basing your diet on animal-based products, complaining that you have to chop vegetables is still not a viable excuse. *Everyone* should be eating vegetables—not just vegans.

CHALLENGE YOUR THINKING: Our threshold for chopping vegetables has become completely distorted.

CHANGE YOUR BEHAVIOR: Change your barometer, and create a new measuring stick. Decide what is a reasonable amount of time to spend on chopping vegetables each day, with 15 minutes being the minimum.

CHALLENGE YOUR THINKING: If we don't have time to be sick, then we have to make time to be healthy.

Fifteen to thirty minutes is a reasonable amount of time to spend on making healthful food for our families and ourselves, and it's not only possible, it's imperative. Taking fifteen to thirty minutes a day to nurture ourselves, to nourish our bodies, and to feed our families is really no time at all. In fact, whatever we're doing that we think is more important than taking care of ourselves or our loved ones will mean nothing when we're not well enough or not here to enjoy it. If we think we can't find a few minutes a day to take care of ourselves or those who depend on us, then perhaps we need to reexamine our priorities.

The bottom line is if we don't have time to be sick, then we have to make time to be healthy.

WE HAVE THE TIME. WE DON'T MAKE THE EFFORT.

However, I think we *do* have the time. Although everyone complains about busy schedules, if we were honest with ourselves, we'd admit that we *do* have the time to cook; we just don't *use* our time to make the effort.

If we have the time to pack the family into the car, drive to a restaurant, find a parking spot, stand in line to wait for a table, decide what to order, wait for the food, eat the food, wait for the bill, pay the bill, then drive back home, we have *time* to chop some vegetables.

The goal is to make healthful, delicious, plant-based meals in a reasonable amount of time—not spend countless hours in the kitchen. With that in mind, let's look at a number of ways to make this a reality.

1. Chop Vegetables in Advance

Most of us can identify with this scenario: you go to the grocery store and stock up on vegetables; you come home and store the vegetables in the refrigerator. When it's time to eat, you return to the fridge, stare into its great abyss, and declare, "There's not a thing to eat." You lament that it would take too long to cut up the veggies in time for dinner, so instead, you call the pizza guy (for whom you have to wait!) or heat up a frozen dinner, while said vegetables begin to break down without being eaten, eventually ending up in the trash can instead of in your belly.

Now picture this: You arrive home from the farmer's market or grocery store and instead of shoving all the vegetables in the fridge, you take 15 minutes to chop them—at least some of them. You store the chopped veggies in bags and containers, and *then* place them in the fridge. Hours later, you return for something to eat. Looking at the ready-to-use chopped peppers, sliced onion, and minced garlic, you're inspired to make a stir-fry. The shredded lettuce and sliced fennel make a quick salad. You snack on the sliced carrots while you put it all together, and the cooking process itself becomes enjoyable and stress-free.

For some reason, if the tops are still on the carrots, the broccoli is still joined at the stem, or the cauliflower is still in its head, we have a mental block. We complain that it will take us *forever* to chop them up, and so we leave them to compost in the refrigerator and wonder why we're always throwing vegetables away.

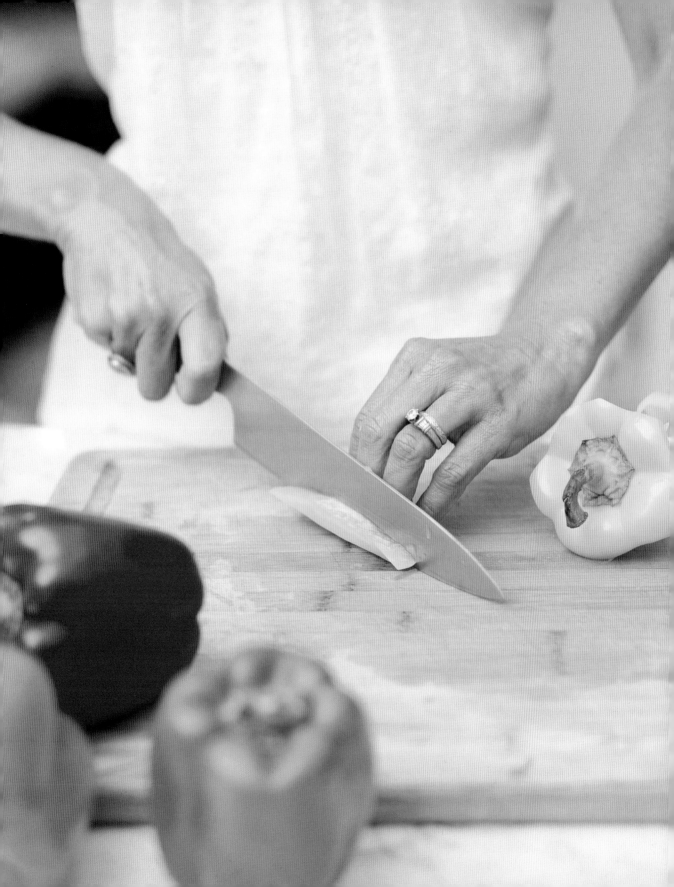

"If we chop them, we will eat them," says me. We know this works with kids, and it works with adults, too.

Once the vegetables are stored, it begs the question, "How long will they keep in the fridge before they start to lose their freshness?" The answer is about five days or so, but here's a secret: *don't let them sit in the fridge.* Eat them! The idea is to get them into your belly—not see how long they keep before they start to break down.

Store these Veggies in Water: If root vegetables and tubers, such as potatoes, yams, beets, sweet potatoes, and winter squash (butternut, acorn, and kabocha) are not kept in water, they'll turn brown.

Store these Veggies in Sealed Containers: Carrots, celery, bell peppers, broccoli, cauliflower, and onions stay fresh in a well-sealed container or bag.

Store these Veggies Wrapped in Towels in a Bag: Green leafy vegetables, including kale, collard greens, chard, beet greens, and lettuce can be chopped in advance, but they need to be wrapped in a dish towel or paper towels and then stored in an airtight plastic bag. Their fridge life is a little shorter, particularly the more delicate lettuces, which will start to oxidize (turn brown) after two or three days.

Store these Veggies in Jars: Garlic, ginger, and shallots are perfect for mincing up in the food processor and storing (separately) in glass jars.

Many grocery stores sell cut-up vegetables, which is also an option. If that helps you eat more vegetables, then do it! They cost a little more, but we always have to decide whether we want to spend our time or our money. You can decide on any given day, which you want to invest. To those folks who assert that vegetables lose their nutrients once they're cut up and stored: it's an unfounded concern. You may be sacrificing a little flavor and freshness, but you're not sacrificing nutrition. Let's keep things in perspective: *vegetables chopped in advance are better than no vegetables at all.*

2. Don't Wait Until Dinnertime to Decide What to Have for Dinner

Because I argue that our blocks to eating healthfully and compassionately are mostly mental, I'm absolutely convinced that the secret to eating well and consuming more vegetables is *planning* in advance.

Giving our meals just a little forethought can make all the difference, and that doesn't require anything more than *thinking.* You don't have to *do* anything. Most people decide what they're going to eat once they're already hungry, and at that stage, we don't make decisions based on nutrition; we make decisions based on speed, convenience, or cravings.

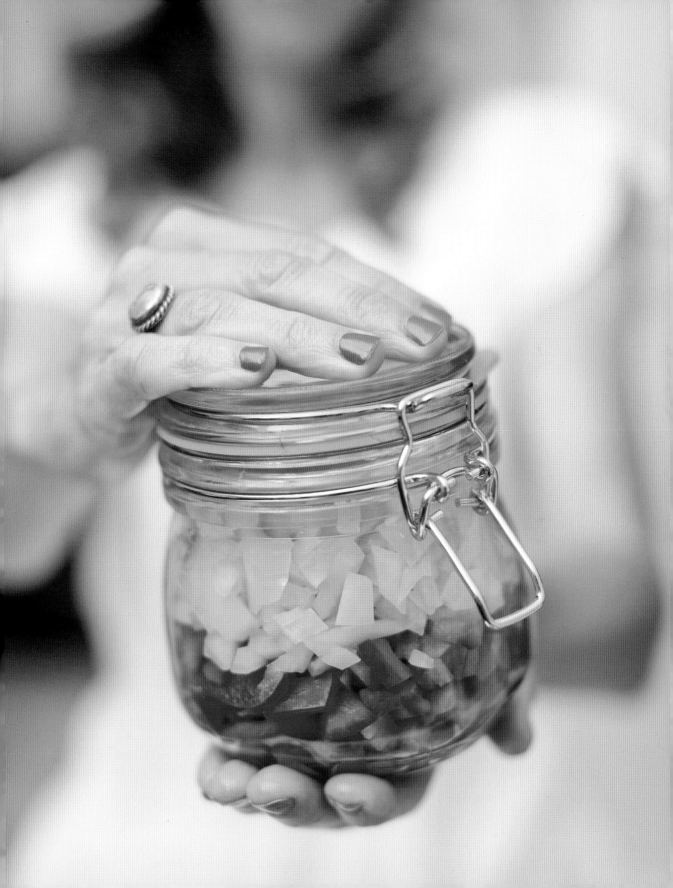

Though we can be a little more flexible with breakfast (since it tends to be the simplest meal of the day), when it comes to dinner in particular, we should know the *night before* what we're going to have for dinner the following night. We should know what we're eating for dinner long before that time arrives.

Here's how it plays out:

► As you lie in bed tonight, think about what you have in the refrigerator. Decide to wake up 10 minutes earlier than usual, and take that time to chop a few veggies: a bunch of carrots, two potatoes, and an onion for a soup; bell peppers for chili; or lettuce, cauliflower, and celery for a salad.

► If you decide you want a grain dish tomorrow night, throw some rice, quinoa, or barley into a saucepan tonight, along with water and a vegetable bouillon cube. Turn on the heat, set the timer, and before you know it, half of tomorrow night's dinner is already prepared.

► When you're preparing dinner tonight and your recipe calls for a chopped onion, chop *two* onions. Use one for your recipe, and store one in a container. You already have the cutting board and knife out, and it will take less than two minutes to chop up the second onion.

► Before you leave for work in the morning, soak your favorite vegetables or tofu in a marinade, and leave them all day. When you come home, roast or grill them.

► While you're getting ready for work, throw lentils, spices, a chopped onion, and garlic into a slow cooker, and turn it to the low setting. Come home to a dinner ready to eat.

3. Cook More Than You Need

Though I stand by my recommendation for taking fifteen to thirty minutes a day to cook, if you're always planning, you'll find that you may not even need to take that much time or that you may skip a day or two. One night you might eat out, one night you may have leftovers, another night you may eat food you prepared in advance and froze, in which case all you need to do is thaw and re-heat.

I've often heard single people lament that most recipes tend to be created for two or four people and that they're forever searching for recipes for *one*. I *encourage* people to cook for two if they're just one person or for four if they're just a couple. The idea is always make more than you need to have leftovers to eat the next day or to freeze for the coming week. That way, you won't have to prepare meals *every day*. Sure, you may have to reheat them or throw together a quick salad, but the bulk of the meal is already made.

4. Create a Meal Schedule

We humans are fierce creatures of habit, which can work in our favor or against us. Habit connects us with the familiar, making us feel comfortable and safe. We appreciate the predictable. We seek out routine. Our food rituals and traditions bear this out, as do our meal rotations.

A memory I cherish from my childhood is pizza night. Every Friday night was pizza night—and not pizza we ordered from a pizzeria. I mean pizza we made ourselves, using our favorite base: English muffins. I could count on these nights like clockwork, and each member of the family made his or her own variations: sauce on top of the cheese, sauce on the bottom of the cheese, shredded cheese, sliced cheese, chunky sauce, puréed sauce. It was serious work, and it always preceded our weekly jaunt to the movie theatre.

A meal schedule doesn't have to be rigid, and it may not work for everyone, but having a general guide might be helpful. You might decide that:

- Monday nights are for soups or stews
- Tuesday nights are dedicated to stir-fries
- Wednesday nights are for Mexican cuisine
- Thursday nights are sandwich nights
- Friday nights are for pasta or pizza

The options are endless. Once you know how you want to break things down, you can create a list of favorite recipes or dishes you already have that fit into these categories. Hang these lists on the refrigerator door.

Knowing exactly what you plan to eat for the week enables you to go to the store with a game plan instead of wandering aimlessly around, spending more money than you want to or planned on. Shopping with a list means you're more likely to stick to it and not buy unnecessary ingredients for dishes you're not even planning on cooking.

With a game plan, you've already tackled the hardest part of cooking: deciding what to make!

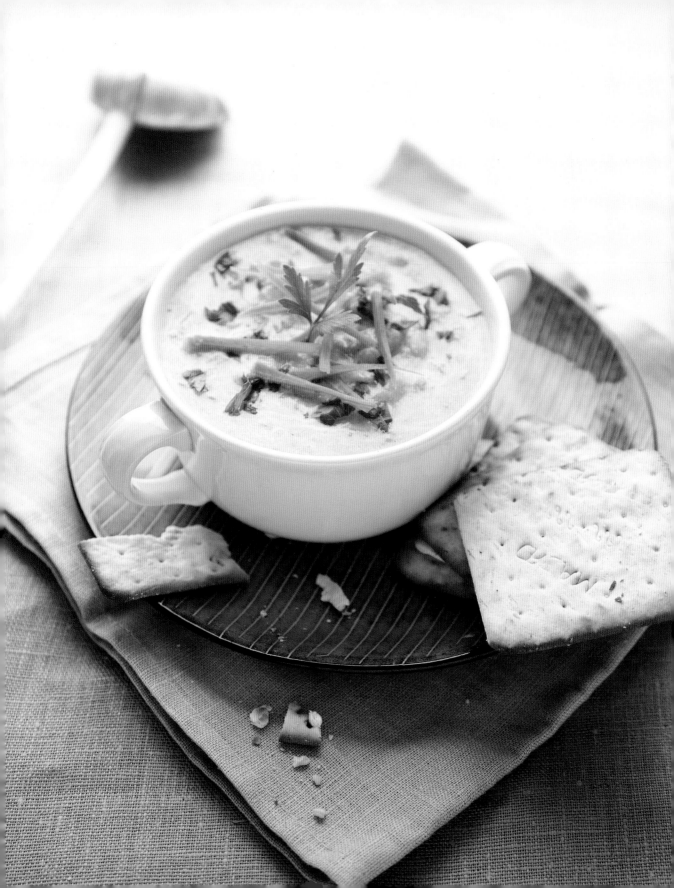

Smoky White Bean Chowder

YIELD Serves 4 as a main dish; 6 as a starter

ALLERGY Gluten-free, wheat-free, oil-free (if using water to sauté), soy-free (if using a non-soy creamer)

INGREDIENTS

1 tablespoon nondairy butter, olive oil, or water for sautéing

1 medium yellow or white onion, chopped

6 cloves garlic, peeled and finely chopped

3 stalks celery, diced

3 medium carrots, peeled and diced

2 bay leaves

2½ cups (600 ml) vegetable broth

2 large yellow potatoes, peeled and diced

1 cup (240 ml) plain soy creamer

3 cups or two 15-ounce cans (420 g) navy, Great Northern, or cannellini beans, drained and rinsed

½ to 1 teaspoon liquid smoke

½ teaspoon smoked paprika or red chili flakes

Salt and black pepper, to taste

Extra broth or creamer, as needed

Parsley and shredded carrots, for garnish

You will love the flavors and simplicity of this thick chowder.

DIRECTIONS

➲ Heat the butter, oil, or water in a large, flat-bottomed soup pot.

➲ Add the onion and garlic, and sauté over medium heat until they are softened and slightly caramelized, about 4 minutes.

➲ Add the celery and carrots; stir well. Add the bay leaves, broth, and potatoes.

➲ Cover and simmer for 20 minutes, or until potatoes are soft. Check occasionally, and give the soup a stir.

➲ Stir well, and mash slightly using a potato masher, breaking up the potatoes a bit. You may also use an immersion blender to do this, but I wouldn't purée the potatoes completely; you want the result to be thick but chunky.

➲ Add the creamer, beans, liquid smoke, smoked paprika, salt, and pepper. Simmer for another 15 minutes, uncovered.

➲ Stir well. The soup should be chowder thickness. If it's too thin, simmer uncovered for 10 minutes more. If it's too thick, add a small amount to broth or creamer. Add garnish, and serve with Saltine crackers (yes, they're vegan!). Or top with the Coconut Bacon on page 113.

**PER SERVING
(USING OIL TO SAUTÉ):**
Calories: 322, **Protein:** 12 g, **Fat:** 5.7 g, **Carbohydrates:** 56 g, **Fiber:** 9.8 g, **Cholesterol:** 0 mg

**PER SERVING
(USING WATER TO SAUTÉ):**
Calories: 302, **Protein:** 12 g, **Fat:** 3.5 g, **Carbohydrates:** 56 g, **Fiber:** 9.8 g, **Cholesterol:** 0 mg

FOR YOUR
MODIFICATION

The Homemade Almond Milk on page 207 can be used in place of the soy creamer. Regular almond or soy milk won't be as thick as homemade almond milk or a commercial soy creamer.

Lemon Artichoke Tapenade

YIELD Serves 8 to 10 as an appetizer (about 2 cups) **ALLERGY** Gluten-free, wheat-free, soy-free

INGREDIENTS

10 canned or frozen (and thawed) artichoke hearts, drained well and quartered (about 13 ounces [370 g] drained)

½ cup (70 g) pitted Kalamata olives

3 garlic cloves, peeled

½ to 1 tablespoon capers, drained

3 tablespoons freshly squeezed (Meyer) lemon juice (1 to 2 lemons)

Zest from 2 lemons

3 to 4 tablespoons extra-virgin olive oil

¼ teaspoon chili powder

Salt, to taste

Baguette, crackers, Ciabatta, or pita bread

PER SERVING (2 TABLESPOONS):
Calories: 55.0, **Protein:** 0.8 g, **Fat:** 4.7 g, Carbohydrates: 3.8 g, **Fiber:** 2.1 g, **Cholesterol:** 0 mg

I must be honest here. Regular Eureka lemons will make this tapenade good, but Meyer lemons will make it great. Meyer lemons are sweeter and perfectly delicious.

DIRECTIONS

- In the bowl of a food processor, pulse the artichoke hearts, olives, garlic, capers, lemon juice, lemon zest, and olive oil until almost smooth, but still chunky. Stop the machine and knock down from the sides any of the ingredients that didn't make it under the blade. Pulse again until thoroughly combined.

- Taste. Add the chili powder, salt, and additional lemon juice, if desired. You may do this while the ingredients are still in the food processor or once you've transferred everything to a separate serving bowl.

- Serve with toasted slices of baguette, any bread you prefer, or crackers. The tapenade will keep for up to one week in the refrigerator.

FOR YOUR MODIFICATION

You can certainly use lemons other than Meyer, but if you do, I would recommend cutting back on the amount of lemon juice a little bit. Meyer lemons are much sweeter than the larger, sourer Eureka lemons.

Although they won't have the punch that Kalamata olives do, green or black olives are also perfectly fine to use here.

FOR YOUR EDIFICATION

Zest your lemons first (a microplane works beautifully), then squeeze them to get the juice.

Herbed Lentil Soup

YIELD Serves 6 to 8 **ALLERGY** Gluten-free, wheat-free, oil-free (if using water to sauté), soy-free

INGREDIENTS

2 tablespoons olive oil or water, for sautéing

3 carrots, coarsely chopped

1 large yellow onion, coarsely chopped

1 medium fennel bulb, chopped

8 ounces (230 g) (about 15) cremini mushrooms, sliced

3 garlic cloves, minced

2 teaspoons dried parsley

2 teaspoons dried tarragon

2 teaspoons dried oregano

2 teaspoons dried thyme

½ teaspoon fresh rosemary, chopped

1 teaspoon Dijon mustard

8 cups (2 liters) vegetable broth or water

3 dried bay leaves

2 cups (410 g) Puy or brown lentils

1½ teaspoons salt

Truffle oil, for garnish

PER SERVING (USING OIL FOR SAUTÉING):

Calories: 257, **Protein:** 14 g, **Fat:** 5.0 g, Carbohydrates: 40 g, **Fiber:** 13 g, **Cholesterol:** 0 mg

PER SERVING (USING WATER FOR SAUTÉING):

Calories: 215, **Protein:** 14 g, **Fat:** 1.7 g, Carbohydrates: 37 g, **Fiber:** 13 g, **Cholesterol:** 0 mg

When fully cooked, Puy lentils remain intact but still absorb the flavor of whatever ingredients they're cooked with. If you can't find Puy, use larger brown lentils; just don't overcook and turn them mushy.

DIRECTIONS

- Heat the olive oil or water in a large soup pot over medium-high heat.
- Add the carrots, onion, fennel, mushrooms, and garlic; sauté until the onions are translucent and the mushrooms are soft, about 5 minutes.
- Add the parsley, tarragon, oregano, thyme, and rosemary, and stir to combine with the vegetables. Then, sauté for about 1 minute. Add the mustard, and cook for another 30 seconds, stirring to combine it with the vegetables and herbs.
- Add the vegetable broth or water (with a veggie bouillon cube for added flavor), bay leaves, and lentils. Cover and bring to a boil, then turn the heat to medium. Keep covered, and cook until the lentils are tender, about 40 minutes. (You may find that it's also helpful to keep the lid half-on and to check the soup periodically to make sure the water doesn't evaporate and burn the lentils.)
- Add the salt and pepper once the lentils are cooked, and stir to combine.
- If the lentils need more time, continue cooking, but check every 10 minutes. If the broth is evaporating, you can add more, or only add enough to make it a thick consistency rather than a stew with a slight broth. It's up to you.
- When the lentils are done, remove the bay leaves and discard them. Taste the lentils and adjust the seasonings. Serve them in a shallow bowl, season with freshly ground pepper, drizzle a little truffle oil on the top of each soup before serving, and garnish with some fresh parsley.

FOR YOUR EDIFICATION

A small amount of truffle oil elevates recipes to a completely new level.

Socca (Chickpea Crepes) with Balsamic Mushrooms and Kale

YIELD Makes 8 crepes using an 8-inch pan **ALLERGY** Wheat-free, gluten-free

INGREDIENTS *SOCCA*

2 cups (250 g) chickpea flour

1 teaspoon salt

1 teaspoon favorite herbs
   and/or spices

2¼ cups (540 ml) water

Olive oil, for cooking

INGREDIENTS *MUSHROOMS*

2 tablespoons olive oil

4 garlic cloves, finely chopped

1 pound (450 g) cremini
   mushrooms, roughly chopped

Salt and freshly ground black pepper

1 tablespoon balsamic vinegar

2 tablespoons finely chopped
   fresh basil or parsley

INGREDIENTS *KALE*

1 tablespoon olive oil

2 garlic cloves, finely chopped

⅓ cup (35 g) pine nuts
   (toasted or raw)

2 bunches Lacinato kale, chopped

Salt and freshly ground black pepper

Herbed Cashew Cheese on page
   168 (optional)

PER SERVING:
Calories: 325.8, **Protein:** 8.3 g, **Fat:** 24.4 g,
Carbohydrates: 20.9 g, **Fiber:** 5.0 g,
Cholesterol: 0 mg

Socca (pronounced soak-ah*) is a popular street food in Nice and other areas along the south coast of France.*

DIRECTIONS *SOCCA*

- Place the flour, salt, and herbs and/or spices in a large bowl, and whisk briefly to break up any lumps. While whisking, pour in the water, and whisk until smooth. Cover and let sit for at least 15 minutes while you prepare the veggies. (You can let it sit in the fridge for up to 24 hours before using.)

- Place an 8-inch nonstick sauté pan over medium-high heat. When the pan is hot enough for a drop of water to dance, add a tablespoon or two of oil. Pour enough batter to cover the pan surface about ⅛ inch thick.

- Cook until the bottom is lightly browned, about 2 minutes or so. Gently use a spatula to separate the edges of the crepe from the pan. Carefully flip to lightly brown the second side. Prepare for the first one to not be as pretty as the rest.

- Transfer to a plate. Repeat with remaining batter.

DIRECTIONS *MUSHROOMS*

- Heat the oil and garlic in a sauté pan over medium heat until the garlic is golden brown. Add the mushrooms, stir, and season with salt and pepper. Cook until mushrooms are glossy, about 7 minutes. Turn off heat, stir in the vinegar and herbs, and set aside.

DIRECTIONS *KALE*

- Heat the olive oil in a large sauté pan over medium-low heat. Add the garlic and cook until golden brown, about 2 minutes. Stir in the pine nuts and kale, season with salt and pepper, and cook, stirring until just wilted, about 1 minute.

- To serve, top each socca with a little of the greens and mushrooms, and a dollop of Herbed Cashew Cheese, if using. Alternatively, you can add the Cashew Cheese first, then top with the mushrooms and kale. Using kitchen shears, cut into triangles.

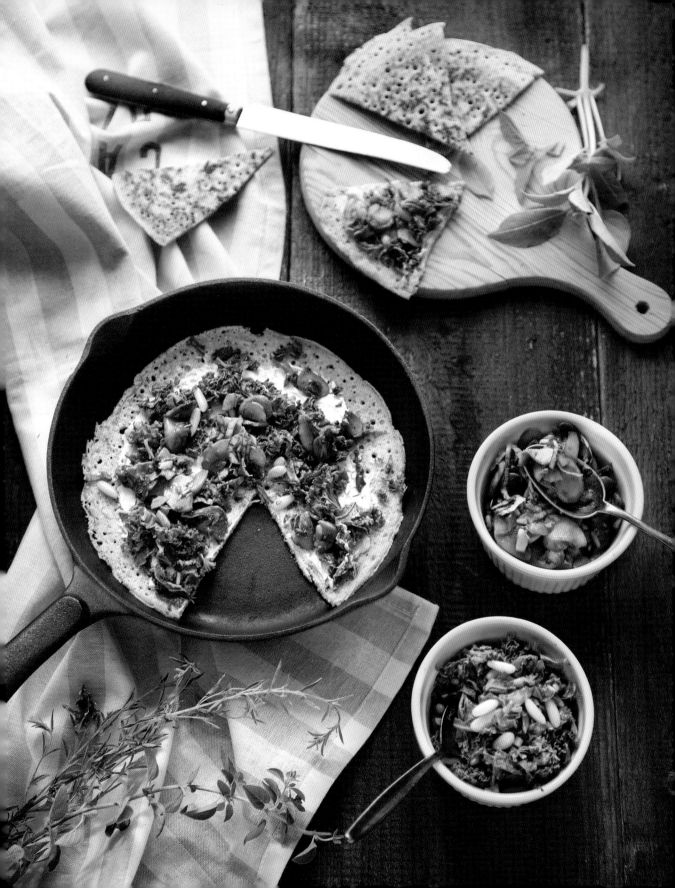

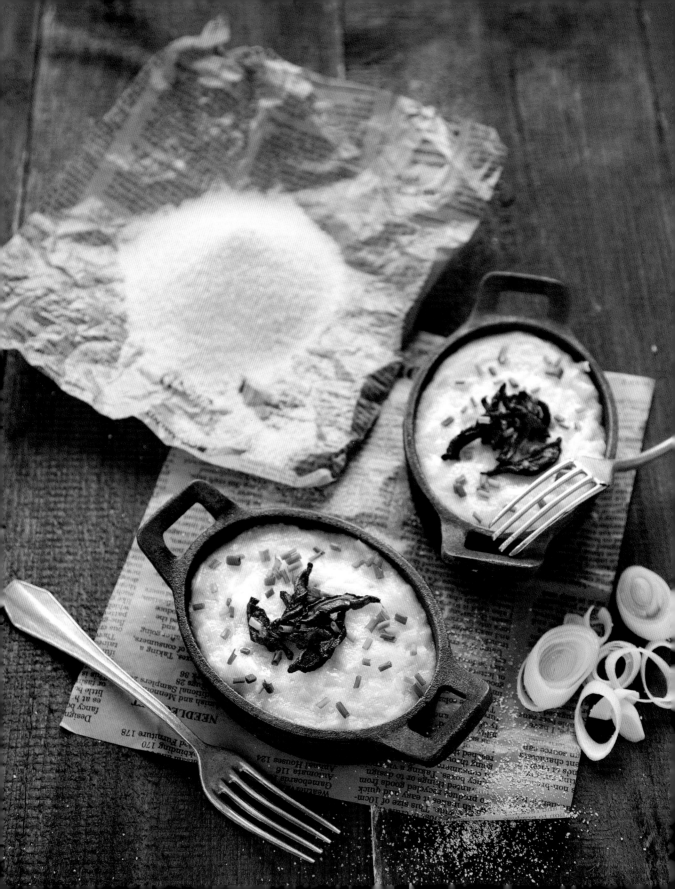

Creamy Leek Polenta

YIELD Serves 4 as a main dish, 6 as a side dish

ALLERGY Gluten-free, wheat-free, soy-free (if using soy-free nondairy butter and milk)

INGREDIENTS

2 tablespoons nondairy butter, divided

3 large leeks (white and pale green parts only), thinly sliced and diced

2 cups (480 ml) water, more if needed

2¼ cups (540 ml) vegetable broth

1 cup (170 g) coarse cornmeal (polenta)

½ to ¾ cup (120 to 180 ml) nondairy milk (almond, soy, rice, hemp, oat, hazelnut)

1 teaspoon salt, added gradually (and you may not use all; depends on your taste)

Freshly ground pepper, to taste

PER SERVING:
Calories: 128, **Protein:** 3.1 g, **Fat:** 3.2 g, **Carbohydrates:** 23 g, **Fiber:** 2.2 g, **Cholesterol:** 0 mg

Dedication

From: Liz and Nick
To: Marilyn Dee
With love and gratitude for keeping our bellies and hearts full

The buttery texture of the leeks and soft texture of the polenta culminate in creamy perfection.

DIRECTIONS

- Melt 1 tablespoon of the nondairy butter in a 4-quart saucepan over medium heat.
- Add the leeks, and stir to coat. Cover and cook until the leeks soften, stirring occasionally, for about 7 to 10 minutes.
- Add the water and broth, cover, and bring to a boil. Reduce heat to medium-low, and slowly pour in the polenta, while whisking simultaneously. Whisking is essential, or the cornmeal will clump up. Cook until the mixture is thick and creamy.
- At this point, you'll want to switch to a wooden spoon, stirring often. As it begins to thicken, add some of the milk, stir, and continue cooking. Add about ¼ teaspoon salt. Continue stirring, cooking, and adding more milk and salt, until you have a creamy mixture.
- Remove the saucepan from the heat, and stir in the remaining tablespoon of nondairy butter. Season with salt and pepper, to taste. Divide the polenta among plates.

Suggestions for Serving

- Slice up some mushrooms, sauté them in a little olive oil with some tamari, and add to the top of each serving of polenta.
- Sauté some of your favorite greens (chard, kale, collards) in olive oil and garlic, and serve on top of the polenta. The color contrast is striking.

FOR YOUR **EDIFICATION**	FOR YOUR **MODIFICATION**
To cut leeks, first cut off the root stem, then the tougher green tops. What you're left with are the more tender white parts. Slice lengthways first, then across.	If you have creamy polenta left over, pour it into a serving dish and store it in the fridge overnight to set up. Then, you can cut it into squares and fry, bake, or grill it.

Giambotta (Vegetable Stew)

YIELD Makes 4 servings **ALLERGY** Gluten-free, wheat-free, oil-free (if using water to sauté), soy-free

INGREDIENTS

1 tablespoon oil or water, for sautéing

1 large yellow onion, chopped

3 medium carrots, peeled and diced

2 stalks of celery, diced

3 cloves garlic, peeled and finely chopped

1 medium globe eggplant, chopped into 1-inch pieces

½ cup (120 ml) water or vegetable broth

1 (28-ounce) can fire roasted diced tomatoes

2 large yellow potatoes, peeled and chopped

2 red bell peppers, seeded and diced

2 medium zucchini or any summer squash, unpeeled and diced

2 bay leaves, fresh or dried

1 teaspoon dried thyme

1 teaspoon dried oregano

1 teaspoon dried parsley

1 teaspoon dried tarragon

1 teaspoon salt

Freshly ground pepper

½ cup (10 to 12 leaves) chopped basil

Although this is called a "stew," it is thick enough to be served as a side dish or first course (prima). Also spelled Ciambotta, *this traditional dish, hailing from southern Italy, is comfort food at its finest—and simplest.*

DIRECTIONS

- Heat the oil or water in a soup pot over medium-high heat for just about 1 minute. Add the onion, carrots, celery, and garlic, and cook for about 10 minutes until all the veggies begin to soften. Stir occasionally.
- Add the eggplant and water, and cook, covered, until the eggplant is slightly softened, about 10 minutes.
- Add the canned tomatoes with their juice, potatoes, bell peppers, zucchini, bay leaves, thyme, oregano, parsley, and tarragon. Stir, then reduce heat to low and cook uncovered for about 25 minutes, stirring occasionally, until all the vegetables are soft. (If water/broth evaporates while the vegetables are still cooking, add a little extra.)
- Stir in the salt and pepper, along with the chopped basil. Serve immediately with a hearty, rustic loaf of bread.

PER SERVING (USING OIL FOR SAUTÉING):
Calories: 280, **Protein:** 7.3 g, **Fat:** 4.7 g, **Carbohydrates:** 58 g, **Fiber:** 9.7 g, **Cholesterol:** 0 mg

PER SERVING (USING WATER FOR SAUTÉING):
Calories: 248, **Protein:** 7.3 g, **Fat:** 1.2 g, **Carbohydrates:** 57 g, **Fiber:** 9.7 g, **Cholesterol:** 0 mg

FOR YOUR MODIFICATION

Add your favorite vegan Italian sausage to the stew at the end.

FOR YOUR EDIFICATION

Mirepoix is a mixture of chopped onions, carrots, and celery, and to reduce some prep time, you can often find prechopped mirepoix in such grocery stores as Trader Joe's and Whole Foods.

Dedication

From: David Goudreau
To: Mom and Dad, the best parents in the world

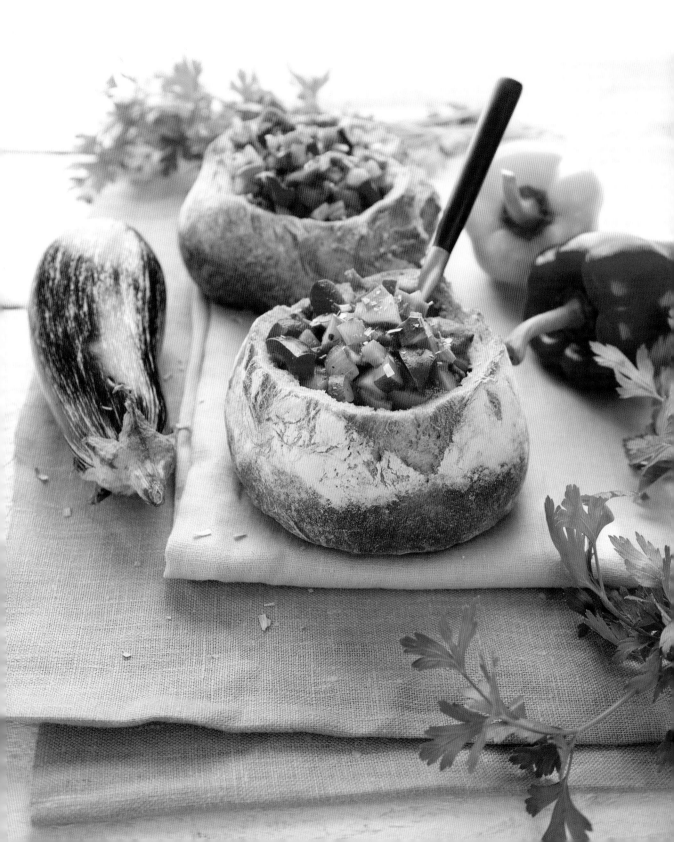

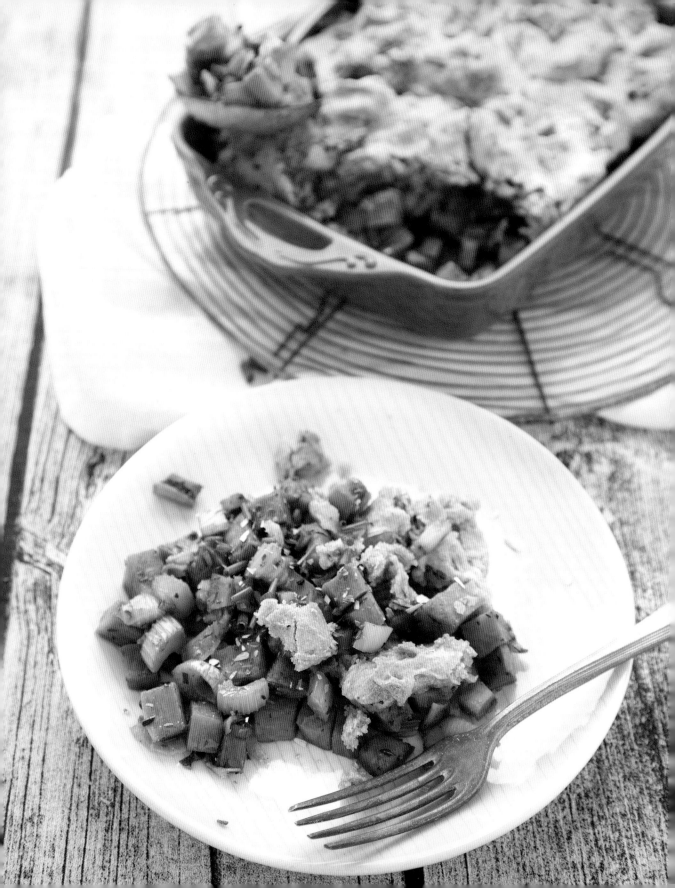

Vegetable Pot Pie

YIELD Makes 6 servings **ALLERGY** Oil-free (if sautéing in water), soy-free

INGREDIENTS

2 tablespoons olive oil or water
   for sautéing

1 large yellow onion, diced

2 sweet potatoes, peeled and diced

2 carrots, peeled and diced

2 stalks of celery, diced

1 fennel bulb, diced

1 tablespoon each dried
   tarragon and dried oregano

1 teaspoon each dried thyme and
   dried sage

3 garlic cloves, minced

½ teaspoon salt, plus more to taste

Freshly ground pepper, to taste

½ cup (120 ml) white wine

1½ cups (360 ml) vegetable broth

3 tablespoons all-purpose flour,
   whisked into a few
   tablespoons of water

1 Chive and Black Pepper Cobbler
   Crust (recipe on page 100)

**PER SERVING
(USING OIL FOR SAUTÉING):**
Calories: 382, **Protein:** 6.6 g, **Fat:** 18 g,
Carbohydrates: 48 g, **Fiber:** 6.4 g,
Cholesterol: 0 mg

**PER SERVING
(USING WATER FOR SAUTÉING):**
Calories: 342, **Protein:** 6.6 g, **Fat:** 13 g,
Carbohydrates: 48 g, **Fiber:** 6.4 g,
Cholesterol: 0 mg

This variation relies on a delicious and easy-to-make cobbler crust (rather than a roll-out crust) that saves you time and effort.

DIRECTIONS

- Grease a 9-by-9-inch baking dish

- Add the oil or water to a large sauté pan and turn the heat to medium-low. Add the onion and cook for 2 minutes. Add the sweet potatoes, carrots, celery, and fennel. Sauté, stirring often, until all the vegetables are soft, about 20 minutes. If the water has evaporated and the vegetables are sticking to the pan, add more water.

- (Prepare your cobbler crust while the veggies are cooking.)

- Once the veggies, especially the sweet potatoes, are fork-tender, add the tarragon, oregano, thyme, sage, garlic, salt, and pepper, and cook for another two minutes. Give the vegetables another stir.

- Pour in the wine, broth, and flour/water mixture, and raise the heat to medium-high. Bring to a boil, then simmer, stirring occasionally, until the mixture has thickened and reduced, about 8 minutes. If the initial broth begins to soak into the veggies, and they start to stick to the pan, add about ¼ cup more veggie broth to deglaze the pan. Stir, taste, and add salt, as needed.

- Transfer the filling into the prepared baking dish.

- When you're ready to assemble and bake, preheat the oven to 375°F. Spoon your cobbler dough on top of the vegetables. You don't need to spread it out to cover the vegetables completely. You can plop them randomly on top; when they cook, they'll spread somewhat. Bake for 15 to 20 minutes or until the cobbler crust is golden brown.

- Serve hot right out of the oven. (Great as leftovers, too!)

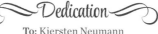

Dedication
To: Kiersten Neumann

Chive and Black Pepper Cobbler Crust

YIELD Makes 6 to 8 biscuits or enough to top a 9-by-9-inch casserole, such as the Vegetable Pot Pie on Page 99. **ALLERGY** Soy-free, if using a plant milk other than soy

INGREDIENTS

1 cup (125 g) unbleached, all-purpose flour

⅔ cup (75 g) whole-wheat pastry flour

1 tablespoon aluminum-free baking powder

¼ cup (55 g) minced chives

½ teaspoon freshly ground pepper

½ teaspoon salt

⅔ cup (160 ml) plant-based milk (preferably unsweetened)

⅓ cup (80 ml) olive, canola, or coconut oil (melted Earth Balance butter is also an option)

PER SERVING (1 BISCUIT):
Calories: 180, Protein: 3.2 g, Fat: 9.8 g, Carbohydrates: 21 g, Fiber: 1.9 g, Cholesterol: 0 mg

Although you could leave out both the pepper and the chives to make a simple biscuit dough, the inclusion of both—or either—makes the crust just a little more special.

DIRECTIONS

- In a mixing bowl, stir together the all-purpose flour, whole-wheat pastry flour, baking powder, chives, freshly ground pepper, and salt until fully combined. You never want to over-stir cobbler or biscuit dough, since it could result in a dense final product, so always mix your dry ingredients first, then add the wet and stir just enough to combine.

- Add the milk and olive oil, and stir until the dry ingredients are just combined with the wet ingredients. The result is a sticky—not smooth—dough. You can either make biscuits using this dough, baking them in a 450°F oven on a parchment-lined or greased cookie sheet for 8 minutes, or use it as a cobbler topping for the Vegetable Pot Pie. Follow the instructions above to use for the pot pie.

FOR YOUR MODIFICATION

This recipe is perfectly delicious if you left out the chives or used (finely chopped) rosemary instead, or even minced green onion. Don't let the absence of chives in your refrigerator stop you from making this delicious recipe!

Everyday Vinaigrette

YIELD ½ cup **ALLERGY** Gluten-free, wheat-free, soy-free

INGREDIENTS

1 clove garlic, peeled and minced

½ teaspoon salt

½ teaspoon ground pepper

1 teaspoon Dijon mustard

1 teaspoon agave nectar

¼ cup (60 ml) acidic liquid (lemon juice, lime juice, apple cider vinegar, white wine vinegar, or balsamic vinegar)

¼ cup (60 ml) oil (sesame, olive, canola, walnut, grapeseed)

1 teaspoon dried or 1 tablespoon finely chopped fresh herbs (any combination of basil, thyme, tarragon, oregano, chives, parsley, etc.)

PER SERVING (2 TABLESPOONS):
Calories: 131.6, **Protein:** 0.2 g, **Fat:** 13.6 g, **Carbohydrates:** 3.2 g, **Fiber:** 0.3 g, **Cholesterol:** 0 mg

Everyone needs a basic vinaigrette they can throw together in a jiffy, and now you have one of your own!

DIRECTIONS

⊙ Place the garlic and salt into a bowl, wide jar, blender, or small bowl of a food processor. Add the pepper, mustard, and agave nectar. Stir or shake well, or blend/process for about 30 seconds.

⊙ Add your acidic liquid and oil of choice, along with the herbs. Stir or shake well, or blend/process for another 30 seconds until the dressing is opaque.

⊙ Store in the refrigerator, and use within one week.

Spicy Red Bell Pepper Soup

YIELD Serves 6 **ALLERGY** Gluten-free, wheat-free, oil-free (if sautéing in water), soy-free

INGREDIENTS

1 tablespoon extra-virgin olive oil, nondairy butter, or water, for sautéing

4 red bell peppers, seeded and roughly chopped

3 medium carrots, chopped

1 yellow onion, roughly chopped

4 cloves garlic, chopped

6 cups (1500 ml) vegetable broth

¼ teaspoon cayenne pepper

¼ teaspoon curry powder

¼ teaspoon crushed red pepper flakes

1 teaspoon salt, or to taste

1½ cups (225 g) raw cashews

½ teaspoon ground black pepper

Parsley, for garnish

An easy soup to prepare and make, it's even better when made in advance and stored in the fridge overnight to let the flavors meld.

DIRECTIONS

◦ Heat the olive oil, nondairy butter, or water in a large soup pot over medium heat.

◦ Stir in the bell peppers, carrots, onion, and garlic. Cook, and stir the vegetables until they're soft, about 10 minutes. Add the vegetable broth, cayenne pepper, curry powder, red pepper flakes, and salt, and bring the mixture to a boil. Reduce heat, cover, and simmer until the vegetables are tender, about 20 minutes. Remove from heat.

◦ Add the cashews to a blender (high-powered is best), and blend on high power. Add about ¼ to ¾ cup of the broth from the soup, and continue to blend until you have a thick cashew cream. When you do, add the rest of the soup contents to the blender, and blend until smooth.

◦ Test for seasoning, and add more salt, if needed, as well as the ground pepper. Blend again, and then return to the soup pot to heat up.

◦ Garnish each individual serving with parsley, serve hot, and pair with a fresh loaf of Ciabatta or other Italian bread.

**PER SERVING
(USING OIL FOR SAUTÉING):**
Calories: 213, **Protein:** 6.2 g, **Fat:** 14 g, Carbohydrates: 18 g, **Fiber:** 2.5 g, Cholesterol: 0 mg

**PER SERVING
(USING WATER FOR SAUTÉING):**
Calories: 198, **Protein:** 6.2 g, **Fat:** 13 g, Carbohydrates: 18 g, **Fiber:** 2.5 g, Cholesterol: 0 mg

FOR YOUR EDIFICATION

Blending hot soups can be a tricky business. To keep things safe and clean, let the soup cool a bit before adding it to the blender. And hold on tightly to the lid; steam has been known to push open blender lids, shooting hot soup all over the kitchen!

FOR YOUR MODIFICATION

If this soup packs too much heat, just cool it down with a little nondairy sour cream (or use less cayenne pepper).

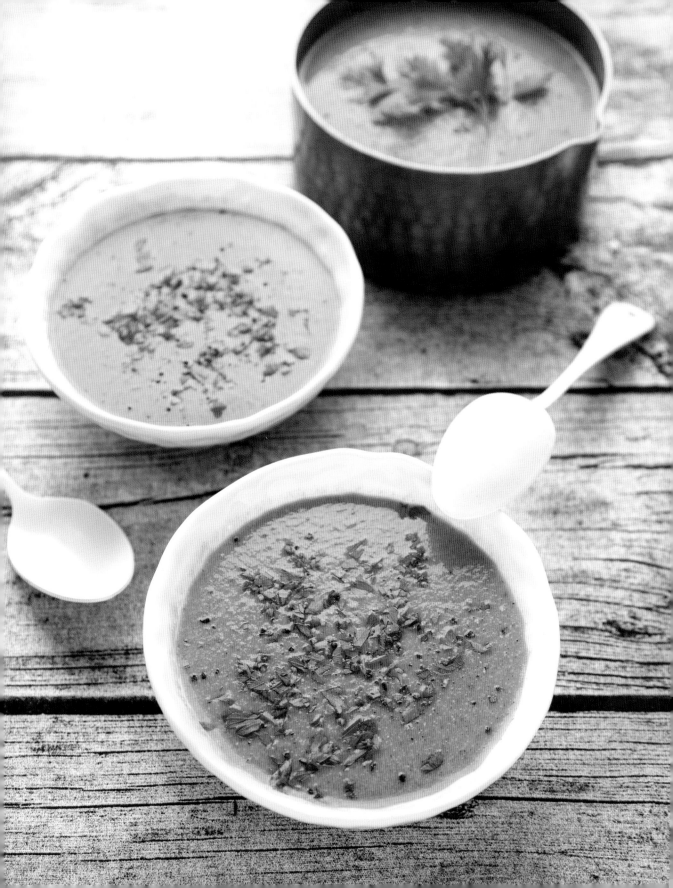

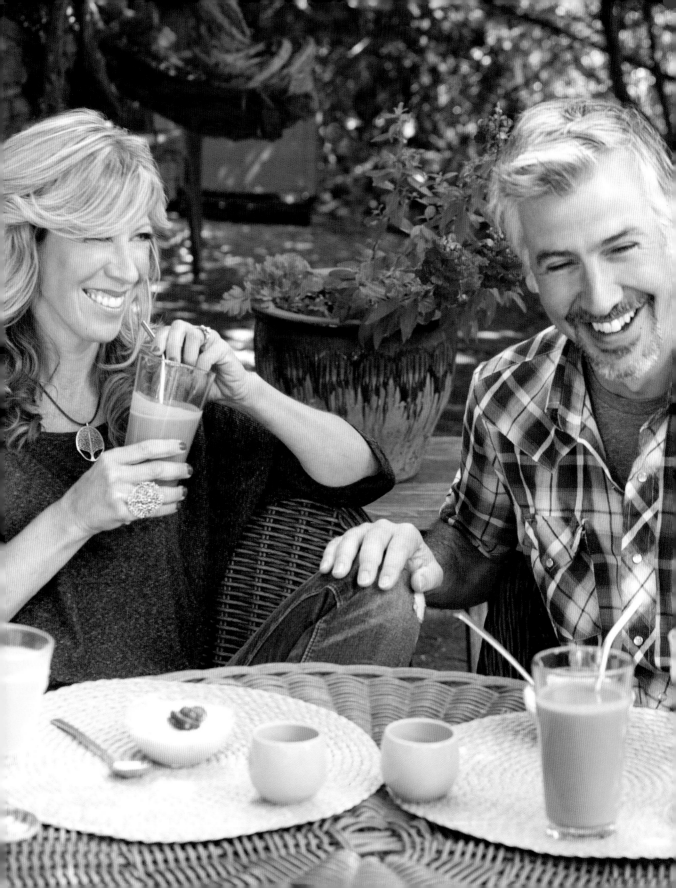

Starting the Day on the Right Foot: A Bevy of Breakfast Ideas

With seven days of breakfast behind you, I imagine you're recognizing how familiar "vegan food" actually is. But, to show you how many options you have, I'm providing a huge range of breakfast ideas here. As with all of our food choices, there is a spectrum in terms of nutrient-density; though plant-based breakfasts are more healthful than any animal-based version, the best thing we can do is choose the most nutrient-rich foods that are high in fiber and low in calories.

WHATEVER YOU DO: DON'T SKIP BREAKFAST!

If you've heard it once, you've heard it a million times: *don't skip breakfast; it's the most important meal of the day*.

A quick glance at the word itself should tell you why this is so; it's a blend (or "portmanteau") of the words "break" and "fast," and that's quite literally what you're doing: *breaking a fast*. After having gone without food for 10 to 15 hours (depending on when you ate dinner and how long you've slept), your body awakes in low gear and needs fuel to help you start your day. Your blood sugar has dropped, your metabolism has slowed, and your pistons aren't exactly firing at their optimum level. By eating—nutrient-dense—food, you create a solid foundation on which the rest of your day can be built.

CHALLENGE YOUR THINKING: People who skip breakfast tend to have a higher body mass index than those who eat it. If weight loss is a goal, skipping breakfast is counterproductive.

CHANGE YOUR BEHAVIOR: Eat breakfast!

Numerous studies strongly link skipping breakfast with being overweight and lacking the ability to concentrate. This applies to children, adolescents, and adults. In fact, if weight loss is a goal of yours, skipping breakfast is counterproductive. When your body fasts, it goes into conservation mode during which your metabolism slows down and remains slow until you give your body a message that it can stop conserving energy. That message is food. Calories. Energy. One of the other reasons people who skip breakfast tend to be overweight is they make up for it later and eat more throughout the day.

So, what will you eat?

Most people—vegan or not—tend to rotate the same things every day. It's not that we don't have a bevy of options to choose from, but our desire for routine and familiarity tend to supersede anything else. That's fine. In fact, even within our regular repertoires, we can find a lot of variety, depending on the type of milk we drink, the kind of bread we choose, or the kind of spread we use. You might also find that you change your breakfast depending on the season—if it's warm or cold—and according to the day of the week. Most of us eat lighter during the week than we do on the weekends.

All of the suggestions below can be applied to kids or adults.

COLD BREAKFASTS

▶ **Fruit smoothies**—Nutritious, filling, and super versatile, homemade smoothies provide the best bang for your caloric and monetary buck whether you drink them at home or take them on the road. See page 111 for the recipe for Green Machine Smoothie, which David and I are enjoying in the photo that opens this chapter.

A couple things to say about smoothies:

» You don't necessarily need a high-powered blender like a Vitamix, but it's nice to have. You can use just a regular blender, but a high-powered blender makes a creamier smoothie—and it's easier to use the tamper that comes with it rather than stopping the blender to scrape off the sides and restart the machine. If you already have a blender, take it out of the closet, and put it on your kitchen counter. We tend not to use appliances that are not visible. So, make them visible.

» Freezing bananas is a great option especially when you have ripe bananas or when stores sell ripe/brown bananas at a discount. Remove the peel, break the banana into pieces, throw them in a bag or container, and keep them in the freezer. This ensures frozen treats or smoothies anytime. You can freeze bananas whole, but it's difficult to work with them because they're extremely hard when you take them out of the freezer.

Moving on...

- ▶ **Nondairy yogurt with fresh fruit and/or nuts**—You have many options here, depending on the yogurt you use (soy, rice, almond, or coconut milk) and what kind of fruit, cereal, granola, nuts, or seeds you add. Return to Day 3: Stocking a Healthful Kitchen, to see the different brands and to remind yourself that *yes*, nondairy yogurts have all the probiotics that dairy-based yogurts have.

- ▶ **Cereal**—Skip the sugary brands and choose those that are made with whole grains. Pour on your favorite nondairy milk (almond, oat, coconut, soy, rice, hazelnut, or hemp), and mix in some fresh fruit.

- ▶ **Muesli**—Muesli is a general term for a combination of uncooked rolled oats, fruit (dried and/or fresh), and nuts. Add ground flaxseeds or hulled hemp seeds, and your favorite nondairy milk for a hearty, healthful breakfast.

- ▶ **Granola**—Typically added to yogurts, cereal, muesli, or fresh fruit, some commercial granolas are heavily sugar-laden. Check out the bulk section of a large, natural food store for more healthful varieties.

- ▶ **Fresh fruit**—There is nothing more beautiful and nutrient-dense than a plate of fresh fruit, which can vary according to the season. If it's not enough to fill you up, add nuts, rolled oats, or peanut butter for more sustenance.

- ▶ **Sliced banana and apple with peanut or almond butter**—One of my common breakfasts—depending on the season—is a sliced banana and apple with peanut or almond butter. I prefer to slice up an apple rather than just bite into it whole. Somehow, it feels more satisfying and substantial.

- ▶ **Banana with a handful of nuts**—This is quick and transportable for one of those on-the-run breakfasts.

- ▶ **Peanut butter and jam sandwich**—Who sanctioned peanut butter and jam sandwiches for lunch only? With banana slices tucked in, this standby is actually a very healthful meal any time of the day, including breakfast.

- ▶ **Leftovers**—Some dishes taste even better as leftovers—cold, right out of the fridge. If you're in a hurry and have the choice between grabbing a container of leftovers and eating nothing at all, choose the former.

- ▶ **Energy Bars**—Though most don't have animal products, some are healthier than others. (Day 3: Stocking a Healthful Kitchen lists some brands under Snacks.)

HOT BREAKFASTS

Not all hot breakfasts are meant for the weekends or special occasions; hot porridges like oatmeal can be prepared in a jiffy and are perfect in the colder months.

▶ **Oatmeal/Porridge**—Whether you make them from cooked oats, cornmeal, grits, quinoa, barley, rice, or cream of wheat, the components are the same: nondairy milk, cinnamon, sweetener, dried fruit (such as raisins or dried cranberries), and additional fresh fruit.

▶ **Baked Oatmeal**—Check out page 118 for a delicious Baked Oatmeal with Blueberries and Bananas that can be made the day before it's served.

▶ **Tofu scramble**—Choosing a firmly textured tofu is the secret to the perfect scramble. A little turmeric turns the tofu a beautiful yellow color, leading many people to never notice that they're eating tofu and not scrambled eggs. You can find my Tofu, Mushroom, and Sausage recipe on page 117.

▶ **Tempeh scramble**—Take my Tofu Scramble, and replace the tofu with tempeh. Steam and crumble the tempeh first, then proceed with directions.

▶ **Mushroom scramble**—Chop up several different types of mushrooms, sauté them in just a little olive oil, season with salt and fresh herbs, and you've got a low-calorie breakfast that can be served with toast or atop polenta.

▶ **Scrapple**—Recipes for vegan scrapple can be found on the Internet. (If you don't know what scrapple is, just revel in the bliss of your ignorance!)

▶ **Breakfast burrito**—Either make it bean-based just like a typical lunchtime burrito, or roll up a tofu, tempeh, mushroom, or polenta scramble in a flour or corn tortilla, along with salsa, chopped avocado, and lettuce.

▶ **Baked beans**—A typical British breakfast item, you can also include tomato slices, and toast with Marmite (or Vegemite).

▶ **Vegan Sausage**—"Breakfast links" made by Gimme Lean, Field Roast, Tofurky, or Yves provide the fat, salt, and mouthfeel people identify with animal-based sausage.

▶ **Canadian bacon**—Yves brand makes a Canadian bacon, which is great for those special weekend brunches when you want an old-fashioned English Muffin sandwich—use tofu scramble, Daiya cheese, Rudi's English Muffins, and Yves Canadian bacon, and you've got a hearty breakfast or brunch.

▶ **Coconut bacon**—See page 113 for the recipe. Serve the bacon as a side dish with a vegetable scramble or pancakes.

- ▶ **Hash browns**—Make them from scratch using shredded potatoes, or buy frozen hash browns. (Brands that are more "natural" will only contain potatoes and sometimes oil.)

- ▶ **Home fries**—Chop (but don't peel) a few potatoes, steam them, and then fry (or roast) them with diced onions in a little oil. Serve with ketchup or nondairy sour cream.

- ▶ **French Toast and Blueberry Pancakes**—French Toast, Pancakes, and other breakfast recipes can be found in *The Vegan Table*. Biscuits, scones, and muffins can be found in *The Joy of Vegan Baking*.

- ▶ **Crepes**—Crepes are simply thin pancakes, and yes, they can be made deliciously and fluffily without eggs! I have a crepe recipe in *The Joy of Vegan Baking*.

- ▶ **Socca**—Socca is a crepe made with chickpea flour. Serve for breakfast with any of your favorite toppings—especially fruit! (See page 92 for my Socca recipe.)

BREAD-BASED BREAKFASTS

- ▶ **Enjoy whole-wheat toast with your favorite spreads:** nondairy butter, peanut butter, almond butter, fruit preserves, Vegemite, or Marmite. For more nutrients, add banana or apple slices. For additional flavor, sprinkle cinnamon on top.

- ▶ **Schmear a bagel with nondairy cream cheese or peanut butter.** Top with a sliced banana or strawberries.

- ▶ **Biscuits and Gravy** are a heavier meal perhaps more conducive to a special occasion; make the Drop Biscuits from *The Joy of Vegan Baking* and serve them for breakfast. Also check out the Chive and Black Pepper Crust on page 100, which can also be made into biscuits.

- ▶ **English Muffins** with your favorite nut butter spread and fruit slices. Some commercial brands contain whey, but vegan English Muffins are available. Rudi's is one brand to look for. *rudisbakery.com*

PASTRIES & CAKES

- ▶ Check out my Lemon Poppy Seed Muffins on page 121.

- ▶ See page 114 for my Apple Breakfast Cake.

- ▶ Vegan muffins, donuts, and other pastries can be homemade or found online and in many large natural food stores. You'd be surprised what you can find when you ask.

BREAKFAST BEVERAGES

▶ **Juice**—In terms of vegan options, beverages abound; in terms of nutrient-density, be aware that some commercial fruit juices may be laden with sugar. (See page 120 for my Carrot Ginger Apple Juice.)

▶ **Coffee**—especially as a replacement for breakfast—is not health food, and exotic coffee drinks (as well as what may appear to be healthful fruit shakes sold in specialty cafes and restaurants) may be incredibly calorie-dense. Better to spend your calories on healthier options.

▶ **Tea and Herbal Infusions**—As a self-described and proud tea junkie, I would be remiss if I didn't recommend it as a perfect way to start the day and herbal infusions as a delightful way to end it. My favorite teas are in the categories of green (Dragonwell, Cloud Mist, Sencha, Gyokuro), oolong (Dong Ding, Bao Zhong), and white (Silver Needle, White Peony). My favorite infusion, especially when I'm feeling a cold coming on, is grated fresh ginger steeped in hot water, along with some agave nectar. I also love mint leaves steeped in hot water. So simple.

▶ **Milk**—Of course, fortified nondairy milks can be drunk as beverages, though I tend not to drink them straight. To increase my intake of nutrients, I always throw them in a blender, and then add my favorite fruit—usually blueberries. Blueberry milk is a daily staple in my home! (See page 207 for my Homemade Almond Milk.)

▶ **Hot cocoa**—Some (not all) commercial hot cocoa powder mixes include cow's milk. Make your own hot cocoa by combining unsweetened cocoa powder with sugar, nondairy milk, and a little vanilla extract. It's inexpensive, and you can determine exactly how sweet to make it. You can make hot *chocolate* by melting dark chocolate into nondairy milk, along with a little vanilla extract. Whisk, and serve.

Green Machine Smoothie

YIELD Serves 2 **ALLERGY** Soy-free, wheat-free, gluten-free, oil-free

INGREDIENTS

1 large ripe fresh or frozen banana

2 cups (480 ml) almond milk,
    vanilla or plain, sweetened
    or unsweetened

1½ cups (250 g) fresh or frozen
    mango, peaches or pineapple

2 fresh pears or apples, peeled
    and cored

2 cups chopped chard (75 g,
    1 bunch should do it), washed

1 teaspoon natural vanilla extract

1 tablespoon hemp, chia,
    or ground flaxseeds

1 to 2 cups (140 to 280 g) ice,
    necessary if using only fresh
    (not frozen) fruit

PER SERVING:
Calories: 391, **Protein:** 4.7 g, **Fat:** 5.0 g,
Carbohydrates: 88 g, **Fiber:** 12 g,
Cholesterol: 0 mg

Technically, you can eat this any time of the day, but it's a particularly lovely way to start the day.

DIRECTIONS

- Add all of the ingredients to your blender—preferably a high-powered one. Start on low, then slowly turn it up to high, and let it run for about 1 minute, until all of the ingredients are thoroughly blended.
- Taste, and add sweetener, if desired.

FOR YOUR
MODIFICATION

- Any combination of fruits will work fine, but I think the tropical pineapple and/or mango complement the chard beautifully. Chard is not as bitter as kale, but typically, with greens, any acid will cut the bitterness, and the pineapple does the job here.

- If you add blueberries, they will be delicious and nutritious, but they will turn your beautiful green smoothie a muddy purple-brown color.

FOR YOUR
EDIFICATION

Accelerate the ripening of bananas by placing them in a paper bag. The paper bag traps the ethylene gas. To ripen them even more quickly, add an avocado or apple to the bag, which increases the amount of ethylene gas.

FOR YOUR
INFORMATION

The more frozen fruit you use, the better. The ice will make it cold but not necessarily thick.

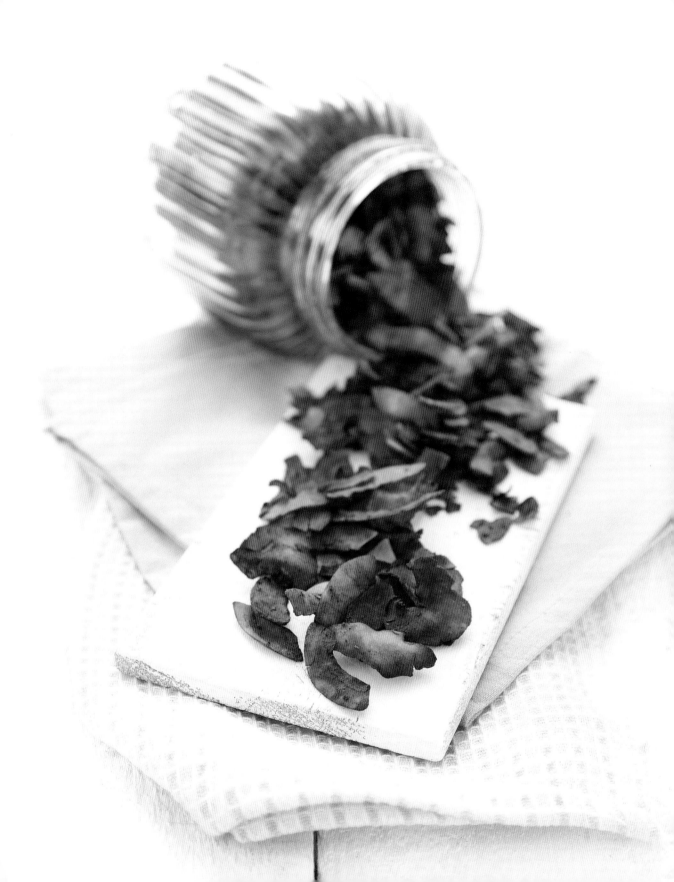

Coconut Bacon

YIELD Makes 3½ cups **ALLERGY** Gluten-free, oil-free, wheat-free

INGREDIENTS

2 tablespoons liquid smoke

2 tablespoons tamari soy sauce

1 tablespoon maple syrup or
agave nectar

1 tablespoon water

3½ cups (200 g) unsweetened
coconut flakes

PER SERVING (2 TABLESPOONS):
Calories: 50, **Protein:** 0.6 g, **Fat:** 4.6 g,
Carbohydrates: 2.2 g, **Fiber:** 1.2 g,
Cholesterol: 0 mg

FOR YOUR EDIFICATION

Liquid smoke adds a wonderful
depth of flavor to so many dishes,
and a little goes a long way. It's a
great staple to keep in the cupboard,
and you'll find yourself using it
often to add a smoky flavor to your
favorite recipes.

FOR YOUR INFORMATION

Look for unsweetened coconut
flakes in the bulk section of your
grocery store; packaged brands
include Edward & Sons/Let's Do
Organic and Bob's Red Mill.

The coconut provides the fat, the liquid smoke provides the smokiness, the tamari provides the salt, and all together, it's incredibly flavorful!

DIRECTIONS

- Preheat the oven to 325°F. Line a baking sheet with parchment paper.
- In a large bowl, stir together the liquid smoke, tamari soy sauce, maple syrup or agave nectar, and water.
- Add the coconut flakes to the bowl, and using a rubber spatula, gently toss together the coconut with the liquid mixture until the coconut flakes are thoroughly coated.
- Transfer the coated coconut flakes onto the prepared baking sheet, spreading them out in a single layer so they cook evenly, and place the baking sheet in the preheated oven. Bake for 20 to 25 minutes, and stay close by.
- After 10 or 15 minutes and every 5 minutes thereafter, you will want to toss and flip the flakes using a spatula. This is not only to make sure the flakes cook evenly but also to ensure that they don't burn, and they will burn if you don't regularly toss them.
- Depending on your oven, you may also need to turn the baking sheet around to ensure they cook up evenly.
- As you continue to check, feel free to taste to make sure they're nice and crispy. They will be a nice brown color when they're done, and if you test them, you'll notice the coconut flavor is pretty much gone.
- Remove from the oven, and let cool before storing in a sealed bag or container. (They continue to crisp up as they cool.)

Suggestions for Serving

- Top a baked potato or twice-baked potato with a couple tablespoons.
- Serve as a topping for a green salad.
- Use as a garnish for the Smoky White Bean Chowder (page 89) or Pasta Alfredo (page 169).

Apple Breakfast Cake

YIELD Makes 6 to 8 servings **ALLERGY** Soy-free, if using a plant milk other than soy

INGREDIENTS

2 cups (250 g) all-purpose flour

2 teaspoons baking powder

1 cup (225 g) light brown
  sugar, packed

½ teaspoon cinnamon

½ teaspoon cardamom

⅛ teaspoon nutmeg

¼ teaspoon salt

1 large or 2 small apples, peeled
  and diced

½ cup (120 ml) canola oil

1 cup (240 ml) plant-based milk
  (soy, rice, almond, oat,
  hazelnut, coconut, or hemp)

2 teaspoons pure vanilla extract

3 tablespoons brown sugar, packed

¼ teaspoon nutmeg

PER SERVING:
Calories: 391, **Protein:** 4.3 g, **Fat:** 15 g,
Carbohydrates: 62 g, **Fiber:** 1.5 g,
Cholesterol: 0 mg

~Dedication~

From: Nazanin Hosseini
To: Sidney Honeycomb
Thank you for all the hummus, vegan
ribbon-cutting ceremonies,
and trips to Disneyland

Whereas a cobbler features fruit baked with a biscuit-dough crust, and a crumble features fruit baked with an oat-streusel topping, and a buckle traditionally features a "cakey" batter underneath the fruit, *rising around the fruit as it bakes, our breakfast cake features the fruit baked* within!

DIRECTIONS

➲ Grease an 8-by-8-inch baking dish, and preheat the oven to 350°F.

➲ In a large mixing bowl, stir together the flour, baking powder, 1 cup of brown sugar, cinnamon, cardamom, nutmeg, salt, and diced apples until fully combined.

➲ Create a well in the center of your flour mixture and pour in the oil, milk, and vanilla extract. Stir to combine the wet and dry ingredients until fully combined. The resulting mixture will be fairly thick—not pourable like liquid.

➲ Transfer the mixture to your prepared baking dish.

➲ In a small bowl, combine together the 3 tablespoons of brown sugar and ¼ teaspoon of nutmeg. Sprinkle on top of the cake batter.

➲ Bake in the oven for 30 minutes, check the center, and bake for 10 to 15 minutes longer or until a fork inserted in the center comes out clean. Let cool (or not), and serve.

FOR YOUR MODIFICATION

Add the batter to greased or lined muffin tins instead of a cake pan, and adjust the cooking time to between 17 and 20 minutes, and you've got yourself more than a dozen muffins.

FOR YOUR INFORMATION

My favorite apples for this cake would be a firm, sweet variety, such as Fuji, but you can't go wrong with whatever your favorite.

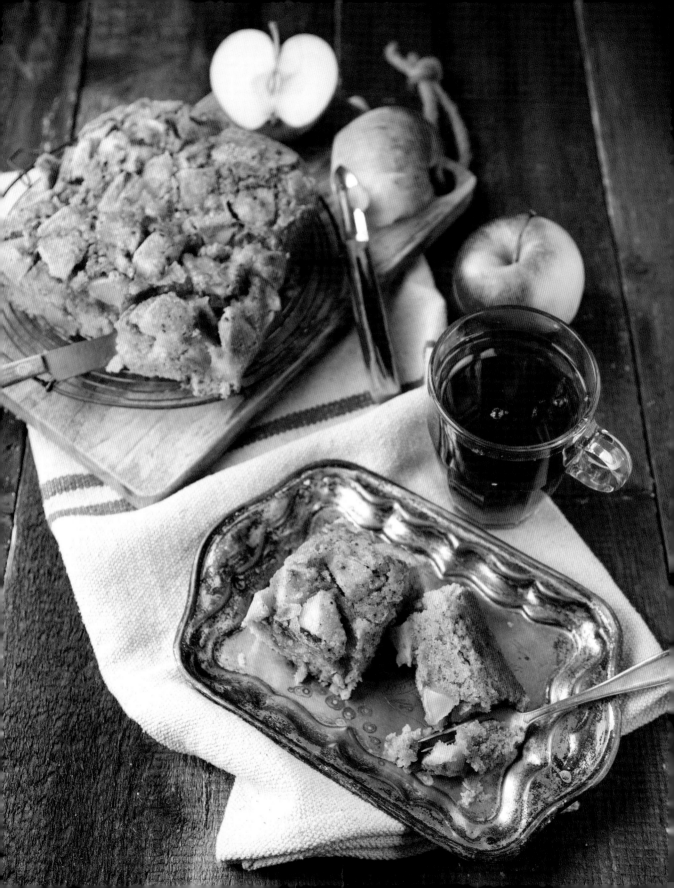

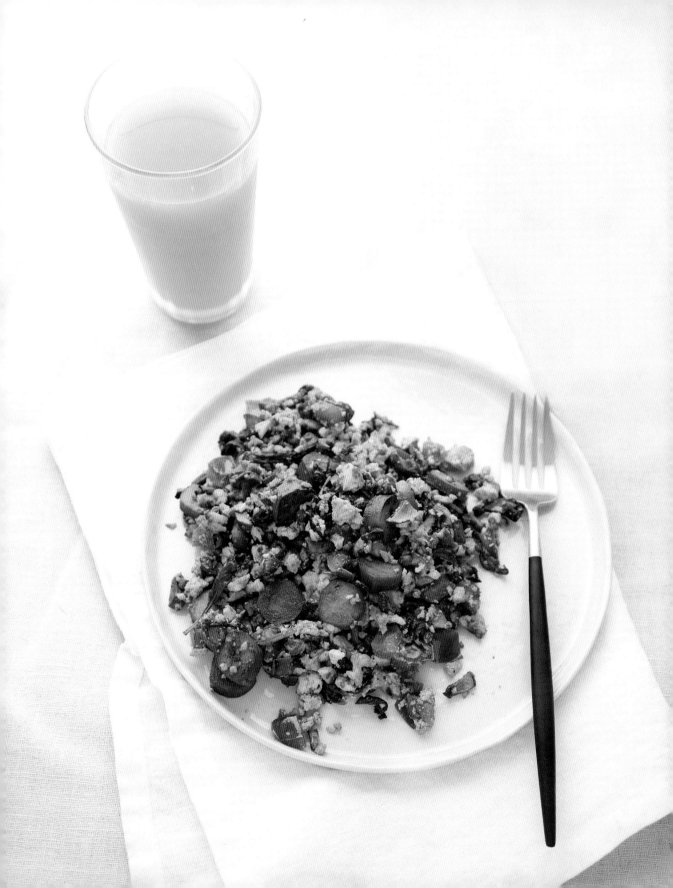

Tofu, Mushroom, and Sausage Scramble

YIELD Makes 6 servings **ALLERGY** Wheat-free, gluten-free (if using wheat-free sausage)

INGREDIENTS

¼ cup (60 ml) water for sautéing

4 cups (350 g), about 15 sliced cremini/brown mushrooms

2 teaspoons olive oil, divided

2 to 3 vegan sausage links, sliced into rounds or crumbled; try Field Roast or Tofurky brands

28 ounces (790 g, about two tubs) extra firm tofu, drained

3 cloves garlic, pressed or minced (or 1 teaspoon garlic powder)

3 tablespoons nutritional yeast flakes

1 teaspoon cumin

½ teaspoon turmeric

2 teaspoons tamari soy sauce

¼ teaspoon hot sauce

2 Roma tomatoes, diced

2 cups (60 g) fresh spinach

Salt and pepper, to taste

2 teaspoons minced chives

PER SERVING:
Calories: 202, Protein: 18 g, Fat: 11 g, Carbohydrates: 9.5 g, Fiber: 3.3 g, Cholesterol: 0 mg

Although I have a fantastic Tofu Scramble in my cookbook, The Vegan Table*, I asked my dear friend Tami Wall to create a new scramble just for this Challenge. And that she did! Try it—it's fabulous!*

DIRECTIONS

◉ Heat the water in a large skillet over medium heat. Add the mushrooms and stir until coated with the water. Sauté until the mushrooms begin to shrink, about 5 to 7 minutes, stirring as needed. Sprinkle with a pinch of salt. Transfer to a bowl.

◉ Add 1 teaspoon of olive oil to the still-heated skillet; add the sausage and brown for about 2 minutes on each side (or about 5 minutes total for crumbled). Remove the sausages from the skillet and add them to the bowl with the mushrooms.

◉ Add the remaining teaspoon of olive oil to the skillet. With your hands, crumble the tofu into the pan (or crumble the tofu in a bowl first, then add it to the heated oil). Cook over medium-high heat for 5 to 7 minutes to brown the tofu.

◉ Add the garlic, nutritional yeast, cumin, turmeric, tamari, and hot sauce, and stir to combine.

◉ Add the tomatoes, spinach, and cooked sausages and mushrooms. Cook for about 5 minutes more to get everything combined and heated through, then season with salt and pepper. Throw the chives in at the very end, stir to combine, and serve.

FOR YOUR MODIFICATION

If you'd like to leave out the veggie sausage, feel free to do so. This scramble is delicious without it, but you may just have to adjust the seasonings.

Dedication

From: Terri Davis
To: My son, Michael.
You are forever in my heart.

Baked Oatmeal with Blueberries and Bananas

YIELD Serves 6 **ALLERGY** Gluten-free, wheat-free, oil-free, soy-free

INGREDIENTS

2 medium or large ripe bananas, sliced into ½-inch pieces

1½ cups (220 g) fresh or frozen blueberries, divided

1½ cups (120 g) uncooked quick-cooking or rolled oats

1 cup (120 g) chopped walnuts, divided

1 teaspoon baking powder

1 teaspoon cinnamon

¼ teaspoon salt

1½ cups (360 ml) plant-based milk (soy, rice, almond, hazelnut, oat, hemp)

¼ cup (60 ml) maple syrup or agave nectar

1 flax egg: 1 tablespoon ground flaxseeds + 3 tablespoons water, blended in a food processor or blender for about 1 minute or until thick and gooey

1 teaspoon vanilla extract

PER SERVING:
Calories: 339, **Protein:** 8.5 g, **Fat:** 16 g, **Carbohydrates:** 45 g, **Fiber:** 6.4 g, **Cholesterol:** 0 mg

This delicious recipes can be made the night before and baked the next morning—an especially lovely treat for guests, brunch, or a special holiday morning.

DIRECTIONS

- Preheat the oven to 375°F. Lightly spray a 9-by-9-inch ceramic or glass baking dish with cooking oil.
- Arrange the banana slices in a single layer on the bottom of the prepared dish. Sprinkle half of the blueberries over the bananas.
- In a large mixing bowl, mix together the oats, half of the walnuts, the baking powder, cinnamon, and salt. Stir well to thoroughly combine.
- In another mixing bowl, whisk together the plant-based milk, maple syrup, flax egg, and the vanilla.
- Cover the bananas and blueberries with the oat mixture. Next, slowly pour the milk mixture over the oats so it's evenly distributed. Sprinkle the remaining berries and the remaining walnuts across the top.
- Bake for 35 minutes, or until the top is nicely golden, the oat mixture has set a bit, and some of the blueberries are bubbling from underneath.
- Remove from the oven and let cool for a few minutes. Drizzle with additional maple syrup if you want it a bit sweeter.

FOR YOUR EDIFICATION

I prefer frozen to fresh blueberries because they retain their shape beautifully when baked in this dish.

FOR YOUR MODIFICATION

Use any combination of fruits and nuts – or add unsweetened dried coconut flakes!

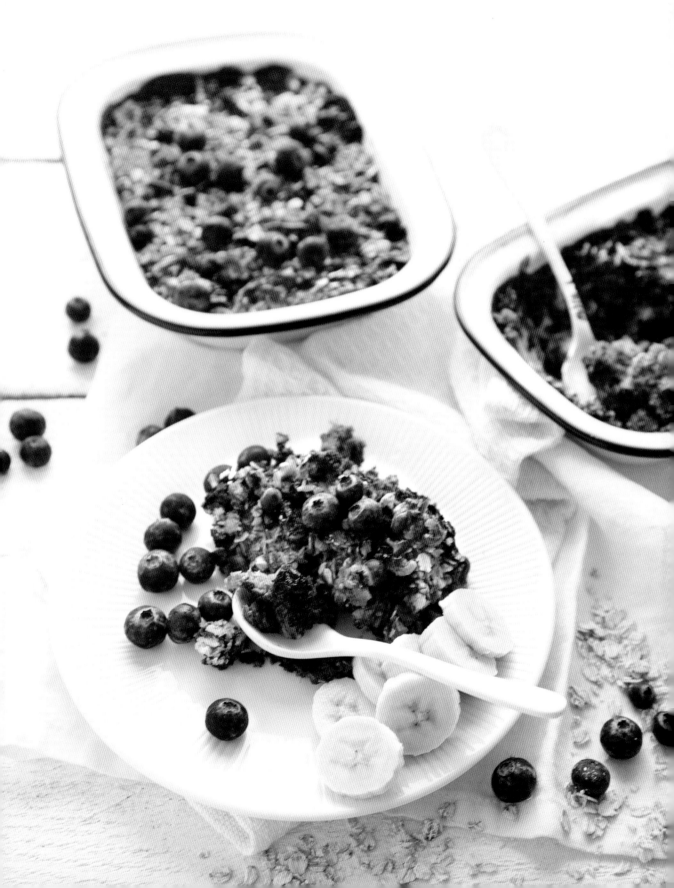

Carrot Ginger Apple Juice

YIELD One 10-ounce glass **ALLERGY** Gluten-free, wheat-free, oil-free, soy-free

INGREDIENTS

6 medium carrots, root stems cut off

1 apple or pear, unpeeled and quartered

1 beet, peeled and quartered (optional)

1-inch fresh ginger, peeled

Juice of 1 medium orange

PER 10-OUNCE GLASS (WITHOUT BEET):
Calories: 338, Protein: 5.6 g, Fat: 1.5 g, Carbohydrates: 79.9 g, Fiber: 3.7 g, Cholesterol: 0 mg

PER 10-OUNCE GLASS (WITH BEET):
Calories: 356, Protein: 6.0 g, Fat: 1.7 g, Carbohydrates: 83.8 g, Fiber: 3.7 g, Cholesterol: 0 mg

---

FOR YOUR INFORMATION

Using a juicer will yield more juice than if you use a blender. It's more powerful than you are in being able to extract the juice from the pulp.

I tend not to include "recipes" for juices in my books because I don't want readers to feel they have to have special equipment to make my recipes. But since this juice is a staple in my home, I really wanted to share it with you. So, I compromised and came up with two versions: one for a juicer and one for a blender. The beet is optional, but it adds a gorgeous color and earthy flavor if you choose to include it. Just don't wear a white shirt!

DIRECTIONS *WITH A JUICER*

- For this juicer version, keep the carrots whole and include the apple or pear core. Add the carrots, apple or pear, beet (if using), and ginger to your juicer, alternating between the carrots, apples, beet, and ginger. When all the ingredients are juiced, transfer to your favorite serving glass, and stir in the orange juice. I find it just adds a little extra sweetness to balance the spicy ginger or earthy beets!

- I prefer to chill mine in the refrigerator for about an hour before drinking, but if you can't wait and prefer it chilled, add some ice to your glass, drink immediately, and enjoy!

DIRECTIONS *WITHOUT A JUICER*

- For this blender version, cut the carrots into chunks, and discard the apple core. Place all the ingredients in a high-powered blender, and blend until smooth. If you don't have the juice from one orange but do have orange or apple juice (in a jar), add about ¼ cup to help move things along.

- Next, place a cheesecloth, or any other fine mesh strainer, over a large bowl. Pour the blender contents into the cheesecloth and squeeze all of the juice out into the bowl. If using a fine sieve or strainer, use a rubber spatula to press the pulp down and press out as much of the juice as possible into the bowl.

- Compost the pulp, and pour the juice into a favorite serving glass with or without ice. I prefer to chill mine in the refrigerator for about an hour, but if you use ice (or don't like it chilled), drink immediately and enjoy!

Lemon Poppy Seed Muffins

YIELD About 20 muffins **ALLERGY** Soy-free, if using soy-free nondairy butter

INGREDIENTS

3 tablespoons ground flaxseed (equivalent of 3 flax eggs)

½ cup (120 ml) + 1 tablespoon water

3 cups (375 g) all-purpose or whole-wheat pastry flour

1¼ cups (250 g) granulated sugar

1½ teaspoons baking powder

3 tablespoons lemon zest (from the 2 or 3 lemons you use for the juice below)

2 tablespoons poppy seeds

1 teaspoon salt

One 13.5-ounce (400 ml) can coconut milk (or any plant-based milk)

⅓ cup (80 ml) fresh lemon juice (from 2 or 3 lemons, depending on the size)

¾ cup (180 ml) canola oil or melted nondairy butter

1½ teaspoons vanilla extract

**PER SERVING (1 MUFFIN)
ALL-PURPOSE FLOUR:**
Calories: 239, **Protein:** 2.7 g, **Fat:** 13 g,
Carbohydrates: 29 g, **Fiber:** 1.1 g,
Cholesterol: 0 mg

**PER SERVING (1 MUFFIN)
WHOLE-WHEAT PASTRY FLOUR:**
Calories: 233, **Protein:** 2.6 g, **Fat:** 14 g,
Carbohydrates: 28 g, **Fiber:** 3.0 g,
Cholesterol: 0 mg

Sweet enough for dessert, flexible enough to be sweetened less and served for breakfast, this is a favorite muffin of mine that is also the perfect accompaniment to a tea party or coffee clutch.

DIRECTIONS

- Preheat oven to 350°F. Lightly oil one or two muffin tins.

- In a blender, food processor, or in a bowl using an electric hand mixer, whip the flaxseed and water together, until you have a thick and creamy consistency. The result should be thick and rather gooey. This can all be done by hand, but high speed in a food processor/hand mixer does a better job in about 1 minute.

- In a large mixing bowl, stir together the flour, sugar, baking powder, lemon zest, poppy seeds, and salt.

- Create a well in the center of the dry ingredients and then add the flax eggs, coconut milk, lemon juice, oil, and vanilla extract. Stir the mixture until smooth, about 1 minute.

- Spoon about two tablespoons of batter into each muffin cup. You will have enough batter for almost 20 muffins, so you can either bake in two batches or use a second lightly oiled muffin tin. (Tip: if you don't fill all of the cups in a muffin tin, add a small amount of water to each cup that doesn't contain batter.)

- Bake for 25 to 30 minutes, or until a toothpick inserted into the center of the muffins comes out clean. Cool in the pans for 10 minutes before removing to a wire rack.

FOR YOUR INFORMATION

When you open a can of regular full-fat coconut milk, you'll notice a solid mass of the coconut fat. This is normal separation, so just stir it in with the rest of the liquid.

FOR YOUR MODIFICATION

You may also make this as bread. Pour the batter into a lightly oiled loaf tin and increase the cooking time to 50 to 55 minutes or until a toothpick inserted into the center of the bread comes out clean.

Eating Out and Speaking Up

Having harnessed in the first week what you need to eat vegan at home, let's address what many people anticipate being challenging about being vegan: eating in restaurants or at the homes of nonvegan friends. You may be surprised at how easy it is.

Since social occasions tend to go hand in hand with food and since we've all been indoctrinated to eat meat, dairy, and/or eggs at every meal, some people are afraid their social lives will suffer when they eliminate animal products from their diet. For anyone who has ever thought it difficult as a vegan to dine out, to eat at the home of a nonvegan friend, or to find food to eat at parties, I can assure you it's just a matter of changing your perception. If you look for lack, that's what you will find; alternatively, if you look for abundance, that is what you will discover. Once you look at the world through a vegan lens, you realize how effortless it is to find an abundance of options in restaurants of all types; you just may have never noticed before because you weren't looking for it. Friends and family members most likely already have "vegan recipes" in their repertoire—they just may not call them "vegan."

FINDING WHAT YOU WANT IN NONVEGAN RESTAURANTS

Though you can find something to eat in every restaurant, the most vegan-friendly restaurants are those that feature non-American fare. That leaves countless options—no matter what town you're in.

- Chinese restaurants offer many vegan dishes, and Buddhist Chinese restaurants serve vegetarian-only fare. Just be sure to tell them to leave out the eggs.

- Thai, Vietnamese, and Burmese restaurants are very vegan-friendly, featuring vegetable, noodle, and tofu dishes. Just ask for no fish sauce. Japanese restaurants feature edamame, vegetable nori/sushi rolls, tempura; salads made of lettuce or sea vegetables with house dressing, vegetable dumplings, and miso soup. Specify no fish sauce.

- Middle Eastern restaurants offer a smorgasbord of delights: baba ghannouj, hummus, olives, tapenade, falafel, tabouli, stuffed grape leaves (dolmas), and pita bread.

- Any pizza place will make a cheese-free pizza for you. Request veggies and fresh herbs for added flavor, texture, color, and nutrients.

- Indian and Sri Lankan restaurants have a bevy of vegan options. South Indian restaurants tend to be vegetarian-only; just be sure to ask them to leave out the ghee (clarified butter).

- Italian restaurants offer lots of pasta (primavera, arrabbiata, and puttanesca), vegetable dishes, salads, and starters such as bruschetta and antipasti. Just specify vegetable broth and no cheese. (Most restaurant pastas are made without eggs, but it still wouldn't hurt to ask.)

- Ethiopian restaurant menus always have a huge selection of vegan selections, including lentils, split peas, greens, and potatoes. Just make sure everything is sautéed in oil—not dairy-based butter.

- Mexican restaurants always have rice, beans, tortillas, salsa, and guacamole. Specify to leave off cheese, make sure the rice isn't cooked in chicken's broth, and ask if refried beans are cooked in lard or vegetable oil. If they're cooked in lard, whole beans are the way to go.

- Sub shops can make a vegetable-only sandwich for you and flavor it with oil, mustard, vinegar, salt, and pepper. (To avoid potential contamination of foodborne pathogens, don't hesitate to ask employees to change their gloves before handling your veggies.)

- Look for all-you-can-eat buffets and salad bars. A good buffet can offer a wide range of healthful options like salad greens, cooked and raw veggies, beans, fresh fruit—even baked potatoes and pasta.

- Many cafes sell chai tea and hot cocoa, using mixes that are often vegan. Also, many authentic chocolate cafes sell "European hot cocoa," which is vegan. Just ask.

- Ice cream stores often have sorbets, which are—by definition—dairy-free, unlike sherbet (which always has dairy). I've also seen many gelato shops offer soy- and fruit-based versions of their gelati. Just ask to be sure.

- Even baseball stadiums, ballparks, and arenas have changed with the times, and many offer many vegan options, including veggie dogs and burgers, pretzels and French fries, burritos and nuts. Visit soyhappy.org for a vegan guide to stadiums around the country.

Of course, vegetarian- and vegan-only restaurants are your best bets for those lucky enough to live near them. (See sidebar at the end of this chapter.)

ASKING FOR WHAT YOU WANT WITH CONFIDENCE

Eating outside of your home is not simply a matter of choosing the restaurant; it's also a matter of communicating your food ethics in a confident, positive, effective way.

1. **BE CLEAR.** Even though the word "vegan" is more familiar than ever before, it's still unknown to some. To avoid any confusion, be clear and specific with your server and ask for exactly what you want. Plenty of people think chicken broth is acceptable for vegans simply because there aren't chicken parts floating around, and some people erroneously think vegans don't eat pasta, bread, or yeast.

   Scenario Suggestion: When eating out, or when invited over a friend's for dinner, it's helpful to state specific foods. Instead of simply saying, "Please make this vegan," you might want to elaborate and say, "I'm vegan, so can you tell me if I unwittingly order something with hidden eggs, dairy products, or animal-based broth?" The more specific you are, the better. Moreover, don't hesitate to send something back if they missed the mark; you are paying for the food and should get exactly what you ask for.

2. **BE POSITIVE.** Most likely, you're making the vegan choice because it makes you feel good—physically, mentally, emotionally, and spiritually. If that's your truth, then that's exactly what you should express to those around you. Your attitude will influence the perception and attitude of others about what it means to be vegan.

   Scenario Suggestion: When ordering in a restaurant, of course it's appropriate to thank the server for accommodating you, but don't apologize to the point of being self-effacing. If you had a food allergy or an aversion to a certain food, you'd do the same. You'd make sure they make your meal without strawberries—or whatever food you don't eat—and you'd just move on. There's no difference here.

3. **BE CREATIVE.** I don't think people realize that you can ask for whatever you want—in general but also in a restaurant! I think the perception that "it's hard to be vegan and eat out" partly stems from the fact that someone looks at a nonvegan menu and says "My goodness—there's nothing to order here!" But you're not looking at the whole picture. You don't have to order exactly what's on the menu! You can modify whatever they already have and ask them to make it differently.

   Scenario Suggestion: You see a pasta dish on the menu with olive oil, basil, capers, and grilled chicken, and you ask them to prepare it for you without the grilled chicken but with grilled squash or peppers or onions (or all of the above)! You'd be surprised how happy chefs are to create something new—and everyone will covet your special dish.

4. **BE TECH-SAVVY.** Many restaurants have websites with their menus online, which means you can check out their options in advance. You'll know right away how friendly they are to vegan customers.

5. **BE HUMOROUS.** Food can be a sensitive subject. We're talking about ingrained habits; we're talking about life and death; we're talking about violence and suffering. Here's something you probably already know: humor diffuses tension. One thing to keep in mind is whenever someone makes a silly joke or insensitive comment about your being vegan, it really hasn't anything to do with you. Responding with levity and humor will be the last thing they expect. It mirrors back to them how passive-aggressive they're being but lightens the mood at the same time.

Scenario Suggestion: If I'm eating at a table where nonvegan food is being served (and everyone knows I'm vegan), invariably someone will apologize for eating the chicken's leg or hamburger they're about to bite into. Instead of lying and saying, "It's okay" or reacting indignantly, I usually say—with a smile—something like, "Don't apologize to me. Apologize to the chickens." It enables me to speak the truth without shaming them, but it also sets a lighter tone.

6. **BE PROACTIVE.** On those occasions when you don't have a say in choosing the restaurant, it's worth calling in advance to find out which menu items can be made meat- and dairy-free.

7. **BE PREPARED.** Sometimes a work or family event centers around meat (like a barbe-cue) or takes place in a restaurant that is unfavorable to vegans (such as a steakhouse). At such times, consider eating something before you go and/or bringing your own food to eat when you get there. This may seem inconvenient, but it's better than not eating at all, and the food you bring will most likely inspire others to try something new.

8. **BE CONFIDENT.** Food is a personal as well as political subject that has been known to bring up people's defenses, and vegans may find themselves on the receiving end of ridicule, criticism, interrogations, jokes, and plain old rudeness. Remaining confident that the attack has nothing to do with you personally will help you take the encounter in stride. Also, don't feel you need to carry the weight of defending *all* the benefits of vegan-ism. If asked why you make the choices you do, speak from your heart, and tell your truth.

Scenario Suggestion: You're at a party, and someone hears that you're vegan and feels the need to confront you about it. He says to you, "I just finished a book by an author who provides a lot of evidence that humans were never pure vegans at any point in our evolution." Many might be tempted to respond with an assertion that the author is wrong, that humans gathered more than they hunted, that we're physically designed to eat plant-based diets, etc., and if your goal is to win an argument, then argue away. But, consider an alternative response that diffuses the attack, speaks to the real issue, and enables you to remain true to yourself. You could say something like, "I haven't read that book so I can't speak to it in particular, but what I do know is that I feel really good about eating this way. It's better for my health and certainly better for the animals. And besides, isn't being human about doing things better than we did in the past, especially as we gain the benefit of more knowledge and more choices?"

9. **BE VOCAL.** When in a group situation, speak up and ask your friends, family, or co-workers to dine at a local vegetarian or vegan restaurant. Not only will you have more than just a few menu options to choose from, *everyone* can eat and experience the abundance and joy of a plant-based menu.

10. **BE GENEROUS.** Bring muffins in for your morning office meeting, leave cookies on your neighbor's porch, make a cake for a special occasion and share it with colleagues. (See my recipes for such goodies on Day 14: Baking Without Eggs.) Co-workers, neighbors, clients, friends, and family all appreciate the gift of homemade goodies. Sharing delicious food can sometimes be more powerful than anything you might say. Anytime nonvegans try your infamous meatless chili or your decadent dairy-free cookies, they are exposed to dishes they may have never chosen on their own, and often they'll walk away with a new perception about "vegan food."

I know some naysayers would say, "Still. It's so much trouble being vegan. You have to spend so much time finding a vegan-friendly restaurant or calling in advance to make sure you'll be accommodated, and to boot, you miss out on the native delicacies in exotic locales."

Well, I just don't agree with that perception. I think there are higher principles than gustatory pleasures, and I am happy to choose nonviolence and compassion over hedonism and gluttony. Knowing I'm trying to make a peaceful contribution to the world and a healthful decision for my body is worth a little inconvenience. In the grand scheme of things, I want to look back on my life and know that I had my priorities straight, that I put my money where my mouth is, that I walked the walk, and that I was true to what I believed in. That means more to me than eating delicately spiced animal parts.

It's not a sacrifice for me to be vegan; it's a matter of living consistently and compassionately, and that feels better going down than any animal-based flesh or fluid.

Restaurant and Travel Resources

Vegetarian and vegan restaurants in cities around the world continue rising in number all the time. These days, you can easily find vegan-friendly restaurants by taking advantage of the many resources available. More than ever, travel books include tips for vegans, but the places to go for the most current information are websites and smart phone apps, most of which are available for different smart phone devices.

WEBSITES AND APPS

🐄 **happycow.net**
Search or browse for vegan and vegan-friendly restaurants all around the world. They rely on reviews from users, so help others by adding reviews of vegan-friendly restaurants you've discovered.

🐄 **vegguide.org**
Search or browse by region, country, or city for veg-friendly restaurants. Boasting a simple, clean interface, it also depends on reviews from its users.

🐄 **vegdining.com**
Is a veg restaurant guide with a focus on international travel.

🐄 **vegcooking.com**
Click on Dining Out in the top menu to access a bevy of helpful information, including Restaurant of the Month, Vegan Eating on the Road, and Vegetarian-Friendly Restaurant Guide. In Vegan Eating on the Road, there's a "Chain Restaurants Guide" so you can see all the vegan options in chain restaurants from Arby's to Taco Bell.

🐄 **yelp.com**
A comprehensive general website for restaurant reviews.

🐄 **veganXpress**
This brilliant app is available for a nominal fee and includes about 100 chain restaurants in the country, listing vegan items that are on the menu. For instance, if you're in the middle of nowhere and have no options other than The Cheesecake Factory or Olive Garden, you can use this app to discover that you will indeed find food to eat. Fast food chain restaurants are also included, as is a list of junk food found in movie theatres. For instance, Skittles are now gelatin-free!

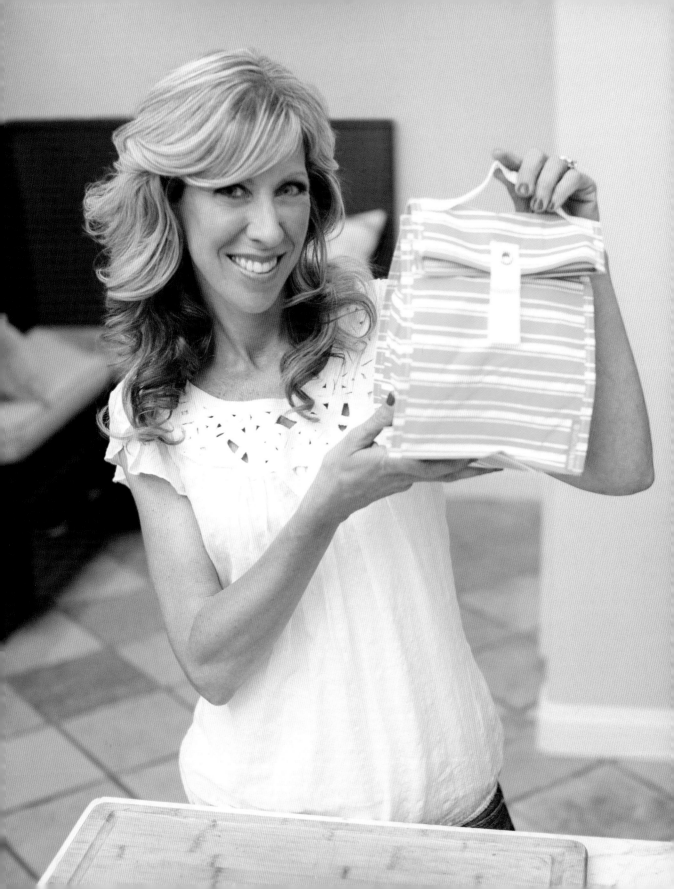

Packing Lunches for School and Work

Now that you have what you need to prepare delicious meals at home with no excuses and no fuss, it's time to apply those principles to preparing delicious meals that you pack up for the road. Whether you're preparing food for a picnic, packing lunches for your children for school, packing a daily work lunch for your partner or yourself, or working outside in such fields as gardening or construction, today is all about making meals that are fast, easy, and transportable. The ground we'll cover today will also apply to when you travel and need food for the car or the plane (though I talk more in detail about traveling in an upcoming day). Of course, all of these suggestions can be applied to eating at home, as well.

Let's start with the easiest of all to prepare and pack: sandwiches.

SANDWICHES

There are as many ideas as your imagination can create. Here are just a few.

1. Deli Sandwich: You'll want to go back to Day 3: Stocking a Healthful Kitchen to review the list of all the delicious deli slices available, or you can just make the sandwich based on whole vegetables. Add your favorite condiments and pile on the veggies: lettuce, tomatoes, roasted red peppers, avocado slices, olives, and alfalfa sprouts.

> **TIP:** *Sandwich spreads and condiments abound, whether they're homemade or store-bought: ketchup, mustard, mayonnaise, relish, mashed avocado, hummus, mashed banana (goes great with nut butters), nondairy cream cheese, baba ghannouj, agave nectar, fruit spreads, pesto, tomato sauce (for an impromptu pita pizza), or Muhammara (store-bought or homemade).*

2. Veggie Subs: Of course, instead of making a basic sandwich with simple bread slices, you can also make a sub sandwich using either rolls, baguettes, or a crusty, rustic Italian bread—then add all your favorite veggies! My preferences for this kind of sandwich include tomatoes, roasted eggplant, roasted peppers, thinly sliced/shredded carrots, thinly sliced/shredded raw beets (peel them first), some lettuce or whatever greens you prefer, and alfalfa sprouts. Of course, for variation, you can also add your favorite vegan deli slices, grilled tofu, grilled tempeh, or grilled mushrooms.

3. Peanut Butter and Jelly: To make it the most healthful PB&J sandwiches, choose high-fiber whole-grain bread, all-fruit jams and jellies sweetened with fruit and not added sugars, and nut butters that don't have added oils and sugars. Remember—peanut butter is just ground peanuts. Buying a version with a little salt is fine, but you don't need the added oils and sugars.

> *VARIATION: Try the other nut and seed butters on the market (or make them yourself at home): almond butter, cashew butter, sunflower seed butter, and hemp seed butter.*

4. Bacon, Lettuce, and Tomato: See page 135 for my Coconut Bacon, Lettuce, and Tomato Sandwich.

5. Burgers: Stick your favorite veggie burger in a bun, and top with your favorite fixings. What's so lovely about plant-based burgers is that they're already cooked, and they're *plants*, so you don't have the risk for contracting foodborne illnesses you do when eating animal-based burgers. Heat them up to make them warm, but it's not like you have to cook them through to the center to kill pathogens, as you have to do with animal flesh.

6. Pita Pockets: Add any and all of your favorite fillings, such as the ones I named above—or whatever you like! A favorite light sandwich of mine is shredded lettuce, chopped apple, and chopped celery in a pita pocket with a light balsamic dressing.

7. Fish-Friendly Tuna Salad: See page 141 for my Fish-Friendly version made with sunflower seeds. You can also replace the sunflower seeds with mashed chickpeas, mashed tofu, or steamed tempeh.

8. Bean burritos: Easy! Open a can of black or pinto beans, rinse and drain, and add some of the beans to a tortilla with lettuce, salsa, avocado or guacamole, and tomatoes.

9. Tofu scramble: Add to a bun or stuff in a pita along with some ketchup and you have a great sandwich for the road.

10. Falafel burgers on a bun or falafel balls stuffed into a pita: You can find falafel mixes in the grocery store or make your own. I have a great Falafel Burger in my cookbook, *The Vegan Table*.

SALADS

Whether they're made of greens, grains, pasta, noodles, lentils, beans, tofu, tempeh, or vegetables, they're fantastic for the road.

1. Green Salad: The most obvious salad to make is a green salad based on your favorite leafy greens. My favorite salad greens are arugula and kale, but you can use romaine, watercress, or even chard—whatever suits your fancy. From there, pile on whatever you love in a salad. It might be a can of beans, chopped or shredded carrots, avocado slices, sliced cucumbers, sliced bell peppers, fresh herbs, raw cauliflower, raw broccoli, nuts, seeds—whatever! Then, just put your dressing in a separate container (or have a couple bottles of your favorite salad dressing with you at work), and dress the salad once you're ready to eat it. (See page 199 for my Green Goddess Dressing and page 101 for Everyday Vinaigrette.)

2. Lentil Salad: There is so much variety when it comes to making lentil salads, and they're so easy to make. Cook lentils with a 3:1 ratio of water (or vegetable broth) to lentils. Add some sautéed chopped garlic, onion, mushrooms, carrots, along with dried herbs such as thyme, oregano, and tarragon while the lentils are cooking. When the lentils are done, let them cool a bit, then stir in a little Dijon mustard and chopped fresh parsley, squeeze in a little fresh lemon juice, and sprinkle on a little salt. Stir it up, and pack it up. See page 147 for Lentil Salad with Beets and Citrus Vinaigrette.

3. Bean Salad: These are even easier than lentil salads because you can just open the can of beans, drain and rinse them, and then make a quick salad (though canned lentils are also available these days). Vary your bean salad with different beans (red kidney, white kidney/cannellini, black, soy, pinto, or chickpeas), different vinegars (rice, balsamic, or apple cider), olive oil, chopped raw veggies, lemon juice, fresh herbs, or even easier—premade, store-bought fresh salsa! Guacamole or chopped avocado and cooked rice will add even more substance, flavor, and nutrients.

4. Fruit Salad: Chop up your favorite seasonal fruits, sprinkle on some cinnamon, a drizzle of agave nectar, and a squeeze of lemon juice. Add some chopped dates or raisins.

5. Pasta Salad: My favorite quickie pasta salad is made with bowtie pasta (many gluten-free pastas are also available), a little eggless mayo, chopped olives, some corn kernels, some chopped bell pepper, and salt and pepper to taste. Or, use your favorite oil and vinegar combination.

6. Noodle Salad: I think noodle salads lend themselves well to Asian flavors, so you can use udon, soba, or vermicelli noodles with peanut sauce, shredded veggies, or sesame oil and sesame seeds with edamame beans.

7. Tex-Mex Salad: I've talked about using beans a lot, but to make a Tex-Mex salad, you can use substitute the beans for vegan chicken, seitan (see page 50 for Homemade Seitan), chopped tofu, or crumbled tempeh (steamed for 10 minutes will always make it better). Whatever you choose, sauté in a little water or oil, and add an envelope of taco seasonings or your own combination of cumin, chili powder, and salt, then add some extra water. Cook until everything is heated through and a thicker sauce is created from the water and spices, and you have a hearty, flavorful mixture. Pack up some tortillas and whatever fixings you like, and you're good to go!

8. Grain Salad: Make your own grain salad by mixing and matching with

- cooked grains: quinoa, barley, bulgur, or couscous (even though it's technically a pasta and not a grain)

- chopped raw veggies: carrots, bell peppers, tomatoes, scallions/green onions, red onion, corn, snow peas, chopped broccoli, or chopped cauliflower

- dried and fresh fruit: raisins, currants, dried cranberries, dried apricots, apples, or oranges

- nuts and seeds: almonds, walnuts, or peanuts (and toast them first if you prefer), pine nuts, sunflower seeds, sesame seeds, or poppy seeds

- herbs and spices: dried ginger, curry powder, turmeric, cardamom, coriander, cumin or fresh basil, fresh parsley, or fresh cilantro

- dressing: salsa, combination of sesame oil and rice vinegar, an Italian Salad dressing, a favorite creamy salad dressing from the bottle, a combination of garlic, lemon juice, and olive oil—or olive oil and balsamic vinegar—or just lemon juice

That enables you to create endless grain salads depending on the combination you choose. Also, check out page 138 for Southwestern Quinoa Pilaf.

9. Potato Salad: Wash and cube potatoes, steam or boil them until they're cooked through, and let cool. Toss with eggless mayonnaise, raw chopped vegetables, fresh herbs, salt, and pepper.

10. Bread Salad: See page 136 for a delicious Panzanella (Bread Salad).

BEVERAGES AND SNACKS TO PACK

In terms of beverages and snacks, the most obvious are:

Fresh Fruit: The most healthful and transportable snacks are fresh fruit (apples, apricots, pears, bananas, blueberries, cherries, figs, mango, papaya, grapefruit, grapes, kiwi, melon, nectarines, orange sections, peaches, pineapple, plums, raspberries, and strawberries). In a separate container, bring peanut, almond, apple, or pumpkin butter as a dip/spread for the fruit.

Raw Veggies with Dip: Carrot, celery, or bell pepper slices pair well with hummus or nut butter.

Dried Fruit: Dried dates, prunes, raisins, and apricots are road foods by definition.

Nuts, Seeds, and Trail Mix: Toasted or raw nuts and seeds, mixed with dried fruit are great for snacking. Buy premade (Trader Joe's specializes in these mixes), or make them yourself.

Popcorn: Make your own and divide the batch up into little bags or containers. I make popcorn with an air popper, spritz on a little oil from a spray-oil can, and toss with salt, cumin, chili powder, and nutritional yeast. If it's for the little ones, skip the chili powder. Otherwise, most already-popped bagged popcorn you buy in the store tends to be vegan, unless it's a variety that features cheese. Check out page 185 for a recipe for Truffle Popcorn.

> *TIP: Most popcorn at movie theatres is made with oil—not dairy-based butter. Just ask for "no butter" when you order—and even bring your own little baggie of nutritional yeast to sprinkle on yourself. Or, make your own popcorn at home and bring it with you to the theatre.*

Pita Bread with Hummus or Tabouli: Make your own hummus/tabouli or buy premade.

Crackers with Peanut Butter: I think I've officially revealed my peanut butter addiction, but it's so delicious and keeps well unrefrigerated. Other nut or seed butters can be used as well.

Vegan Jerky: A few different companies make vegan jerky—processed, yes, but good when you're in a pinch. Turtle Island (makers of Tofurky) makes Tofurky Jurky; Primal Spirit makes a variety of "Primal Strips," including Teriyaki, Texas Barbeque, Smoked, and—my favorite—Hot and Spicy Mushroom; Stonewall's makes Jerquee; and Tasty Eats makes Soy Jerky. Check out fakemeats.com for a great selection.

Energy Bars: Great for a quick refuel, many—if not most—energy bars are vegan. 22DaysNutrition, Clif Bar, Luna, Lara, Organic Food, ProBar, Kind Bar, Raw Revolution, 18 Rabbits, and Vega bars are some of the brands to look for.

Olives: A healthful, surprisingly low-cal snack, olives make great road food.

Cereal/Granola: Throw your favorite cereal or granola in a bag to enjoy as a hand-to-mouth snack, or even bring along some nondairy milk for the whole shebang.

Snack-Size Apple Sauce: Individually packaged healthful snacks such as applesauce are available in many stores.

Bagged Crisps: Not as healthful as fruit and veggies, but not as greasy as potato chips: pretzels, tortilla chips, crackers, Veggie Booty (aka Pirate Booty: Veggie), and Tings by Robert's American Gourmet are great treats for the lunch box.

Dark Chocolate Bars: Good pick-me-ups for a midday snack, vegan chocolate bars are available in stores everywhere. Good brands that carry vegan chocolate bars include Chocolove, Endangered Species, Dagoba, Equal Exchange, Tropical Source, Green & Black, and many more. I'm lucky enough to have Tcho in my backyard.

> *TIP: So that our compassion is consistently reflected across the board for all beings, I encourage you to choose chocolate labeled "fair trade." Check out foodispower.org for a list of the most ethically sourced cocoa beans.*

Smoothies and Fruit Drinks: Certainly, you can make your own and transport them in a thermos or portable cup, but many companies make good, healthful bottled smoothies to pack for lunch, including Odwalla, Naked Juice, Bolthouse Farms, and Sambazon.

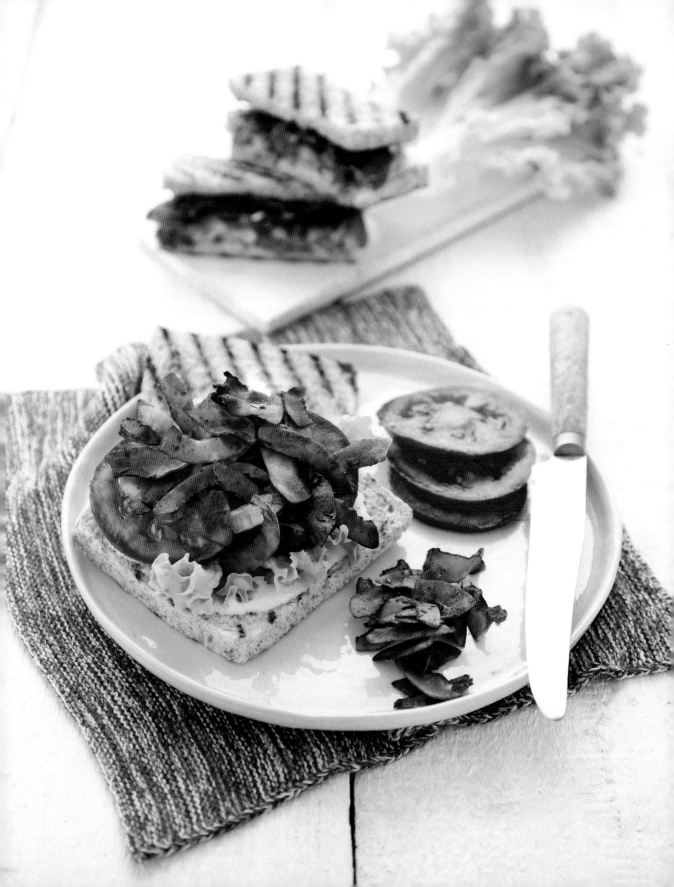

Coconut Bacon, Lettuce, and Tomato Sandwich

YIELD 2 sandwiches **ALLERGY** Gluten- and wheat-free, depending on bread

INGREDIENTS

4 slices whole grain bread

4 tablespoons eggless mayonnaise (Wildwood, Just Mayo, Vegenaise)

1 large tomato, sliced

4 lettuce leaves

½ avocado, seeded, peeled and sliced

Coconut Bacon (see page 113 for recipe)

⅛ teaspoon salt

PER SERVING (1 SANDWICH):
Calories: 487.7, **Protein:** 15.7 g, **Fat:** 27.5 g, Carbohydrates: 48.0 g, **Fiber:** 12.8 g, Cholesterol: 0 mg

This healthful and kind version leaves the other in the dust. It's got salt, fat, texture, flavor, and familiarity – all the components a good meal needs without anyone getting hurt!

Note: *Since you'll want to make the Coconut Bacon (see page 113) first, you will want to factor that into your total prep time for this recipe.*

DIRECTIONS

◐ Spread 1 tablespoon of the mayonnaise on one side of each slice of bread.

◐ For each sandwich, stack two slices of the tomato, two lettuce leaves, ¼ of the avocado slices, and a generous helping (about 3 tablespoons) of the Coconut Bacon between two slices of bread. Season with salt.

◐ Close the sandwich, cut in half, and serve.

⟩Dedication⟨

From: Tim Anderson and Ellen Kim
To: Our beloved Jeb. We miss you.

Panzanella (Bread Salad)

YIELD 8 servings **ALLERGY** Soy-free

INGREDIENTS

5 to 6 medium tomatoes, cut into large chunks

4 to 6 cups (360 to 540 g) day-old crusty bread (Italian loaf or French baguette), cut into cubes the same size as the tomatoes (a full loaf or baguette should be fine)

1 medium hothouse cucumber, unpeeled, seeded, and coarsely chopped

1/2 small red onion, finely chopped

2 to 3 medium cloves garlic, minced

3 tablespoons capers, drained

20 large basil leaves, coarsely chopped

2 to 3 tablespoons high-quality balsamic vinegar

1/4 cup (60 ml) high-quality extra-virgin olive oil

Salt and freshly ground pepper, to taste

PER SERVING:
Calories: 181, **Protein:** 4.2 g, **Fat:** 8.1 g, **Carbohydrates:** 24 g, **Fiber:** 2.5 g, **Cholesterol:** 0 mg

Instead of discarding that hearty Italian loaf that's going stale, make this delicious bread salad that is absolutely divine in the summer when tomatoes, cucumbers, and basil are at their peak.

DIRECTIONS

- Add the tomatoes, bread, cucumber, red onion, garlic, capers, and basil to a large bowl, and toss together. Drizzle in the balsamic vinegar and 1/4 cup olive oil, and toss some more. Add salt and pepper to taste, and add additional olive oil, if desired.

- Set aside and marinate, covered, at room temperature for at least 30 minutes, up to 12 hours. I would avoid marinating the salad in the refrigerator, since the tomatoes tend to become somewhat "mealy" in the fridge.

- Serve at room temperature.

FOR YOUR EDIFICATION

Panzanella is a bread salad (*pan* means "bread") that was most likely invented as a way to use stale bread, along with fresh vegetables from the garden. The earliest written reference is from the 1500s in a poem by the famous artist, Bronzino. The tomato hadn't yet been introduced to Italy, so the original recipe wouldn't have included tomatoes.

FOR YOUR INFORMATION

If you don't have stale bread, take a fresh loaf of hearty bread, cut it into large cubes, spread them on a baking sheet, and bake in a 300°F-degree oven for about 10 to 15 minutes. You don't want to completely toast the bread; you just want to dry it out. It's essential that you dry out the bread first before soaking it in the oil and vinegar; otherwise, it will just become soggy.

FOR YOUR MODIFICATION

Add other ingredients that pair well with the traditional classic, such as olives, sundried tomatoes, capers, red wine, parsley, mint, roasted bell peppers.

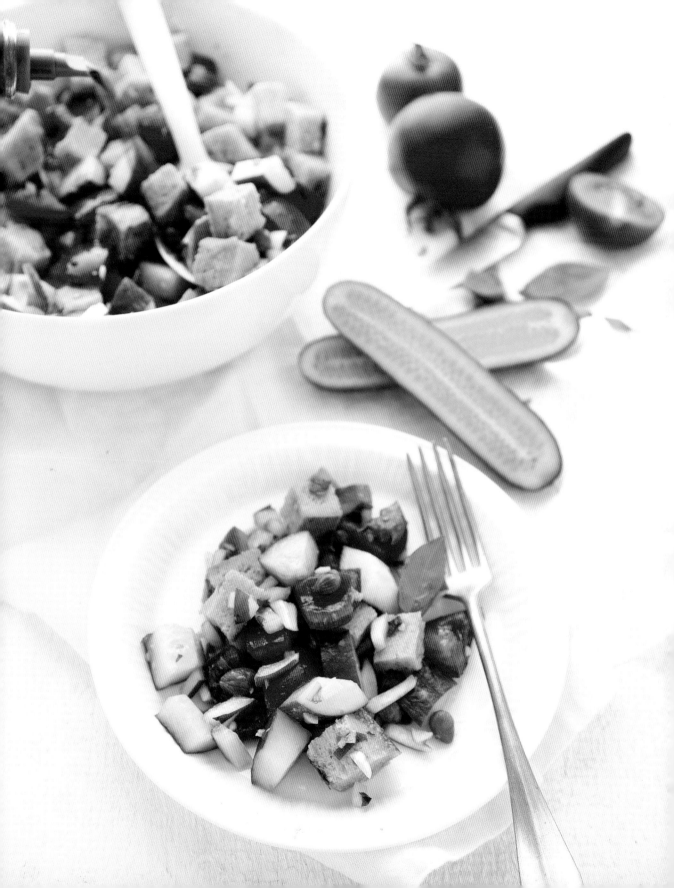

Southwestern Quinoa Pilaf

YIELD 6 to 8 servings as a side **ALLERGY** Gluten-free, wheat-free, oil-free (if you eliminate the oil), soy-free

INGREDIENTS

1 cup (170 g) uncooked quinoa

1 tablespoon extra-virgin olive oil

1 small red onion, finely chopped

1 jalapeno pepper, seeded or not
(depending on your heat
preference), minced

3 cloves garlic, peeled, and finely
chopped or sliced

1 teaspoon cumin

¼ teaspoon cayenne pepper

2 cups (480 ml) vegetable broth
or 1½ cups (360 ml) water
+ vegetable bouillon cube

½ teaspoon salt, or to taste
(depends on how salty
your broth is)

1 cup frozen (160 g) corn
kernels, thawed

1 15-ounce can black beans, rinsed
and drained

Enjoy this marriage of Mexican (corn, beans), Mediterranean (cumin), and Peruvian (quinoa) cultures.

DIRECTIONS

→ Rinse the quinoa using a fine colander, shake dry, and set aside.

→ Heat up the oil in a 3-quart saucepan over medium-high, and add the onion and pepper. Sauté for about 2 to 3 minutes until the onion begins to brown a bit. Next, add the quinoa, and cook for about 2 minutes, until the quinoa begins to toast. You will smell a delightful nutty aroma.

→ Add the garlic, and stir into the quinoa mixture, cooking for about 1 minute before adding the cumin, cayenne pepper, and vegetable broth or water/bouillon cube.

→ Cover, reduce heat to medium, and cook for about 12 to 15 minutes, until the broth is absorbed into the quinoa, causing it to expand and become translucent.

→ Test, and add salt, as needed. Stir in the corn and beans, and season with additional salt, if necessary. Remove from heat, but keep covered for about 5 more minutes before serving. It is also delicious at room temperature or right out of the fridge!

Suggestion for Serving

↳ Use as a filling for burritos or tacos. Add guacamole, chopped lettuce, and tomatoes.

PER SERVING:
Calories: 192, **Protein:** 7.5 g, **Fat:** 4 g,
Carbohydrates: 33 g, **Fiber:** 6 g,
Cholesterol: 0 mg

FOR YOUR INFORMATION

Quinoa, an ancient grain from the mountains of Peru, contains all the amino acids, making it a complete protein. 1 cup of cooked quinoa yields 8 to 9 grams of protein. The reason some people like rinsing it is because it tends to be coated with a phytochemical called saponin, which can taste bitter.

FOR YOUR MODIFICATION

Roasted corn adds additional flavor to this dish. Either roast the corn yourself, or look to Trader Joe's (and probably other brands) for their roasted corn kernels in the freezer section.

Chipotle Roasted Chickpeas

YIELD 6 servings **ALLERGY** Soy-free, gluten-free, wheat-free

INGREDIENTS

Two 15-ounce cans (about 3 cups (850 g) cooked) chickpeas, rinsed and drained

2 tablespoons olive oil

1 teaspoon cumin

1 teaspoon dried thyme or oregano

1½ teaspoons chipotle powder

1½ teaspoons smoked paprika

½ teaspoon salt

Zest and juice of half a lemon

PER SERVING (½ CUP):
Calories: 163, **Protein:** 6.2 g, **Fat:** 6.9 g, **Carbohydrates:** 21 g, **Fiber:** 5.9 g, **Cholesterol:** 0 mg

These smoky little gems make the perfect snack—healthful and delicious—and they're also great to use as "croutons" for a big green salad.

DIRECTIONS

- Preheat the oven to 425°F.
- Use a salad spinner or a dishtowel to make sure the chickpeas are as thoroughly dry as possible.
- Lay them flat on a nonstick baking sheet. Roast in the oven for 10 minutes, then shake to redistribute them, and roast for another 10 minutes.
- Meanwhile, combine the olive oil, cumin, thyme or oregano, chipotle powder, paprika, salt, lemon zest, and lemon juice in a large bowl, and stir to combine. Remove the chickpeas from the oven, and add them to the bowl, mixing until they are fully coated.
- Return the chickpeas to the baking sheet, and roast in the oven for 5 more minutes.
- Serve warm and crispy right away or at room temperature. Once you store them in Tupperware in the fridge, they will lose their crispiness but retain their flavor.

FOR YOUR
MODIFICATION

If these are too spicy for the little ones, just eliminate the chipotle and rename the recipe to Cumin Roasted Chickpeas!

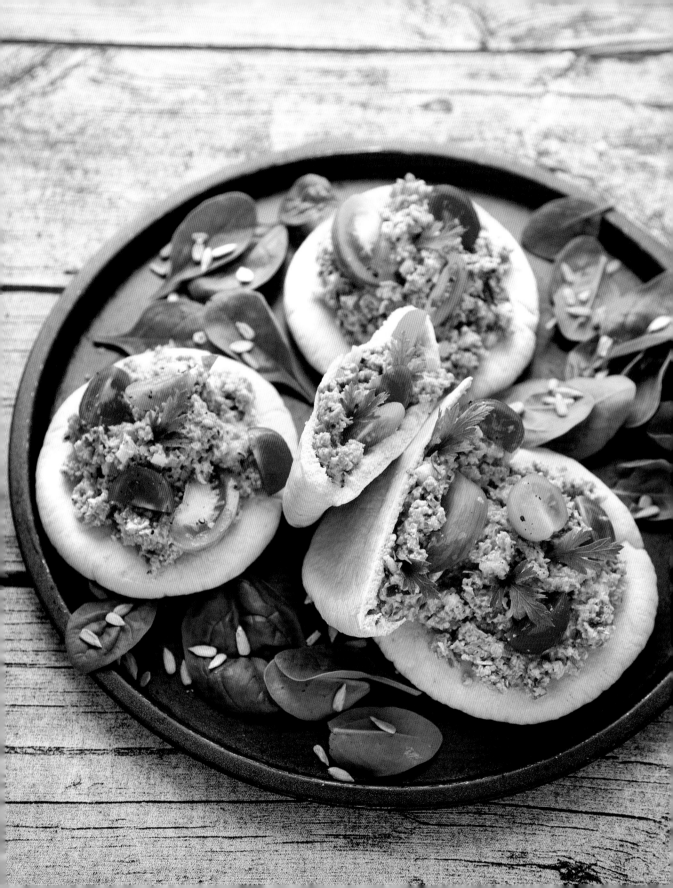

Fish-Friendly Tuna Salad

YIELD About 4½ cups **ALLERGY** Gluten-free, soy-free (depending on oils used in the mayo), wheat-free

2 cups (260 g) raw sunflower seeds (soaked for 2 hours to overnight)

2 cloves of garlic, peeled but left whole

¼ cup (25 g) chopped green onions (scallions)

½ red onion, finely chopped

2 stalks celery, finely chopped

2 carrots, finely chopped

2 kosher dill pickles, finely chopped

3 tablespoons finely chopped parsley

½ cup (60 g) roughly chopped walnuts

1 tablespoon Dijon mustard

¼ cup (50 g) eggless mayonnaise

½ to 1 teaspoon salt

Freshly ground pepper

PER SERVING (¾ CUP):
Calories: 392, Protein: 13 g, Fat: 33 g, Carbohydrates: 17 g, Fiber: 6.2 g, Cholesterol: 0 mg

Dedication

From: Dianne Waltner

To: My beloved feline companion, Mandi, who rescued me and has brought so much love, joy, and laughter into my life

I grew up on tuna salad sandwiches; from childhood through to young adulthood, they were one of my go-to lunches—until I stopped eating the critters of the sea. This version has a similar texture and the same satisfying fat content while leaving the animals alone.

Note: *Because the seeds need to soak for anywhere from 2 hours to 24, you'll want to factor that into your start-to-finish timing for this salad.*

DIRECTIONS

- After the sunflower seeds have soaked for at least 2 hours (up to 24), drain and rinse the seeds.
- Add the sunflower seeds and garlic to a food processor, and pulse until the seeds are a textured paste. Scrape the sides with spatula, as needed. Transfer to a large bowl, add the green onions (scallions), red onion, celery, carrots, pickles, parsley, walnuts, mustard, mayonnaise, salt, and pepper to the bowl, and stir to thoroughly combine. Taste, and add more salt, pepper, or mayonnaise, as needed.

Suggestions for Serving

- Serve on whole-wheat toast with lettuce, alfalfa spouts, sliced tomato, and/or avocado slices.
- Wrap in romaine lettuce leaves or large chard or collard leaves.
- Use as a dip for raw veggies such as carrots, bell peppers, cucumber, or celery.
- Spread on crackers and serve as an appetizer.
- Serve on a bed of mixed greens.

FOR YOUR EDIFICATION

As I discuss in the sidebar about supplements on page 250, you want to get your vitamin E from food—not pills—and sunflower seeds are an excellent source of this fat-soluble antioxidant.

FOR YOUR INFORMATION

Because sunflower seeds have a high fat content and are prone to rancidity, it's best to store them in an airtight container in the refrigerator.

Edamame Ginger Hummus

YIELD 2 cups **ALLERGY** Wheat-free, gluten-free, oil-free

INGREDIENTS

2 cups (310 g) cooked edamame
(shelled soybeans)

3 peeled garlic cloves

½-inch-piece of fresh ginger,
peeled and minced

1 tablespoon raw tahini (sesame
seed butter) or almond butter

3 tablespoons freshly squeezed
lime juice (the juice from
1 small lime)

1 teaspoon salt

½ teaspoon ground coriander

¼ teaspoon red pepper flakes

3 to 4 tablespoons water

Black sesame seeds, chopped
chives, or chopped scallions,
for garnish (optional)

PER SERVING (2 TABLESPOONS):
Calories: 53, **Protein:** 4.0 g, **Fat:** 2.6 g,
Carbohydrates: 4.4 g, **Fiber:** 1.5 g,
Cholesterol: 0 mg

Dedication

From: Sam Muñoz
To: My dog, Striker, who rescued me
as much I rescued him

The word hummus is an Arabic word for "chickpea," so technically, this isn't hummus in the literal sense of the word. However, this beautifully colored, incredibly fresh-tasting purée can be served and eaten just as you would the chickpea version.

DIRECTIONS

→ Place the edamame, garlic cloves, ginger, lime juice, tahini, lime juice, salt, coriander, red pepper flakes, and 3 tablespoons of the water in a food processor, and process or blend until smooth, stopping the machine and scraping down the sides with a rubber spatula, if necessary. If it's too thick, add one or two more tablespoons of water, and blend again until smooth.

→ Garnish with sesame seeds, chopped chives, or chopped scallions.

→ Serve with crackers or assorted raw vegetables, such as carrots, fennel, cucumbers, cherry tomatoes, broccoli, cauliflower, or snow peas. Or, use as the dip for pita bread or tortilla chips.

FOR YOUR INFORMATION

⚬ You can find shelled edamame in the frozen section of many grocery stores, including Trader Joe's. If you use frozen beans for this recipe, just remember to thaw them first.

⚬ I find that a food processor works better than a blender to get the perfect consistency; it also makes it easier to get all the hummus out of the bowl. With a blender, much of the hummus gets stuck under the blade.

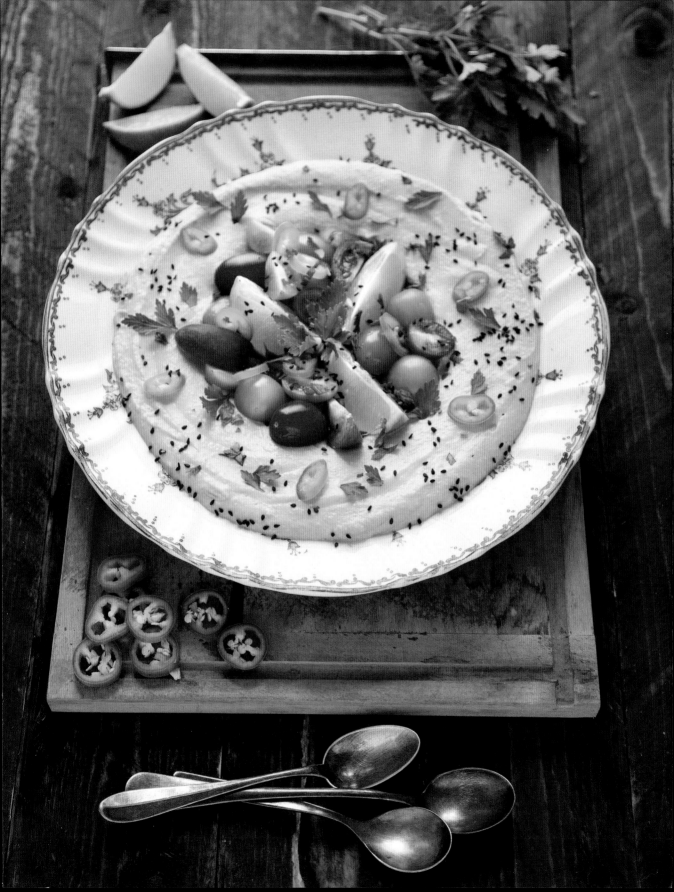

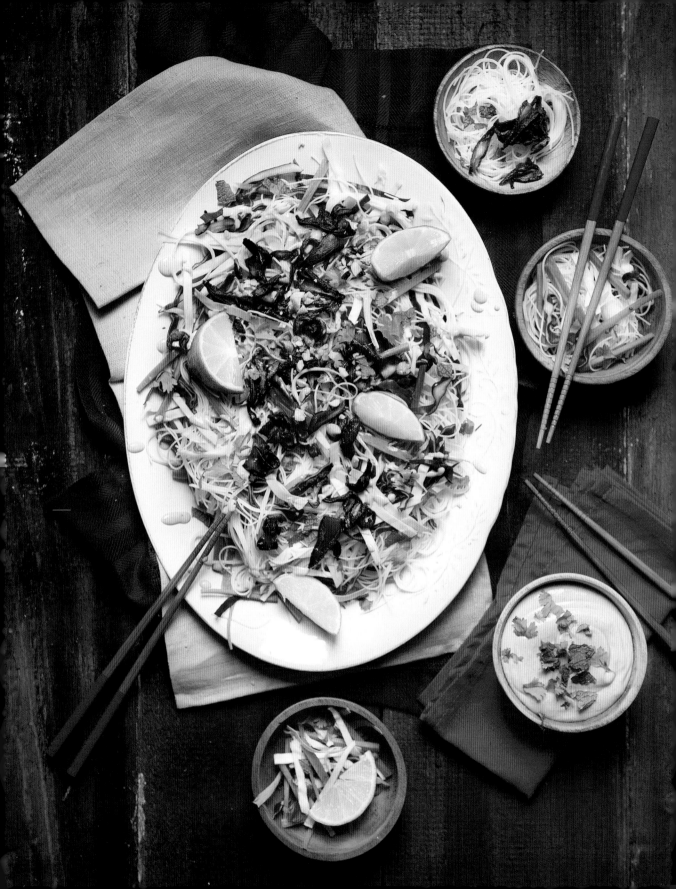

Spring Roll Salad

YIELD 8 servings

ALLERGY Wheat-free, gluten-free (depending on rice noodles), oil-free (if not using the mushrooms)

INGREDIENTS

4 ounces vermicelli rice noodles

Coconut Peanut Sauce (see
    page 146 for recipe)

1 pound fresh shitake mushrooms,
    thinly sliced

2 tablespoons tamari soy sauce

1 tablespoon toasted sesame oil

½ small head green cabbage,
    thinly sliced/shredded

¼ head red cabbage, thinly
    sliced/shredded

4 medium carrots, shredded

¼ small red onion, thinly sliced

¼ cup (10 g) minced fresh basil
    leaves (Italian or Thai)

¼ cup (5 g) minced fresh
    mint leaves

¼ cup (12 g) minced fresh
    cilantro leaves

1+ tablespoon rice vinegar

Salt

¼ cup (33 g) roasted peanuts,
    chopped

**PER SERVING
(WITHOUT PEANUT SAUCE):**
Calories: 155, **Protein:** 4.5 g, **Fat:** 4.3 g,
Carbohydrates: 26 g, **Fiber:** 4.2 g,
Cholesterol: 0 mg

All the freshness and flavor of spring rolls—deconstructed. This salad is even better after it sits for a few hours to marinate and tenderize the veggies.

DIRECTIONS

- Preheat the oven to 375°F. Cook the noodles according to package directions. Prepare the Coconut Peanut Sauce.

- Add the shitakes to a bowl, along with the tamari and sesame oil.

- Next, spread them out on a parchment-covered baking sheet, and transfer to the oven. Roast, stirring once or twice, until the mushrooms are shrunken, browned, and somewhat crisp, about 20 to 30 minutes, depending on your oven. Remove from the oven, and let cool.

- While the mushrooms are roasting, bring a medium-size pot of water to a boil. Add the noodles, cook for 5 minutes. Test for doneness, then drain and rinse the noodles for at least 30 seconds under cold water to prevent sticking. Set aside.

- Add the green cabbage, red cabbage, carrots, onion, basil, mint, and cilantro to a large bowl. Toss to combine. At this point, add the rice vinegar and a dash of salt. I like to use a pair of tongs at this point to toss the vegetables and coat them with the vinegar, but also to tenderize the cabbages a bit.

- Mound some of the noodles on a plate, then add the vegetables. Drizzle with the peanut sauce, and top with the mushrooms and peanuts.

FOR YOUR MODIFICATION

Add some sautéed or baked tofu cubes.

FOR YOUR EDIFICATION

Tamari is a Japanese soy sauce that tends to be wheat-free.

Dedication

From: Jenn Bridge
To: My wonderful parents,
Grant and Carol Bridge

Coconut Peanut Sauce

YIELD 2 cups **ALLERGY** Wheat-free, oil-free

INGREDIENTS

One 13.5-ounce (200 ml) can
    unsweetened coconut milk

½ cup (125 g) creamy natural
    peanut butter

2 tablespoons light brown sugar

½ to 1 teaspoon cayenne pepper
    (depends on how spicy
    you want it)

3 tablespoons tamari soy sauce

2 tablespoons fresh lime or
    lemon juice

1½ teaspoons red curry paste

PER SERVING (¼ CUP):
Calories: 209, **Protein:** 5.8 g, **Fat:** 18 g,
Carbohydrates: 8.8 g, **Fiber:** 1.1 g,
Cholesterol: 0 mg

Don't say I didn't warn you: this is a very addictive sauce! You're going to have to fight the temptation to eat it with a spoon!

DIRECTIONS

- Combine the coconut milk, peanut butter, brown sugar, cayenne pepper, tamari, lime/lemon juice, and red curry paste in a saucepan. Whisk ingredients to smooth them out, and cook over medium-low heat for 3 to 4 minutes, stirring occasionally.
- Let cool before storing in an airtight container.
- The sauce will keep in the refrigerator for up to a week. Before serving, I recommend you bring it to room temperature, or warm it up.

Suggestions for Serving

- Use for the Spring Roll Salad on page 145.
- Use as a pasta sauce, drizzled over steamed or roasted vegetables, or as the sauce for a veggie wrap.

Lentil Salad with Beets and Citrus Vinaigrette

YIELD Serves 4 as a main dish, 6 as a side **ALLERGY** Soy-free, wheat-free, gluten-free

INGREDIENTS *SALAD*

1 cup (200 g) French green (Puy) or brown lentils

4 cups (960 ml) water or vegetable broth

3 oranges, peeled and cut into sections (squeeze extra juice into a bowl and set aside)

2 large red beets, washed

1 fennel bulb, chopped

¼ cup (5 g) fresh dill, finely chopped

¼ cup (15 g) fresh parsley, finely chopped

4 leaves lacinato kale, finely chopped

½ cup (65 g) walnuts, toasted

Dressing (recipe follows)

INGREDIENTS *DRESSING*

1 clove garlic, minced

3 tablespoons extra-virgin olive oil

3 tablespoons champagne vinegar

2 tablespoons lemon juice

2 tablespoons reserved orange juice

2 teaspoons agave nectar

1 teaspoon salt

½ teaspoon black pepper

PER SERVING:
Calories: 338, **Protein:** 13 g, **Fat:** 14 g,
Carbohydrates: 43 g, **Fiber:** 12 g,
Cholesterol: 0 mg

If you can't find the French Puy (pronounced pwee*) lentils, the larger brown lentils work just as well, as long as you don't overcook them and make them mushy. Thanks to Chef Alicia Smiley for developing this recipe.*

Note: *Because the beets have to be roasted, you'll want to factor that into your total prep time for this recipe.*

DIRECTIONS

◉ Preheat the oven to 400°F.

◉ Roast the beets (see instructions below).

◉ While the beets are roasting, cook the lentils in the water or broth at a simmer, uncovered, until tender, approximately 20 to 30 minutes, until they are soft but not mushy.

◉ Meanwhile, add the dressing ingredients to a small bowl, and whisk to combine. You may also use a small food processor.

◉ Drain the lentils well, and place in a large bowl. Set aside to cool. When cool, add the orange sections, beets, fennel, dill, parsley, kale, and walnuts.

◉ When the beets are done roasting, peel and dice them. Add them to the bowl with the other salad ingredients. Pour on the dressing, and toss to combine.

FOR YOUR EDIFICATION

To roast beets: Pierce the unpeeled beets with a fork in several places to release steam while cooking. Place on the center oven rack at and cook for 1 hour at 400°F, until a fork can pierce through to the center. Let cool completely, cut the tops off, and peel off the skin.

FOR YOUR MODIFICATION

For a shortcut, use canned mandarin oranges stored in juice (not syrup). Roughly chop and use in place of the 3 oranges. If you go this route, you're going to need some orange juice for the dressing.

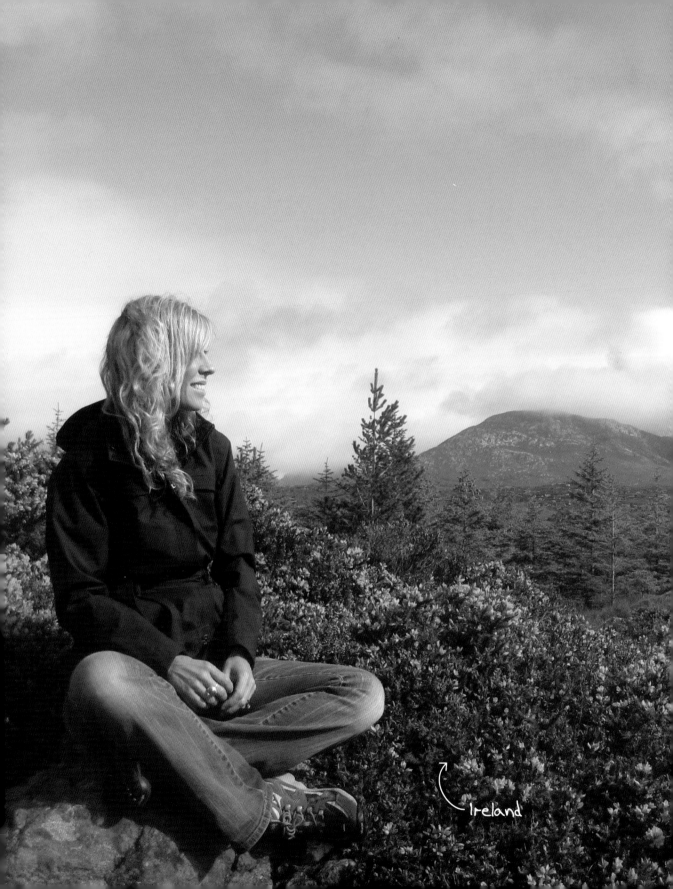
Ireland

Finding Abundant Food Options While Traveling

Whether you travel frequently for work or periodically for pleasure, you've no doubt observed how easy it is to find junk food everywhere you look; to find good *healthful* food on the road, however, requires a little more effort. Healthful options are available in more places than ever before, but I think it's important to understand that fast food joints, tourist destinations, airports, and even restaurants—by their very nature—cater to people who are either indulging themselves or are (for whatever reason) choosing convenience over health. In other words, it's not the fault of "being vegan" that makes it challenging to find nutrient-dense food on the road. The problem is that as individuals and as a society, we have not made eating well a priority—whether we're at home or traveling.

The truth is that eating vegan on the road is easy in most places and a little challenging in others. It's just a matter of knowing what to look for and taking the time to prepare.

We know how important food schedules are for infants and children, but at some point as adults, we stop making this a priority for ourselves. Parents never leave the house without having snacks for their kids, and we need to honor this need in ourselves, too. Instead, we create helter-skelter lives without routine or order, and this is exacerbated when we travel. Personally, I eat my meals at the same times every day, which means that I know exactly what's wrong with me if my mood or energy level drops. One

CHALLENGE YOUR THINKING: It's not the fault of being vegan that it's challenging to find nutrient-dense food on the road. The problem is that we have not made eating well a priority—whether we're at home or traveling.

CHANGE YOUR BEHAVIOR: Take some time to prepare for your trip by bringing food with you and knowing where to go once you arrive at your destination.

of the most stressful components of travel is straying from my eating schedule, so I make it a priority to maintain a regular routine when I'm on the road.

No matter how hard I try, when I travel, I accept that I'll be eating less optimally than when I'm home, but I do try to follow some guidelines to make traveling as pleasant as possible.

▶ I try to follow my normal eating schedule, while factoring in different time zones.

▶ I try to avoid getting hungry so my energy level stays consistent and high.

▶ I try to eat as healthfully as possible, but I accept I might have to choose calorie-density over nutrient-density. In other words, eating a meal of French fries, salted peanuts, an apple, and crackers at an airport restaurant is better than going hungry—if those are my only options. And, the truth is there never is a risk of going hungry. There's always *something* to eat *somewhere*.

These goals can be reached no matter where you're traveling to or what your mode of transportation is.

AIRPORTS

Depending on the time of my flight, I try to eat before I leave for the airport, even if I know it's a vegan-friendly airport. With food out of the way, I can focus on just getting through security and onto the plane.

However, the need will most likely arise when you need to eat at an airport. When it comes to vegan food, some airports are most definitely better than others are, but you'll always be able to find *something*. It might be a bean burrito at Taco Bell (their refried beans are made in vegetable oil—not animal lard; just ask for no cheese or sour cream) or a vegetable sandwich at Subway (pile on the veggies and ask for oil and vinegar and mustard instead of mayonnaise). Most airport restaurants have premade food, but there are often vegan options—some more healthful than others.

> **CHALLENGE YOUR THINKING:**
> We know how important food schedules are for infants and children, but at some point as adults, we stop making this a priority for ourselves. Parents never leave the house without having snacks for their kids, and we need to honor this need in ourselves, too.

Nicer sit-down restaurants may not say "vegan" on the menu, but apply the principles you're learning in this book to ask for what you want. If there's a salad on the menu, ask if they can prepare it with all vegetables and a simple oil and vinegar dressing. If there's pasta on the menu, ask if they can sauté vegetables in oil and combine them with the pasta and some oil, salt, and pepper. Or, perhaps they have a basic marinara sauce. The only way you'll know is if you ask.

Each year, the Physicians Committee for Responsible Medicine (pcrm.org) puts out a list of the airports with the best vegan options. They evaluated 15 of the busiest U.S. airports, and you might be surprised to know which airports ranked the highest in terms of offering the most healthful plant-based options. One year it was Orlando

International Airport; another year Detroit Metropolitan Wayne County Airport tied for second with San Francisco International Airport; and a consistent top ranker is Dallas/Fort Worth International Airport. Many vegan options can be found in Denver, Chicago, Newark, Los Angeles, Phoenix, Minneapolis/St. Paul international airports, among others.

Follow the same guidelines on Day 9: Eating Out and Speaking Up in terms of finding vegan food in various types of restaurants, but in addition:

▶ Many cafes sell bagels they will toast for you. Ask if they have peanut butter instead of dairy-based butter, and if not, just spread on some jelly.

▶ Many kiosks sell bagged nuts, seeds, energy bars, trail mix, fruit leather, baked chips, pretzels, bananas, and apples.

▶ Many airports have fruit smoothies or fresh fruit juice stands, such as Jamba Juice, whose default milk for most of their smoothies is soy. Just ask them to replace the frozen yogurt or sherbet with sorbet or—better yet—a banana.

AIRPLANES

Free meals are virtually obsolete on most airlines, unless you're traveling first-class or on an international flight. If you are, be sure to contact the airline at least 24 hours in advance to confirm that your "special meal" request is in the system. The airlines vary in terms of offerings and quality, but I've had the pleasure of enjoying Amy's Organics burritos and fajitas, decent green salads, and vegan cookies. I've also enjoyed some really good Indian meals, which are often called "nondairy strict vegetarian" or even "Hindu nondairy," depending on the airline.

In the coach/economy cabin, sandwiches and snack boxes are often available for purchase, though the former tend to be animal based. As for the snack boxes, check the contents of your various options in the airline's magazine in the seat pocket in front of you. I've often had snack boxes with hummus, crackers, nuts, and olives.

Instead of relying on the airline to be satisfied, however, I plan ahead and bring food on the plane with me, much to the envy of my row-mates. I've learned the hard way that some things travel better than others. In my travel bag, there are always variations of:

🍃 Peanut butter and jam sandwiches

🍃 Hummus and roasted red pepper wrap

🍃 Baggies of cut-up carrots, celery, cauliflower, or snow peas

🍃 A bag of nuts, particularly walnuts, almonds, and pistachio nuts

- A small container of chickpeas. Before you leave for the airport, open a can of chickpeas, drain and rinse, and add to a transportable container sprinkled with a little salt. Or, make the Chipotle Roasted Chickpeas on page 139.

- A bag of trail mix or granola

- Dates, apples, and bananas

- Energy bars

Other convenient travel foods include fruit leather, whole grain crackers, homemade popped popcorn, and vegan beef jerky. It's easy to stock up on these things before leaving home to go somewhere else; the key is making sure to have enough when flying back home.

The other two things you will never find me without are my stainless steel water bottle for cold water and my tea thermos for hot water. Although you can't bring filled water bottles through the security gate, you can bring empty ones, so I just fill them up with water from fountains once I'm at my gate. As for tea, I always travel with my favorite white, green, and oolong teas. My tea thermos has a built-in strainer, enabling me to just add the tea leaves to the thermos and then fill it with hot water, which the flight attendants are happy to do for me. The other option is to use a spoon strainer that you can get at kitchen supply stores. Fill the strainer with loose tea leaves and steep it in a cup of hot water.

For the coffee drinkers out there, I suppose you can do the same thing, but I'm not an authority on the matter. I've never had a cup of coffee in my life!

CAR TRAVEL

Day 10 provides a bevy of options for packed lunches and snacks, which can easily be implemented if you're taking a road trip or camping and bringing along a cooler. To have even more options (and if you're not one to build a campfire), consider buying a portable burner that's fueled by butane cartridges. I've used them in my cooking classes for years, and they're incredibly convenient for car trips, camping, picnicking, and tailgating.

ACCOMMODATIONS

Most chain hotels have something to eat at their buffet, such as bagels and toast with peanut butter and jam, fresh fruit, and cereal. Unless noted, the pastries, pancakes, and waffles all tend to contain animal products. Some large hotel chains also carry soy milk (just ask), which can be used for the cereals they offer. If the hotel doesn't have nondairy milk for the cereal, order fruit salad with cereal, and stir it all together. Or, use orange juice in place of milk for your cereal. Try it.

Bed and breakfasts are a different story. Proprietors of bed and breakfasts often love to show off their creativity by making delicious vegan breakfasts upon request. Some of the most memorable breakfasts

I've ever had were at nonvegan bed and breakfasts. Contact them first before booking, and ask if they can accommodate you. Whenever I contact B&Bs, I always get overwhelmingly positive responses. My favorite experience was when I called a B&B in West Hollywood to ask if they accommodate vegans. The response on the other end of the line was, "Oh sweetheart—oh my goodness—of course we accommodate you being vegan. So no problem, we accommodate vegans. No problem. Now tell me, sweetheart, what is vegan?" How could I not fall in love immediately with someone who says, "Yes" first then asks, "What vegan means" second? Now *that's* customer service!

Never underestimate how joyfully people will rise to accommodate you, but to experience this, you have to ask for what you want.

Whether you're staying in a chain hotel or a bed and breakfast, you always have access to hot water. Packaged oatmeal, dry soups, packaged dry noodle dishes, quick-cooking oats, or premade Indian foods are great to have on hand. Just add hot water and you have a hot, filling meal for the airport or hotel room.

Accommodations don't have to be limited to hotels and B&Bs. Renting an apartment or house in the city you're visiting is a wonderful and often more economical way to travel. One of the many advantages is that you have a kitchen in which to cook and store your own food, so you don't have to eat at a restaurant every single meal. You can simply find a local grocery store and stock up. Websites such as airbnb.com make it easy for you to find and book the perfect accommodation anywhere in the world.

> **CHALLENGE YOUR THINKING:** Never underestimate how positively people will rise to accommodate you, but first you have to ask for what you want— joyfully and with respect.

INTERNATIONAL TRAVEL

All of these principles apply whether you're traveling domestically or internationally. It's true that some cultures/countries are more vegan-friendly than others, but you may be surprised by the number of options you will find. Cities have more vegan and vegan-friendly restaurants than rural areas, but even in the countryside, there are always things to eat. I've never been on the verge of starvation while on vacation.

I think we forget that plant-based foods were once the staples in the diets of people all around the world, so choosing the simple indigenous foods of the countries we're visiting means increasing the chances that they're vegan.

- Tomatoes, corn, and beans are abundant in Mexican and Latin American cuisine.
- Lentils, root vegetables, and grains are staples in African cuisine.
- Tofu, vegetables, and grains are staples in Asian cuisine.
- Legumes and rice are central to Indian and Pakistani cuisine.
- Regional vegetables and breads are staples in European cuisine.

In the United States, we've come to rely on processed foods—even as vegans—but when you travel abroad, you realize that what would be called "peasant food" (versus the "luxury" animal products) is not only the healthiest, it also tends to be vegan. Natively grown fruits and vegetables abound, depending on where you are, and instead of the fancy, expensive bottled salad dressings we've become accustomed to, we can appreciate lime or lemon juice with a little salt or simply oil and vinegar on salads brimming with vegetables.

In terms of communicating your needs in non-English-speaking countries, I've learned that it's much more helpful to know how to say, "without meat, cheese, and eggs" rather than "I'm vegan." Most languages do *not* have a word for "vegan" and some people think vegans eat chicken and fish. It's much more effective to order what looks like a vegan-friendly dish on the menu and then in the language of the country you're visiting, confirm that it has "no butter," "no milk," and "no animal fat." So, in addition to learning the words for *fruit, vegetables, beans,* as well as specific types within these categories, I highly recommend learning the words for *meat, fish, cheese, butter, eggs, and milk.*

One of the most wonderful things about traveling in Italy, for instance, is that—because they value every ingredient that goes into making their dishes—restaurant menus often provide a description of exactly what the dish comprises. For example, if the title of the dish is "White Beans in Tomato Sauce," underneath it, it says, "Beans, olive oil, tomatoes, garlic, and basil." If it is Bruschetta, underneath it says, "Tomatoes, olive oil, garlic, and salt." And amazingly, what you order is exactly what you get. That is very different from my experience in the United States, where cheese is automatically added to everything you order, even if it doesn't say so on the menu. In Italy, when I order something like the "White Beans and Tomato Sauce" and say, "No formaggio, vero?" ("No cheese, right?"), the waiter looks at me like I have three heads, as if to say, "Does it say "formaggio" on the menu? Then, why would you think it would be there?" (Yes, living in Italy is on my bucket list.)

Once you get to know the foods native to the region you're in, it's a lot easier. For instance, Rome, Florence, and other Italian cities have produce stands as well as street vendors that sell *macedonia di frutta,* which is just fruit salad. In Mexico, street vendors sell corn on the cob with lime juice, or baked plantains. In Spain, *horchata* (nut milk made with water and sugar) is easy to find all over the place.

In whatever towns I travel to, one of the first things I do is scope out a health food store, which many large and small cities have. If our hotel doesn't already have nondairy milk, I buy some at the store and ask the hotel to keep it in the fridge. At the health food store, I also stock up on nuts, granola, and other healthful snacks. Many towns—large and small—also have farmer's markets and farm stands, from which I've crafted the most delicious meals based on local produce and fresh breads.

Perhaps the only time you would need to work a little harder to make sure you're accommodated is if you're part of some kind of tour package, going on a cruise, or staying at some kind of resort. I do think things are improving all the time, and if you talk to the kitchen/chef/organizers beforehand, you may be pleasantly surprised.

I've had some of the most memorable meals while traveling, and I've had some that fulfilled only one essential need: filling my belly. Sometimes that's just good enough.

The Power of "Cravings": Fat and Salt Taste Good

I've heard countless well-meaning people say things like "I tried eating vegetarian, but I just craved meat" or "Humans were meant to eat meat—just look at my teeth." Then they point to those dull little eyeteeth that would make any member of the cat family laugh. Have you ever seen the teeth of a true carnivore? They don't resemble human teeth at all. The fangs of obligate carnivores are designed for piercing and seizing flesh and tearing apart their prey; their incisors efficiently strip flesh from bones.

Beyond teeth, when we compare the anatomy of humans with that of herbivorous animals and of carnivorous animals, physiologically, we resemble the herbivores substantially more than we do the carnivores. Not only could we not capture and kill another animal with our jaws and claws and strength (or lack thereof), we don't want to. Blood, guts, carcasses, and corpses disgust most of us, and I think it's fair to say that no one sees "road kill" and starts planning lunch. When we see an animal who has been hit by a car, we tend to feel compassion rather than hunger. Many of us even turn away from the screen when watching a nature show where a predator overpowers his prey.

Humans don't crave the flesh, sinews, tendons, muscles, and blood of animals. Obligate carnivore, such as lions and other members of the cat family, *do*; indeed, they would die without animal flesh. Moreover, they don't grapple with a moral dilemma or find themselves in an ethical quandary when they contemplate their meals. *We do.*

Humans don't see birds, squirrels, or cows and start salivating, but if you've ever watched a domestic cat react when a prey animal is in view, you'd know what it means to "crave" animal flesh. The cat lies down

> **CHALLENGE YOUR THINKING:**
> We do not crave the flesh of another animal, but what we do crave is flavor, texture, salt, fat, and familiarity, and all of these are found in plant foods.

low and flits her tail; her teeth begin chattering and she makes a funny little chirping sound. Her eyes dilate, and she remains completely still and focused on her potential prey. Is that how you react when you see deer grazing on the side of the road or birds flying overhead? My guess is that you don't.

So, I repeat: we *do not* crave the flesh of other animals, but what we do "crave" is fat, salt, flavor, texture, and familiarity, and all of these are found in plant foods.

Unfortunately, we've all been conditioned to think of the *form* of our craving (meat, dairy, and eggs) rather than the *source* of it (fat, salt, flavor, texture, and familiarity), so when we think we're "craving meat," we're most likely craving one or all of these elements. If you identify the actual craving rather than jumping right to the familiar *form* of that craving, you can better fulfill that need. Here are some foods that satisfy the typical "cravings." Some may be new to you; some may be familiar.

FAT

Let's face it: fat tastes good. By now, everyone knows that the fat in plant foods is healthful, whereas the fat in animal products is not. So often, when people think they're "craving meat," they're really just craving something with *fat*. The remedy? Eat fat—*whole plant-based fat* that comes in the form of nuts, seeds, avocados, and other nutrient-rich foods.

- ▶ Toast pine nuts or walnuts with some salt, and pulse in the food processor along with a little nutritional yeast, and sprinkle over your pasta. You get the texture, fat, and salt of "Parmesan cheese," but nobody is harmed in the making or eating of it!

- ▶ Add nuts to your oatmeal.

- ▶ Add your favorite nuts and/or seeds to your salad.

- ▶ Blend peanut or almond butter into your fruit smoothie.

- ▶ Top bean chili with nondairy sour cream, avocado, or guacamole.

- ▶ Cook with a little coconut oil, coconut butter, or coconut milk. Though it's true that the fat in coconuts is saturated, it's molecularly different from that of animal-based saturated fat and does not have the same negative effects on our body.

- ▶ Add guacamole to your burrito or fajita.

- ▶ Add eggless mayonnaise or avocado to your favorite sandwich.

- ▶ Lightly brush your favorite veggies with oil, then grill or roast them.

- ▶ Snack on some olives, or add them to a green salad.

- ▶ Heck, make a peanut butter and jelly sandwich!

SALT

Most of the sodium in people's diets comes from meat, dairy, and eggs, so you're doing yourself a huge favor in terms of reducing sodium and thus blood pressure by getting these things as far away from your mouth as possible. There is naturally occurring sodium (which we need) in many plant foods, but one thing I promise is that you start to crave added salt less and less after you remove the bulk of it from your palate. It's okay to use table salt (preferably iodized sea salt) to bring out the flavor of some foods or tamari soy sauce as a condiment, but I think you'll find your desire for it diminish as your palate becomes less coated with salt from animal-based products (meat, dairy, and eggs).

> *CULINARY NOTE: I have a variety of flavored salts in my cupboard, my favorite of which is truffle salt, which you can find in many gourmet grocers and online. My husband's favorite salts are the Maldon salt flakes, and I admit, he's converted me. Again, you can find them online or in specialty stores.*

FLAVOR

We are the only animals who have to cook other animals before eating them. (We're not equipped to handle the pathogens in raw meat.) We are also the only animals who have to flavor other animals before making them palatable. Think of all the things you've used to flavor meat: ketchup, mustard, barbecue sauce, Worcestershire sauce, steak sauce, relish, vinegars, oils, horseradish, hot sauces, chutneys, jellies, jams, salsa, soy sauce, wasabi, curries, tahini, pickles, garlic, ginger, onions, lemons, limes, and an endless array of spices and herbs. *The flavor is in the plant foods,* as evidenced by all the condiments in your kitchen.

If flavor is what you're "craving," seek out plant-based foods and condiments. It's what you did anyway when you ate meat. You flavored it with plants!

TEXTURE

I've heard naysayers of veganism scoff that because (some) vegans eat what is often called "fake meat," it belies a latent desire to eat animal-based meat. "After all," they argue, "if you don't want to eat animal meat, why try to mimic it with the fake stuff?" I respectfully but completely disagree. People don't necessarily stop eating animal meat because they stopped liking the taste or texture; they stop eating animal flesh because they don't want to contribute to violence against animals or because they want to be healthy.

Indeed, just because we stop eating animal flesh doesn't mean we don't still desire a hearty, chewy texture. The pleasure of food involves mouthfeel as much as flavor. Even the word *meat* doesn't refer only to the flesh of animals. As I discussed on Day 2: Trying New Foods, the Old English word *mete* referred to something that was eaten to distinguish it from something that was drunk. In other words, it simply referred to solid food rather than beverages. There are plenty of options for enjoying a satisfying chewy or creamy texture without eating anything that comes off or out of an animal.

Mushrooms

Ironically, the very thing that draws some people to mushrooms—their meaty, chewy texture—is what repels others. There are many mushrooms to choose from, and each provides a satisfying mouthfeel, though the ones often compared to animal-based meat are portobello mushrooms. Whole, marinated, and properly cooked (grilling is my favorite method), they are fantastic placed on a bun with all the fixin's. Day 2: Trying New Foods provides some suggestions for incorporating them into your repertoire.

CHALLENGE YOUR THINKING: People don't necessarily stop eating animal flesh because they stopped liking the taste; they stop eating animal flesh because they don't want to contribute to violence or because they want be healthy. That doesn't mean they stop wanting a satisfying mouthfeel.

CHANGE YOUR BEHAVIOR: Eat foods, with a hearty, chewy texture, such as thawed tofu, tempeh, seitan, and mushrooms.

Seitan

Seitan is made from gluten, the protein in wheat, and is most commonly used to create the textures we associate with cooked animals. Probably invented by vegetarian monks in China,[42] you'll often see it on Chinese and other Asian restaurant menus as "mock duck" or "mock chicken," etc. Some vegans don't *like* that the texture is so similar to the animal-based meat they once ate. Some vegans *love* that they can have their [vegan] meat and eat it, too! See more about seitan in Day 2: Trying New Foods, and check out the recipe for Homemade Seitan on page 50.

Tofu

As I outline on Day 17: Demystifying Tofu: It's Just a Bean!, the best way to create a satisfying mouthfeel with this versatile food is to *freeze* it. It will be wonderfully chewy, as a result, and have more heartiness than if you didn't freeze and thaw it.

Tempeh

Not as chewy as seitan and tofu, tempeh has a wonderful texture nonetheless. I love it sliced and baked with BBQ sauce or steamed, cooled, crumbled, and mixed with eggless mayonnaise, raw veggies, and herbs to make a tempeh salad or pate.

FAMILIARITY

Some of our attachment to food stems simply from the way it looks. We want to recognize the food that's in front of us. We want to meet it like an old friend. Playing on our desire for the familiar, this is exactly why companies create vegan versions of animal-based foods, but you don't have to be a food scientist to accomplish this goal. It might be as simple as making a sandwich or putting a veggie burger on a bun—with lettuce, tomato, pickles, and other familiar fare. It might mean serving veggie dogs to your kids as you transition them from the animal-based versions or adding tofu crumbles instead of ground beef to the chili you're serving for dinner. The point is, if it's familiar (and delicious), it doesn't even matter what it's made from.

MOUTHFEEL

Mouthfeel, like texture, is another element underneath our "cravings," and I talk about it more in the following chapter: Day 13: Discovering That There is Life After (Dairy-Based) Cheese.

So, just to recap: identify the desire, the "craving," and fulfill it with plant foods.

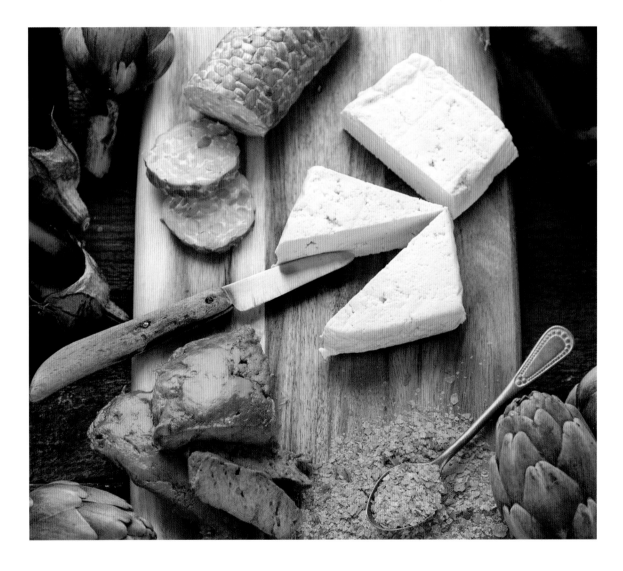

Aren't Humans Designed to Eat Meat?

Whether you're vegan for 30 days or beyond, eventually every vegan runs across the argument that humans are *designed* to eat animal-based meat. I would never claim that humans are *unable* to eat meat; of course, we're *capable* of it, though we're not doing a very good job. (Lions don't get heart disease; we do.) But, it is a mistake to conclude that humans are "carnivores" and "supposed to eat meat," simply because we have what we call "canine" teeth. Let's examine this by comparing the physiology of the herbivorous and carnivorous animals of the world and see where humans fit in.

Since the best place to start is the means by which animals come by their food, let's look at the teeth and nails.

> Herbivores have much shorter and softer fingernails than flesh-eating animals and pathetically small and dull "canine" teeth. In contrast, carnivores have incredibly sharp claws and large incisors called "carnassial teeth," capable of tearing and slicing flesh. In fact, the word *carnassial* is derived from the Latin word *carnis*, which means "meat." Herbivores (and humans) have flat molars that enable them to grind fibrous plants; carnivores lack these.

How about the jaw structure?

> The jaws of carnivores move only up and down, enabling them to slice and tear chunks of flesh; the jaws of herbivores (and humans) move from side to side, enabling them to push food back and forth into the grinding teeth with the tongue and cheek muscles.

What about saliva?

> Because carnivores do not chew their food, they don't need to mix it with saliva to help the digestion process. Thus, unlike that of herbivorous animals, the saliva of carnivorous animals does not contain digestive enzymes. The saliva of herbivores—and humans—contains carbohydrate-digesting enzymes.

The intestines?

> In carnivores, the small intestine is only 3 to 6 times the body length, and the large intestine or colon is very short and doesn't have pouches. The small intestine of plant-eating animals—and humans—tends to be very long (greater than 10 to 12 times body length) to allow adequate time and space for absorption of the nutrients.
>
> In all ways (including even our facial muscles, jaw muscles, mouth size, stomach acidity, and stomach volume), humans resemble herbivores rather than carnivores.

Even if I were not able to illustrate this through our physiological traits, humans have the ability to contemplate our actions and choose what to eat; obligate carnivores do not. So why would we use them as models for our own behavior? The truth is there are more herbivores than carnivores in the world, and yet the herbivorous animals are never used as the example of what is "natural." We never point to our molars and say, "Look at that—just like the herbivores!" Instead, we align ourselves with the carnivorous lion rather than the vegetarian elephant.

And why wouldn't we? When we want to continue doing something that is ethically problematic, it's imperative that we seek a way to justify behavior that stems from habit, tradition, convenience, or pleasure—but certainly not required by nature.

Personally, I believe the real reason we eat animals is simply that we can—certainly not because we have to, but just because we're *capable* of doing something doesn't mean it's the right thing to do. Just because we've done something for a long time doesn't mean we have to keep doing it.

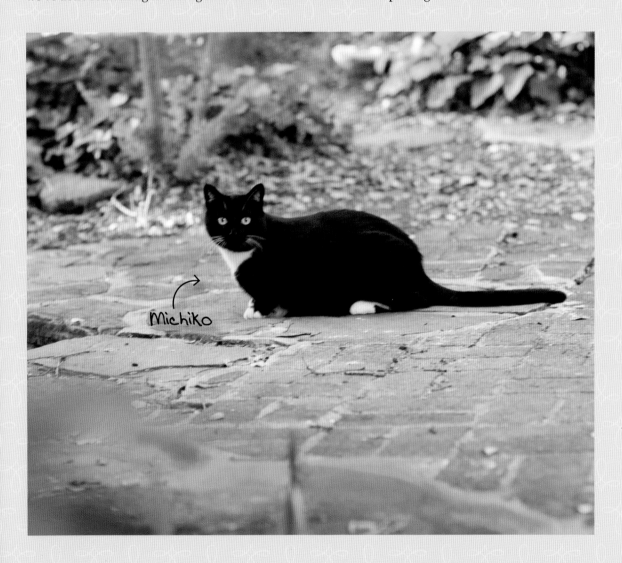

Michiko

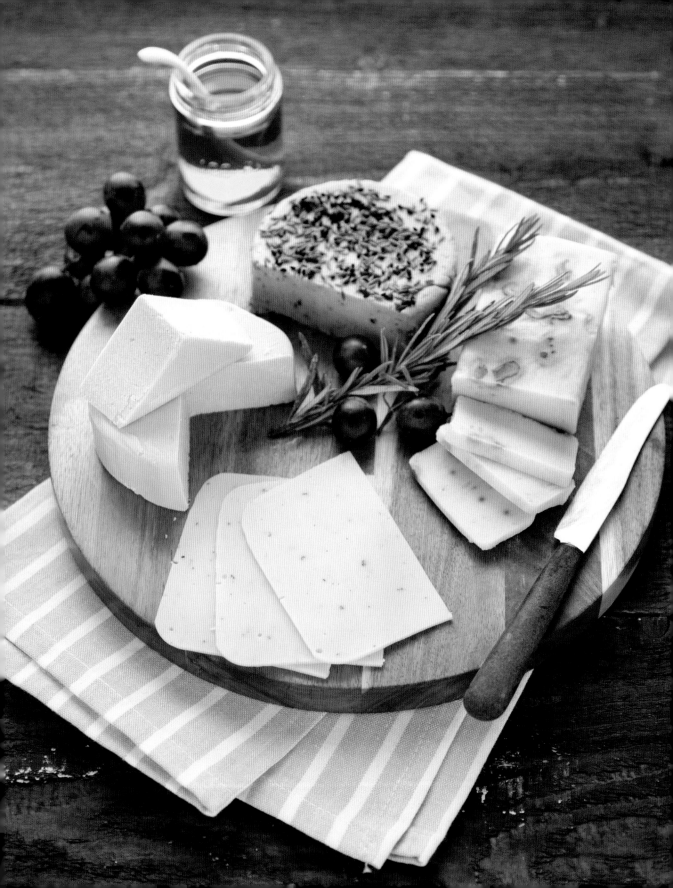

Discovering That There is Life After (Dairy-Based) Cheese

I've guided thousands of people through the process of becoming vegan and if you're like the vast majority of them, you've probably thought that dairy—and specifically cheese—would be the thing you'd miss most. Given the tenacious hold cheese has on people, I'm certain that everyone has muttered a variation of, "I could never live without cheese," at some point in their lives. I'm sure *I* did before I went vegan. My short response is *of course you can live without cheese*—and a healthier, more satisfying life it will be.

But, I think my longer response gets to the heart of why we give so much power to this thing called cheese and provides the key to finally letting go of it.

No doubt, you'll agree that food triggers high emotions in people, and many of us have some serious attachments to certain products that—quite literally—act as a security blanket. With that in mind, it's no wonder that people react so strongly at the thought that these things will be taken away. What I suggest is that it's the *feeling* we get when we eat something like cheese—and not the cheese itself— that keeps us going back for more. Because it triggers an emotional reaction or a pleasant memory, it's that *emotion* we crave—not the cheese itself. Let me explain.

CHALLENGE YOUR THINKING: It's the *feeling* we get when we eat cheese—and not the cheese itself—that keeps us going back for more. Because it triggers an emotional reaction, a pleasant memory, it's that *emotion* we crave—not the cheese itself.

CHALLENGE YOUR THINKING: Comfort is the desire; cheese is just the form that desire takes.

CHANGE YOUR BEHAVIOR: Identify the desire (comfort, nourishment, nostalgia), and meet that desire with a new food for new version of an old favorite.

We tend to be attached to the *form* of something and forget that the form is often just a conduit for the thing we're really seeking. The risk we take in becoming attached to the *form* is that we overlook what we *really* want. We may be seeking comfort—and we happen to find it in cheese. Some may find this comfort in chocolate, some in coffee, and some in a good book. There's nothing wrong with seeking comfort; it doesn't always have to belie some deep, hidden pathology. But, with this perspective, we can see that it's the *comfort* we're seeking—not the *form* of that comfort. Not the *cheese*. The comfort can be found in so many ways that don't involve cheese. So, let's stop giving cheese so much credit. It's just one form of comfort. Comfort is the desire; cheese is the form that desire takes.

Let's illustrate this even further. Maybe eating cheese triggers a nostalgic event for you. Maybe it reminds you of a trip you took or of your grandmother who served you her "famous mac and cheese" when you were young or of your family's cheese-centered dinners when you were growing up.

I would argue that it is the *events*, the *experiences*, the *people*, and the *emotions* that are meaningful for you—not the ingredient called cheese. It's just acting as a trigger. And, because cheese plays such a significant role in our culture, it's no surprise that it plays a significant role in many of our memories. If you grew up in a culture without dairy-based cheese or if you grew up vegan, entirely different foods would be your triggers. So, while it's wonderful to embrace the memories, it's helpful to remember that the food is often just the memory trigger.

> **CHALLENGE YOUR THINKING:**
> If you grew up in a culture without cheese or if you grew up vegan, entirely different foods would be emotional triggers for you.
>
> **CHANGE YOUR BEHAVIOR:**
> Embrace the memories—not the cheese.

> **CHALLENGE YOUR THINKING:**
> When our habits or rituals become devoid of meaning or harm ourselves or someone else, perhaps they need to be reexamined.

FAMILIARITY

As I discussed in the previous chapter, another thing many of us seek out is the feeling of familiarity. We're fierce creatures of habit, and we crave that feeling of the familiar. Let's face it—not many of us openly embrace change very easily. How many of us go to the same restaurants over and over and order the same dish off the menu? How many of us have rituals when we return home, before we eat dinner, or even before we go to bed? When I say rituals—I mean those patterns of behavior regularly performed in a set manner, like the order in which we get ready for bed: wash our face, brush our teeth, and brush our hair—whatever. We love that feeling of familiarity; it grounds us. It makes us feel like we belong to something. It gives significance to or increases our anticipation of whatever it is we're about to engage in.

It also adds order to our lives. Have you ever walked out of the house without your keys because on that morning, a wrench was thrown into your regular routine? You walked out a different door. Or, you got a phone call on the way out. Something threw you off that upset the order of your normal routine.

The need for order and familiarity is very real, but when our habits or rituals become devoid of meaning—or worse yet—when they contribute harm to ourselves or others, it's then I would suggest we need to reexamine these habits.

Food and eating are two components of our lives where we experience ritual and familiarity on a daily basis. We're used to sitting in the same chair at the dinner table. We have a certain glass we like to use. Some of us like our sandwiches cut a certain way. Some of us get used to having a certain meal on Friday nights. Some of us pray before we eat. Some eat food from our plates in a certain order. At the risk of implying that we all have elements of what is now termed "Obsessive Compulsive Disorder," we can't deny that eating is not just a mere act of taking in nourishment for survival. If only it were that simple!

"But wait," you say, "That all sounds really nice, but *cheese tastes good!* It's not just a matter of seeking comfort or creating rituals or finding the familiar." Okay, so you think it tastes good and from *that* standpoint, you think you could never give it up. To that, I would say the following.

I, like many people, stopped eating the flesh and fluids of animals not because I stopped liking the taste but because I didn't want to participate in violence against animals. Once I learned the truth about dairy cows (and goats and sheep), there was no way I could continue eating any product that was made from the milk of those animals. It was that simple for me. Their suffering took precedence over any desire I may have had for the stuff—even my childhood English muffin pizzas, the ice cream I had on a regular basis, or the croissants I loved with my tea. None of it mattered in the face of suffering. Of course, for others, experiencing the health benefits of cutting out dairy is the motivating factor—and a powerful one at that.

So, if you're attached to cheese but are willing to become *unattached*, it may be that simple for you, too. Read, learn, and watch videos about what the cows endure. Educate yourself about the artery-clogging, diabetes-provoking, and cancer-causing properties of cheese. The very least we can do is learn the truth.

The bottom line is if we think we "can't give up cheese," it may be because we're unwilling to. I promise there will come a time when you will not obsess over dairy-based cheese, but first you have to give your body and your palate time to adjust without it. You have to give yourself a chance *not* to eat it.

FINDING SATISFACTION WITHOUT DAIRY CHEESE

In terms of the gustatory pleasure we derive from this substance, when we deconstruct it, it comes down to fat, salt, flavor, texture, familiarity, and mouthfeel, just as with animal-based meat. Think about it:

► Consider the common custom of sprinkling Parmesan cheese onto pasta. What we really get out of that is the satisfaction of salt and fat. With that in mind, try toasting some pine nuts or walnuts along with some salt, pulse them in a food processor, and sprinkle them on your pasta instead.

► Think about the habit of adding sour cream to our favorite Mexican dishes and the role it plays: it has a satisfying creamy texture, it provides some fat, but mostly it's used to cool down a spicy dish. With that understanding, we can accomplish the same things with guacamole, mashed avocado, nondairy sour cream, fresh tomatoes, or shredded lettuce. (A quick sour cream can be made by puréeing silken tofu with lemon juice and some salt.)

▶ Pesto is a great example of something that has been so laden with cheese as to mask the fresh flavors of the garlic, basil, pine nuts, and olive oil. The latter two ingredients give us the satisfaction of fat, and the oil also creates the creaminess. (Try my delicious pesto recipe in *The Vegan Table*.)

▶ When ordering pizza, ask for just sauce and a variety of vegetables and herbs. In fact, the *Marinara* is the original pizza, which is simply tomato sauce spread on thin crust, topped with a little basil. You can always bring nondairy cheese to a pizza place and ask them to make pie for you with your cheese.

COMMERCIAL NONDAIRY CHEESES

Having said all that, commercial nondairy cheeses—which also provide fat, salt, and a satisfying mouthfeel—can certainly play a role in our repertoires, especially when we're first transitioning away from dairy-based cheeses. But, the more you build your diet on whole foods, the less you crave *concentrated* fat, salt, and highly processed foods. You will even become accustomed to familiar dishes without nondairy cheese.

When you *are* trying nondairy cheeses for the first time, let me make a few suggestions:

▶ Judge them on their own merit. Do *not* taste dairy and nondairy products side by side to compare them. They're going to be different, because they're made from *different ingredients*. More significantly, you'll be biased to the old standby—not because it's superior but because that's what you're used to. If you were raised on nondairy milks and cheeses, they would be your preference.

▶ Try nondairy cheese in the context in which it was meant to be eaten. You wouldn't eat dairy-based sour cream from a spoon, so don't do that with nondairy sour cream, either. Add it to a burrito, fajita, or chili.

New cheeses are being introduced all the time; however, here is a list of some popular brands. You should be able to find many of them in large natural food stores and in vegan stores online.

GRATED CHEESES

Parma, by Eat in the Raw: Made from organic walnuts, nutritional yeast, and sea salt, it's essentially a commercial version of what you can easily make at home.

Soymage Vegan Parmesan, by Galaxy Nutritional Foods: A soy-based powdery cheese used for sprinkling on pasta or pizza.

SLICING AND SPREADING CHEESES

Daiya: Daiya offers many types and flavors of cheese, including slices (for grilled cheese sandwiches) and blocks (for crackers), and contains no common allergens such as casein, gluten, nuts, or soy.

Violife: Available mostly in Europe, Violife offers a variety of flavors, and it melts well for grilled cheese sandwiches or pizza.

Dr. Cow's Tree Nut Cheese: Dr. Cow's gourmet nut-based cheeses are outstanding and organic though expensive. All of the cheeses have been aged for three months and come in various flavors.

Sheese, by Bute Island Foods: Several creamy, spreadable flavors are available, including Cheddar, Original, Chives, Garlic & Herb, and Mexican.

Cheese Singles: There are a number of companies that make rice- and soy-based American-style cheese slices (just make sure they are casein-free).

MELTING CHEESES

Daiya: Daiya melts just like dairy-based cheese; it's available in several flavors, including Havarti, Mozzarella, Cheddar.

Teese, by Chicago Soydairy: Teese boasts Mozzarella and Cheddar flavors. Melts well.

Vegan Gourmet, by Follow Your Heart: Best when grated first, this soy-based cheese is best for something like burritos or tacos, whether you're using the Cheddar, Mozzarella, Monterey Jack, or Nacho.

CREAMY CHEESES

A few different brands make boxed vegan macaroni and cheese, so look for them in vegan stores or natural foods stores. (Turn to page 169 for a delicious Alfredo Sauce.)

Sour Cream: Make your own sour cream by puréeing silken tofu or cashews with lemon juice and salt, or check out the many commercial varieties, such as those made by Tofutti, Wayfare, and Galaxy Foods.

Cream Cheese: The commercial versions are very good for spreading on bagels or for making cheese-cake! Brands include Tofutti and Galaxy Foods.

Ricotta: My popular lasagna recipe is in *The Vegan Table*, and the tofu ricotta from that recipe can be used to make stuffed shells and manicotti as well.

The plant-based cheese market is exploding! Miyoko's Kitchen, the first vegan artisan cheese shop is Marin County, CA! If you can't visit, you can order online: miyokoskitchen.com

Herbed Cashew Cheese

YIELD 1½ cups or 12 servings **ALLERGY** Soy-free, gluten-free, wheat-free, oil-free

INGREDIENTS

2 cups (300 g) raw cashews
    soaked in 3 cups (720 ml) of
    water for at least 1 hour or
    as long as overnight

2 tablespoons lemon juice

¾ teaspoon salt

⅛ teaspoon freshly ground pepper

2 tablespoons minced basil

¼ cup (60 ml) water

PER SERVING (2 TABLESPOONS):
Calories: 140, **Protein:** 4.6 g, **Fat:** 11 g,
Carbohydrates: 7.8 g, **Fiber:** 0.9 g,
Cholesterol: 0 mg

I was tempted to call this recipe Basil Cashew Cheese, but I didn't want to limit you. Consider this delicious spreadable cheese a basic foundation to which you can add any variation of fresh herbs or other ingredients.

Note: *Because the cashews have to soak for at least an hour, you will want to factor that into the total prep time.*

DIRECTIONS

- Once the cashews have soaked, drain and rinse them in a strainer.
- Place them in a food processor, along with the lemon juice, salt, pepper, and basil. Turn on the machine, and let it run for a few seconds to start combining the ingredients.
- Add most of the water, and process until the mixture is completely smooth, about 2 to 4 minutes, turning the machine off periodically to scrape down the sides of the bowl. Before adding all of the water, I like first seeing what the consistency is; it's always easier to add more than it is to take any out!
- Salt, to taste. The consistency should be thick but spreadable.

Suggestions for Serving

- Serve as a spread for crackers.
- Use it as the base for the Socca on page 92.
- Use it as the base for the Strawberry Bruschetta on page 170.

FOR YOUR MODIFICATION

- Instead of basil, add chives, dill, parsley, or any combination of herbs you desire.
- Add finely chopped sundried tomatoes and/or olives instead of or along with the fresh herbs.

FOR YOUR INFORMATION

It will keep well in the refrigerator for at least 3 days.

Pasta Alfredo with Walnut Parmesan

YIELD 6 to 8 servings **ALLERGY** Soy-free, oil-free, gluten-free, wheat-free (depending on pasta)

INGREDIENTS *SAUCE*

1 pound of uncooked tubular pasta (penne, rigatoni, ziti, etc.)

2 cups (300 g) of raw, unsalted cashews, soaked in water for 1 hour

2 cups (480 ml) of vegetable broth

2 cloves garlic, peeled

¼ cup (12 g) nutritional yeast flakes

1 tablespoon apple cider vinegar

Salt and pepper, to taste

Chopped fresh basil, for garnish

½ cup Walnut Parmesan (recipe below)

INGREDIENTS

WALNUT PARMESAN

½ cup (60 g) raw walnuts

2 tablespoons nutritional yeast flakes

½ teaspoon salt

½ teaspoon garlic powder

Rich, creamy, and comforting, this dish can also be modified to include favorite ingredients baked into it—such as sundried tomatoes, chopped greens, sliced mushrooms, squash, olives, or whatever you desire.

Note: *Because the cashews need to soak for an hour, you'll want to factor that into the start-to-finish timing for this recipe.*

DIRECTIONS *SAUCE*

- Boil pasta according to package directions, rinse with cold water, and transfer to a large bowl.
- Once the cashews have soaked for an hour, drain them and rinse well. Next, place the cashews, broth, garlic, nutritional yeast, vinegar, and salt and pepper in a high-speed blender, and blend until thick and creamy. (A food processor will do the trick, but a high-powered blender will make the sauce perfectly creamy smooth.) The sauce should be about as thick as pancake batter.
- Taste and adjust seasonings. Pour the sauce over the pasta, and stir to coat.
- Serve the pasta in shallow bowls, sprinkled with fresh basil (or any fresh herbs you prefer) and a couple tablespoons of the Walnut Parmesan.

DIRECTIONS *WALNUT PARMESAN*

- Blend all the ingredients in a food processor until finely chopped but still crumbly. Store in refrigerator for up to a month.

PER SERVING:
Calories: 477, **Protein:** 17 g, **Fat:** 23 g, **Carbohydrates:** 55 g, **Fiber:** 4.7 g, **Cholesterol:** 0 mg

FOR YOUR MODIFICATION

Baked version: Preheat oven to 350°F. Once you've made the sauce, mix it with the pasta in a bowl. Pour into a 9-by-13-inch baking dish. Cover and bake for 10 minutes. Uncover, sprinkle with Walnut Parmesan, and bake for 10 minutes more.

FOR YOUR INFORMATION

If you store the leftovers in the fridge, you might notice that the sauce is a bit congealed the next morning. Just add a little extra milk, mix it up, and re-heat, and you're good to go.

Strawberry Bruschetta

YIELD Makes 20 servings **ALLERGY** Soy-free, oil-free

INGREDIENTS

1 baguette (seeded or plain), cut into 1-inch-thick slices

3 tablespoons light brown sugar

2 teaspoons lemon juice

3 cups (500 g) diced fresh strawberries

Herbed Cashew Cheese (see recipe on page 168) or nondairy cream cheese

4 tablespoons finely chopped basil

Shaved chocolate (optional)

PER SERVING:
Calories: 120, **Protein:** 3.7 g, **Fat:** 6.0 g, **Carbohydrates:** 14 g, **Fiber:** 1.3 g, **Cholesterol:** 0 mg

~Dedication~

From: CPG

To: My beloved mom Arlene, who beautifully models what it means to love and embrace life

I've served this for brunch, as an hors d'oeuvre, and as an after-dinner dessert. For the latter, I've also added chocolate shavings on top. The point is it's incredibly flexible, super delicious, and very pretty!

DIRECTIONS

- Lightly toast the bread in a toaster oven (or in a regular oven) at 250°F.
- Meanwhile, heat a medium skillet or saucepan over medium-high heat. Add the sugar and lemon juice, and cook, stirring, until the sugar melts and the mixture begins to bubble, about 30 to 60 seconds.
- Add the diced strawberries, and stir to combine with the liquid. Allow the berries to cook down a little and get heated through, about 2 minutes. Remove from heat.
- Spread approximately 1 tablespoon of Herbed Cashew Cheese or commercial nondairy cream cheese on each piece of toast. Using a spoon (a slotted spoon will allow you to get strawberries without so much liquid), top the cheese with the warm berries.
- Sprinkle the chopped basil onto each slice. Add a little shaved chocolate along with or instead of the basil, if serving for dessert.

FOR YOUR EDIFICATION

Bruschetta means "burnt toast," so that's an essential component of this dish. You just get more of a texture contrast when the bread is toasted than when it's not. Plus, toasted bread means it will hold up better with the liquid.

FOR YOUR INFORMATION

Bruschetta is an Italian word, which means "ch" is pronounced as a hard "k." The proper pronunciation is "broo-sketta."

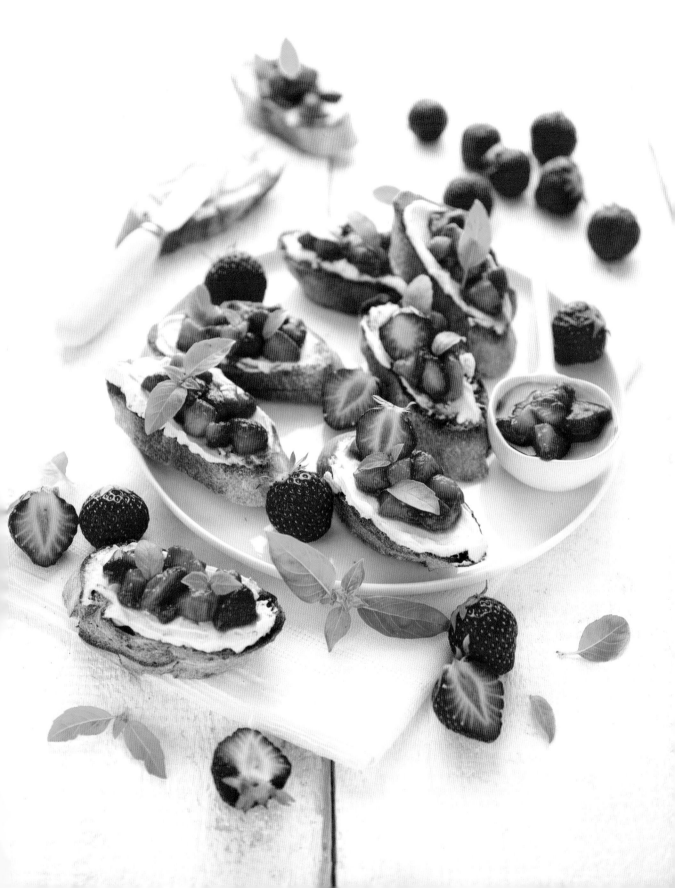

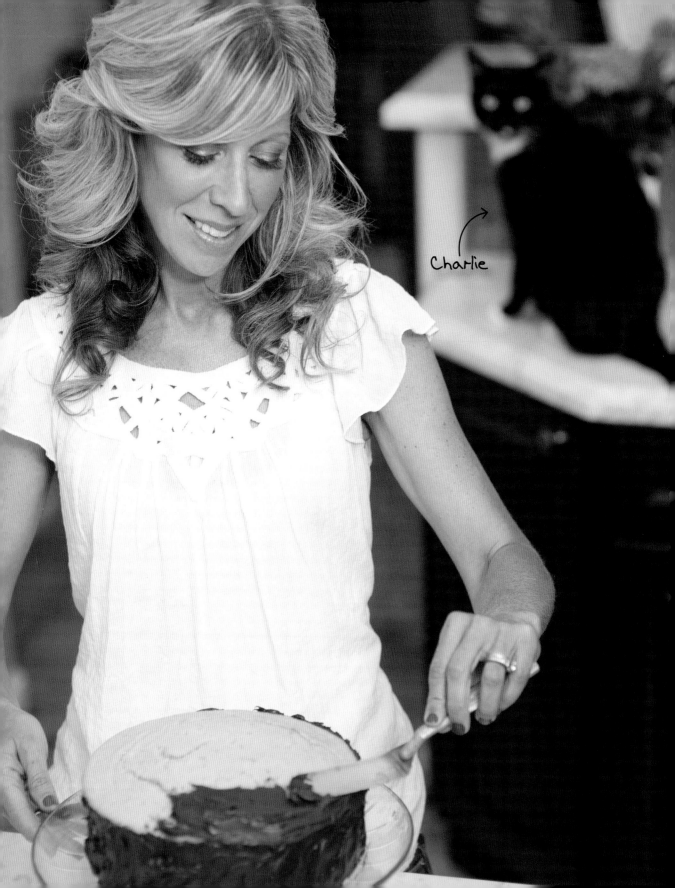

Charlie

Baking Without Eggs (It's Better!)

Having enthusiastically noticed the many commercial baked goods on the supermarket shelves, perhaps by now you're anxious to bake some goodies yourself. So grab the flour, sugar, baking soda, and baking powder, and leave the eggs behind. That's right—you do not need eggs to bake.

One of the factors that led to eggs being used with such abandon was the end of World War II. Prior to and during the war, animal products were considered "luxury items," so they were used only sparingly—even in baked goods. Baking without eggs was common and left us with many "wartime" recipes such as Victory Cake and other eggless desserts. When the war ended, however, Americans had more money than they knew what to do with, and animal products became more available than ever before. To demonstrate their affluence, people purchased meat, dairy, and eggs without thought, and food manufacturers included cow's milk and chicken's eggs in their products—even when they weren't necessary. Animal products equaled wealth—and still do.

Even non-bakers suffer from the misconception that baked goods require chicken's eggs, cow's milk, and dairy-based butter. The fact is, to create delicious, decadent, successful baked goods, you do not need animal products at all. What you need is:

- Binding
- Moisture
- Richness/Fat
- Leavening

You can accomplish all these things with plant-derived ingredients that are better for you and better for the animals! In fact, you do not need a "replacement" for every egg you eliminate. Often, the eggs are superfluous and can be left out and without being "substituted," or if you merely need extra moisture, you could "replace" the egg with puréed banana or applesauce.

Because strongly ingrained habits are hard to change, when you contemplate baking without eggs, you might feel like you'll have to learn all over again how to bake. But, that's the case with any new recipe, cuisine, or technique you're embarking on for the first time. The good news is once you learn the new way, it becomes second nature and replaces the old. I guarantee it. As I say in my cookbook, *The Joy of Vegan Baking,* "baking without eggs will become as natural to you as laying eggs is to chickens."[43]

So let's leave the eggs to the birds and create binding, fat, moisture, richness, and leavening in recipes without them. Once you become familiar with the effect of the different ingredients at your disposal, you will be able to confidently and successfully "veganize" any baking recipe.

Both moisture and fat in baked goods come from oil, nondairy butter, applesauce, bananas, water, or nondairy milk. I write in great length about all the many ways to create "egg substitutes" in my first baby, *The Joy of Vegan Baking,* so I'm not able to repeat it all here. In short, there are a few techniques/ingredients you'll want to be aware of for creating egg-free baked goods.

1. Vinegar and baking soda. The ratio is 1 teaspoon of baking soda with 1 tablespoon of vinegar, and the combination—when heated—creates bubbles that help to lighten the final product or enable it to rise.

2. Ground flaxseeds and water. For the equivalent of "1 egg," blend 1 tablespoon of ground flaxseeds with 3 tablespoons of water to create a thick, gooey, gelatinous mixture. Use a blender or food processor—or even hand-held blender—to create this desired consistency. (Always buy whole seeds and grind them at home using a coffee grinder; refrigerate the ground seeds and use them to make "flax eggs," or just to add omega-3 fats to your diet.)

3. Commercial egg replacer/powder and water. There are a few on the market these days, including Ener-G Egg Replacer and Bob's Red Mill Egg Replacer. Both are based on potato starch, and when mixed with water (blended to become thick, as in the flax eggs), you have an "egg replacement." They're convenient to keep in your cupboard (or refrigerator) for those times when you don't have flaxseeds. Follow the directions on the package, but the ratio tends to be about 1 tablespoon of powder to 3 tablespoons of water. I tend to prefer "flax eggs," but commercial egg replacer comes in handy when you don't want tiny brown specs in your finished product.

The average American eats over 250 chicken eggs every year, making the total egg production in the United States about 76 billion. That translates to over 290 million hens being exploited for their eggs. Every time we replace chicken's eggs with a plant-based food, we're making a compassionate, healthful choice for ourselves—and the chickens—whether we're cooking or baking.

There are many other baked goods/desserts sprinkled throughout these pages, but here are some that are meant to dispel any myths about baking without eggs.

Chocolate Gingersnaps

YIELD Makes about 24 to 30 cookies **ALLERGY** Soy-free, depending on the nondairy butter you use

INGREDIENTS

½ cup (1 stick) nondairy butter, softened

½ cup (100 g) light brown sugar

¼ cup (85 g) molasses

1 tablespoon water

2 tablespoons grated fresh ginger

1½ cups (190 g) all-purpose flour

1 tablespoon unsweetened cocoa powder

1 teaspoon baking soda

1 teaspoon ground ginger

1 teaspoon ground cinnamon

½ teaspoon ground nutmeg

½ cup (85 g) semisweet or dark chocolate, chopped

¼ cup (50 g) granulated sugar

PER COOKIE:
Calories: 92, Protein: 0.8 g, Fat: 4 g, Carbohydrates: 14 g, Fiber: 0.5 g, Cholesterol: 0 mg

These cookies are hard to resist—particularly when served at wintertime with some vegan nog.

Note: *Because the dough needs to sit for a couple hours before baking, you'll want to factor that into the start-to-finish timing for these cookies.*

DIRECTIONS

- Add the nondairy butter and brown sugar to a medium-size bowl, and using an electric mixer, cream until fluffy. Add the molasses, water, and fresh ginger, and continue to mix until combined.

- Next, add the flour, cocoa powder, baking soda, ground ginger, cinnamon, and nutmeg. Stir until well blended. You'll have a nice, thick cookie batter at this point.

- Add the chopped chocolate bits, and stir just enough to make sure they're mixed into your batter.

- Cover the bowl with plastic wrap, and store in the refrigerator for at least 2 hours. (You can leave it overnight if you want to.)

- When it's time to bake your cookies, set the oven to 350°F, and line a baking sheet with parchment paper.

- Shape the dough into 1½-inch balls. Press each ball down to flatten slightly, and "dip" the top in the granulated sugar (added to a shallow bowl). Make sure the top is completely coated with the sugar. Place each coated cookie on the baking sheet.

- Bake for 14 to 15 minutes or until the cookies are just firm to the touch. Transfer the cookies to wire racks to cool. Cool completely before storing in an airtight container.

FOR YOUR INFORMATION

Some gingersnap recipes have you roll the entire dough ball in the granulated sugar, but I've found that the bottoms often burn. And, nobody likes a burnt bottom!

FOR YOUR EDIFICATION

A microplane is the best tool for grating fresh ginger.

Cowboy Cookies

YIELD Makes about 30 cookies **ALLERGY** Soy-free

INGREDIENTS

1½ cups (300 g) light brown sugar, packed

1 cup (220 g) nondairy butter, softened

1 teaspoon pure vanilla extract

1 flax egg or 3 tablespoons water + 1 tablespoon ground flaxseeds

2 cups (180 g) quick-cooking oats

1½ cups (200 g) all-purpose unbleached flour

1 teaspoon baking soda

¼ teaspoon salt

1 cup (180 g) semisweet chocolate chips

1 cup (60 g) broken-up pretzels

PER SERVING (1 COOKIE):
Calories: 174, **Protein:** 1.9 g, **Fat:** 8.1 g, Carbohydrates: 24 g, **Fiber:** 1.1 g, Cholesterol: 0 mg

These goodies are essentially oatmeal cookies with lots of extras. You can add or substitute dried coconut, raisins, cranraisins, dried cherries— or anything you like (short of adding cowboys, cows, or anything that comes out of either!).

DIRECTIONS

→ Preheat the oven to 350°F. Line two baking sheets with parchment paper.

→ In the bowl of an electric stand mixer or a large freestanding bowl, mix together the nondairy butter and brown sugar until fully blended and creamy. You can do this by hand, but for best results use an electric hand mixer. Add the vanilla and flax egg, and beat until light and fluffy.

→ Stir in the oats, flour, baking soda, and salt, mixing just until the dry ingredients are incorporated. Finally, add the chocolate chips and pretzels, and stir to combine.

→ Make balls the size of golf balls and place them at least 2 inches apart on the baking sheet. To create uniform-size cookies, you can also use a small scoop. Lightly wet your hand with some water, and gently press down the top of each cookie to flatten it out somewhat.

→ Bake for 14 to 15 minutes, until the tops of the cookies are firm and the outside edges are golden brown. Let cool 5 minutes on the baking sheets, then transfer the cookies to a wire rack and cool completely.

Dedication

From: Karin Bauer
To: My animal-loving mother, Waltraud Helene Bauer

FOR YOUR EDIFICATION

To break up the pretzels, place a handful in a sealed plastic bag. Use your hand or a heavy kitchen utensil (like a potato masher) to make chocolate chip-sized pieces. Don't pulverize them. Measure after you break them up, and then add more, if necessary.

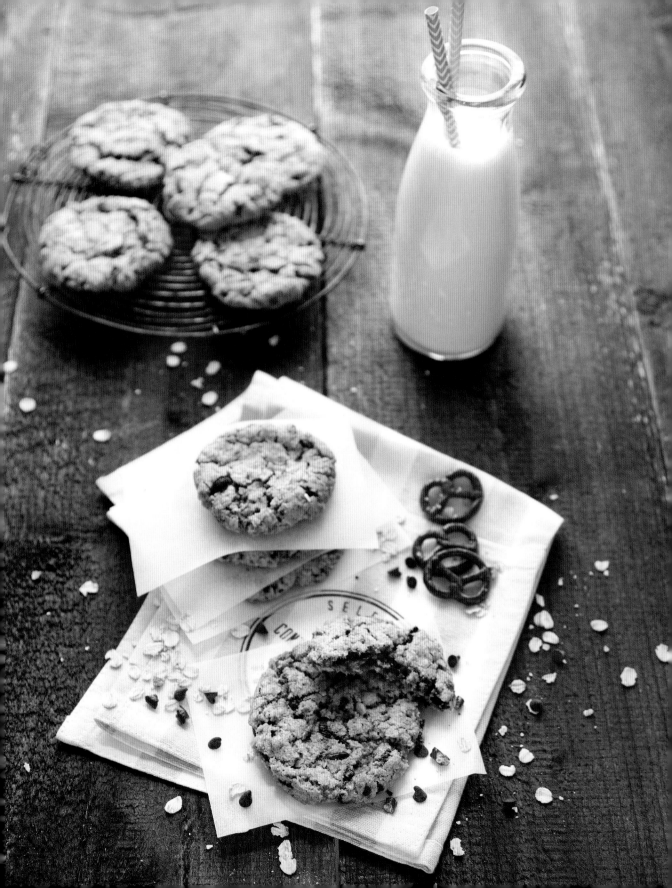

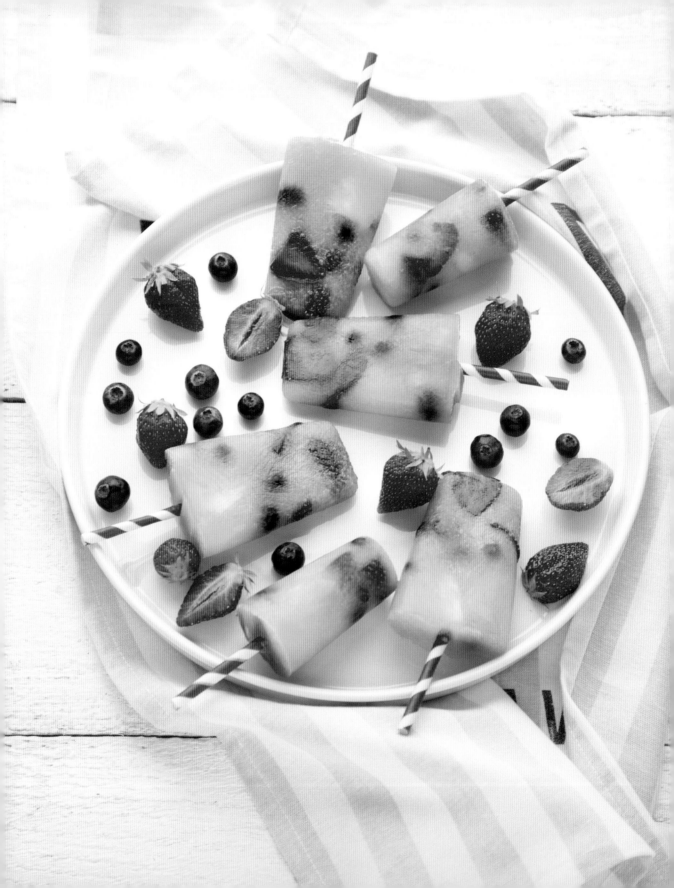

Fresh Fruit Popsicles

YIELD Makes 6 popsicles **ALLERGY** Soy-free, wheat-free, gluten-free, oil-free

INGREDIENTS

Fresh or frozen strawberries, halved or sliced

Fresh or frozen blueberries

Fresh or frozen pineapple chunks

1½ cups (360 ml) of natural fruit punch or 100 percent white-grape juice

---

PER SERVING (1 POPSICLE):
Calories: 89.7, **Protein:** 0.9 g, **Fat:** 0.3 g, **Carbohydrates:** 22.7 g, **Fiber:** 0.8 g, **Cholesterol:** 0 mg

---

Homemade fruit popsicles are so much better than the sugar-loaded ones you would buy at the grocery store. Any combination of fresh or frozen fruit will work; it's a great way to use fresh fruit that you might not have a chance to eat before it's ready for the compost bin, and of course, any frozen fruit chunks will be perfect.

DIRECTIONS

- Combine fruit in a mixing bowl and arrange the mixture into six 3-ounce popsicle molds (depending on which ones you buy). Alternatively, you can create layers for each fruit. First, add the strawberry slices, then the blueberries, then a few pineapple chunks.
- Pour enough juice into each mold to just cover the fruit. Don't overfill.
- Insert the popsicle sticks and freeze until solid (about four hours).

Dedication

From: Rachel Smith

To: Tippie, my sweet old girl; beloved canine yoga buddy and meditation friend who teaches me quiet kindness every day

FOR YOUR EDIFICATION

You can use disposable plastic cups and popsicle sticks for your molds, but the most eco-friendly method for making these delicious healthful treats is to invest a few dollars in reusable popsicle molds you can find online or at any kitchen supply store.

FOR YOUR INFORMATION

You can use as little or as much fruit as you like, so it's hard to give exact amounts, but to keep it manageable, I would say to use about one or two strawberries, six blueberries and four pineapple chunks per individual popsicle mold.

Strawberry Parfait with Vanilla Custard and Candied Almonds

YIELD Serves 6 **ALLERGY** Soy-free, oil-free, gluten-free, wheat-free

INGREDIENTS

VANILLA ALMOND CUSTARD

4 tablespoons cornstarch

6 tablespoons light brown
or granulated sugar

¼ teaspoon salt

3 cups (720 ml) plain or
vanilla almond milk

1 teaspoon vanilla extract

INGREDIENTS

CANDIED ALMONDS

1 cup (100 g) slivered
raw almonds

2 tablespoons granulated sugar

1 tablespoon maple syrup

1 tablespoon organic corn syrup

¼ to ½ teaspoon salt

INGREDIENTS PARFAIT

1 batch of Vanilla Almond Custard

2 pints (680 g) fresh strawberries,
sliced or halved

1 batch Candied Almonds

4 large ripe bananas, sliced

PER SERVING:
Calories: 363, **Protein:** 5.6 g, **Fat:** 9.6 g,
Carbohydrates: 69 g, **Fiber:** 7.2 g,
Cholesterol: 0 mg

DO NOT be intimidated by the number of steps. This is a sophisticated- but fun-dessert to make and eat!

DIRECTIONS VANILLA ALMOND CUSTARD

- In a 3-quart saucepan, whisk together the cornstarch, sugar, and salt. Slowly whisk in a small amount of almond milk, and continue whisking until smooth. Whisk in the remaining milk and vanilla extract.

- Place the saucepan on the stove over medium heat. Whisk continuously until the mixture comes to a full boil. Boil for 1 minute, whisking the entire time as it starts to thicken.

- Remove from heat, and pour into a bowl that is sitting in a larger bowl filled with cold water and ice. Whisk frequently to prevent a skin from forming and to release the heat. Set aside.

DIRECTIONS CANDIED ALMONDS

- Preheat oven to 325°F.

- Mix all the ingredients together and spread onto a parchment-lined cookie sheet. Bake for 5 minutes. Check, and rotate sheet, if needed. Bake for 5 to 8 minutes more, or until the mixture is light brown. Let cool completely on the pan, then break into bite-size pieces.

DIRECTIONS PARFAIT

- Layer in a martini or parfait glass: ¼ cup of custard, a few strawberry slices, a sprinkle of almonds, another ¼ cup of custard, a few banana slices, more almonds, and repeat until glasses are ¾ full. Repeat.

- Refrigerate for several hours until custard is completely set up. Top with few candied almonds right before serving.

Dedication

From: Jennifer Kannegaard
To: My inspirational friend,
Valerie Green

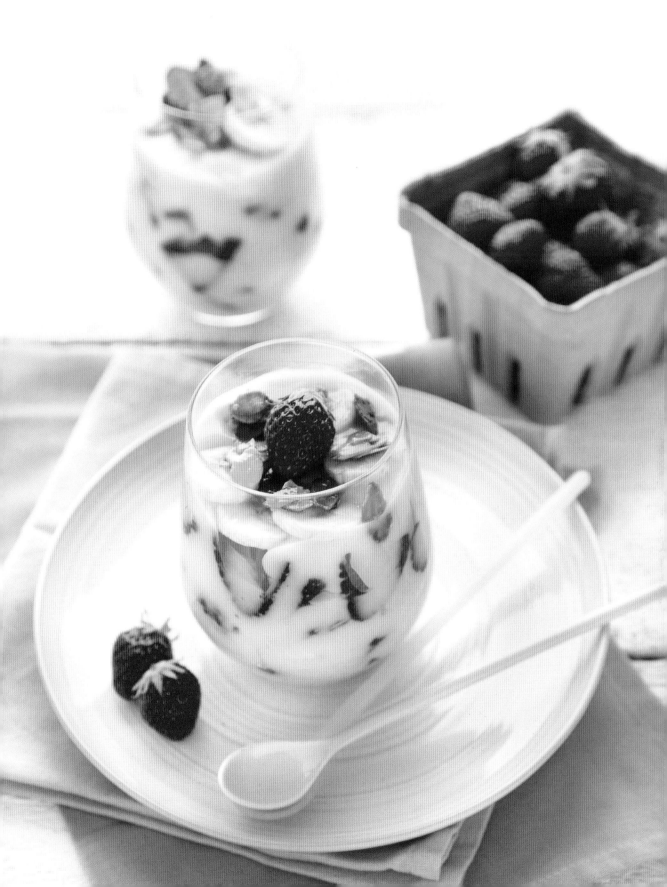

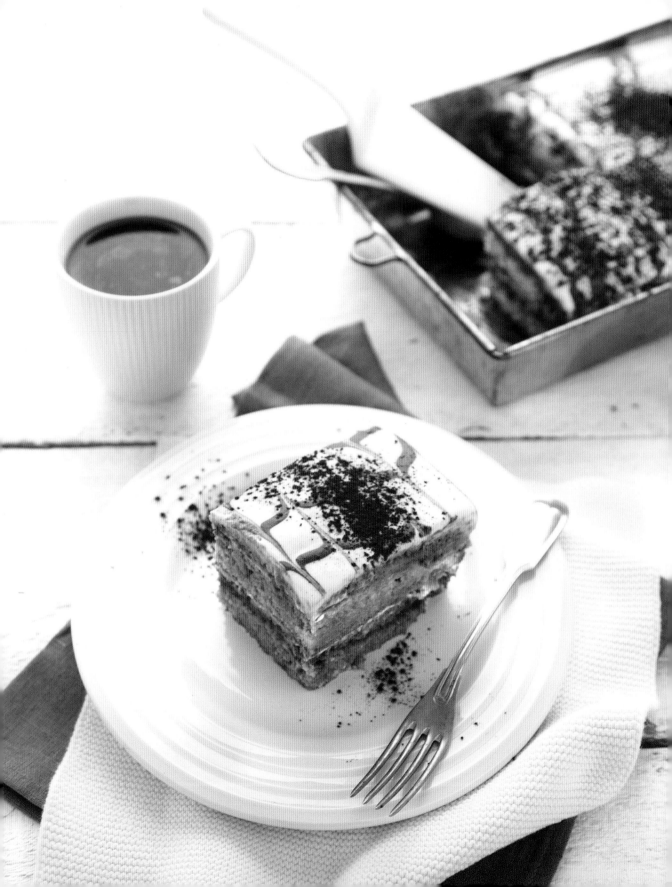

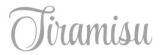

Tiramisu

YIELD Makes one 9-by-13-inch cake or 14 servings

INGREDIENTS *CAKE*

2½ cups (310 g) unbleached
 all-purpose flour

1 tablespoon baking powder

2 teaspoons baking soda

¾ teaspoon salt

1 cup (240 ml) plant-based milk

1 teaspoon apple cider vinegar

⅓ cup (56 g) silken tofu

½ cup (120 ml) water

⅔ cup (160 ml) canola oil

2 teaspoons vanilla extract

1¼ cups (300 ml) maple syrup

1½ to 2 cups (360 to 480 ml) black
 coffee/espresso, cooled

Cocoa powder, optional (for garnish)

INGREDIENTS *CREAM FILLING*

2 12-ounce boxes (680 g) silken tofu

2 8-ounce containers (450 g)
 nondairy cream cheese

2 teaspoons lemon juice

2 teaspoons vanilla extract

½ cup (120 ml) maple syrup

Pinch of salt

INGREDIENTS *GANACHE*

1 cup (240 g) plant-based milk

1 cup (150 g) nondairy
 chocolate chips

½ teaspoon vanilla extract

Pinch of salt

Traditionally, ladyfingers are the base for this "pick me up" cake, but our version relies on a yellow cake, which can be used on its own. This fabulous recipe comes from the wonderful Kristin Kolnacki, pastry chef at peace-food cafe in New York City.

Note: *It's worth purchasing a half-sheet pan; you'll use it for more than this recipe. You also need a 9-by-13-by-2-inch pan.*

DIRECTIONS *CAKE*

- Preheat the oven to 325°F. Lightly oil a half-sheet pan (18-by-13-inch), then place parchment paper on top of the oiled surface.
- To a large mixing bowl, add the flour, baking powder, baking soda, and salt, and stir to combine. Set aside.
- Measure out the milk in a measuring cup, and add the teaspoon of vinegar. Allow it to curdle, creating a nondairy buttermilk. Let this sit for a couple of minutes, while you prepare the rest of the cake ingredients.
- In a food processor or blender, blend the ⅓ cup silken tofu and ½ cup water. Add the oil, vanilla, and maple syrup. Blend until smooth.
- Make a well in the middle of the dry ingredients; pour in the blender mixture, along with the milk/vinegar mixture. Whisk together just until fully combined and smooth. Be careful to not over mix, as you don't want to build up the gluten. You want to cake to be nice and tender.
- Pour the batter onto the prepared half-sheet pan. Bake the cake until lightly golden, 15 to 20 minutes. Test for doneness by pressing your finger in the center of the cake. If it springs back, the cake is done.
- Let the cake cool completely before assembling.

DIRECTIONS *CREAM FILLING*

- In a food processor or blender, blend the two boxes of silken tofu until smooth. Add the cream cheese, and blend again.
- Add the lemon juice, vanilla extract, maple syrup, and salt, and blend again. Check for lumps, scrape down the sides, and blend again, if necessary. Set aside.

PER SERVING (1 SLICE):
Calories: 450.1, **Protein:** 7.6 g, **Fat:** 21.7 g,
Carbohydrates: 57.5 g, **Fiber:** 1.5 g,
Cholesterol: 0 mg

Dedication

From: Laura Yasinitsky
To: Miss Honey LaBronx, The Vegan
Drag Queen, and my dear friend

DIRECTIONS *GANACHE*

- In a small pot, scald the milk; that is, cook it until it bubbles a little around the edges, but remove it from the heat before it boils.

- Place the chocolate chips in a small bowl and pour the scalded milk over them. Starting from the middle, whisk until smooth. Add the vanilla and salt. Let sit until it thickens up a little (just a few minutes) or pour into a squeeze bottle.

DIRECTIONS *ASSEMBLY*

- Use a 9-by-13-by-2-inch rectangular pan to assemble (no need to oil). Glass is preferable, but plastic or metal will work, as well.

- Cut the cooled vanilla cake in half so that each half will fit perfectly into the 9-by-13 rectangular pan you are using.

- Carefully place the first half of the cake in the bottom of the pan, with the bottom of the cake facing up. The cake bottom has lots of air holes that will more easily absorb the coffee.

- Take a brush and generously drench the cake with half of the espresso until it seeps in. You want the Tiramisu to be very moist.

- Next, pour half of the cream filling over the espresso-drenched cake, and smooth it out evenly. Then, drizzle the ganache over the cream. This layer will be covered, so there's no need to make it pretty.

- Take the second half of the vanilla cake, and place it on top of the cream layer—also bottom side up. Drench in espresso. Pour on the remaining cream, and spread it evenly on top.

- For this ganache topping (which will be the top of your cake), you can use a squeeze bottle or a spoon. Start in one corner and drizzle the ganache back and forth diagonally until you reach the opposite corner.

- Create a marble effect by dragging a toothpick or knife tip opposite along the lines (see photo). Sift a little cocoa powder on top, and refrigerate from 3 hours to overnight to firm up.

Truffle Popcorn

YIELD Makes 8 to 8½ cups **ALLERGY** Gluten-free, wheat-free, soy-free (if using soy-free nondairy butter)

INGREDIENTS

AIR-POPPED VERSION

½ cup (220 g) popcorn kernels

1 tablespoon nondairy butter

2 teaspoons white or black
truffle oil

Salt, to taste

Freshly ground pepper (optional)

Nutritional yeast (optional)

INGREDIENTS

STOVETOP VERSION

1 tablespoon olive or canola oil

½ cup (220 g) popcorn kernels

1 to 2 teaspoons nondairy butter

½ to 1 teaspoon black or white
truffle salt

Salt, to taste

Freshly ground pepper (optional)

Nutritional yeast (optional)

PER SERVING (2 CUPS):
Calories: 84, Protein: 2.1 g, Fat: 3.2 g,
Carbohydrates: 12 g, Fiber: 2.3 g,
Cholesterol: 0 mg

My favorite restaurant in my beloved city sparked my inspiration for this delicious popcorn: Encuentro Café and Wine Bar in Oakland, CA.

DIRECTIONS *AIR-POPPED VERSION*

- Using your air popper, add the popcorn kernels, and start popping.
- Meanwhile, in a small saucepan over low heat or in a microwave, melt the nondairy butter. Add the truffle oil, and stir. Remove from heat.
- Transfer the popcorn to a large bowl, and drizzle on the truffle-infused butter, along with the salt, tossing well. Season with additional salt, pepper, and nutritional yeast, if desired. Serve and enjoy.

DIRECTIONS *STOVETOP VERSION*

- In a large pot, heat the oil over medium heat. Once heated, add 4 or 5 kernels to the oil, cover and cook over medium heat until they start popping. Be sure to shake the pot continuously until the popping has stopped. As soon as the test-kernels have popped, add the ½ cup of popcorn to the pot, cover, and shake continuously until the popping slows to a few seconds between pops. Remove from heat.
- Meanwhile, in a small saucepan over low heat or in the microwave, melt the nondairy butter. Remove from heat.
- Transfer the popcorn to a large bowl, and drizzle on the nondairy butter along with the truffle salt, tossing well. Season with additional salt, pepper, and nutritional yeast, if desired. Serve and enjoy.

FOR YOUR EDIFICATION

Because Earth Balance has salt, you will want to adjust your own salt accordingly.

Mexican Chocolate Cake

YIELD Makes one two-layer cake or 18 cupcakes

ALLERGY Soy-free (if using a plant milk and butter other than soy)

INGREDIENTS *CAKE*

2¼ cups (280 g) all-purpose flour

¾ cup (150 g) granulated sugar

½ cup (60 g) unsweetened
   cocoa powder

1½ teaspoons baking soda

1 teaspoon cinnamon

½ teaspoon cayenne pepper

½ teaspoon salt

1 cup (240 ml) unsweetened
   applesauce

¾ cup (180 ml) canola oil

1 tablespoon (15 ml) vanilla extract

1½ cups (360 ml) plant-based milk

2 tablespoons (30 ml) apple cider or
   white distilled vinegar

INGREDIENTS *FROSTING*

½ cup (100 g) or 1 stick nondairy
   butter, somewhat softened

2 cups (400 g) powdered
   (confectioner's) sugar, sifted

⅓ cup (25 g) unsweetened cocoa

1 teaspoon cinnamon

¼ teaspoon cayenne pepper

1 teaspoon pure vanilla extract

3 tablespoons plant-based milk

The "Mexican Chocolate" aspect of this cake has to do with the combination of the spicy cayenne pepper and sweet cinnamon. Pair with a nondairy vanilla ice cream, and book a flight to heaven.

DIRECTIONS *CAKE*

- Preheat the oven to 350°F.
- Lightly oil two 9-inch (round or square) cake pans, or prepare cupcake/muffin tins with paper liners or silicon cups.
- In a large mixing bowl, combine the flour, sugar, cocoa powder, baking soda, cinnamon, cayenne pepper, and salt.
- In a separate bowl, beat together the applesauce, oil, vanilla extract, milk, and cider or vinegar. Add the wet mixture to the dry ingredients, and mix until everything is thoroughly combined. (You can use an electric hand mixer.) It will be a bit of a thick batter.
- Pour the batter into the prepared baking pans or cupcake/muffin tins, and bake for 20 to 30 minutes (cupcakes: between 15 and 17 minutes), or until the cake comes away from the sides of the pans and a toothpick inserted into the center comes out clean. Set aside to cool.

DIRECTIONS *FROSTING*

- Although it can be done by hand, it's much easier to use an electric hand mixer to come up with the fluffiest frosting. Cream together all the ingredients on low speed until smooth. Increase the speed once all the ingredients are combined and you don't risk powdered sugar flying everywhere. Mix until the frosting is light and fluffy (about 3 minutes). Lick the spoon, and frost your cake!

**PER SERVING
(1 CUPCAKE WITH FROSTING):**
Calories: 286, Protein: 3.2 g, **Fat:** 15 g,
Carbohydrates: 36 g, **Fiber:** 2.2 g,
Cholesterol: 0 mg

~Dedication~
From: Kent Gustavson
To: Our sweet Golden Retriever, Jacob.
We miss you.

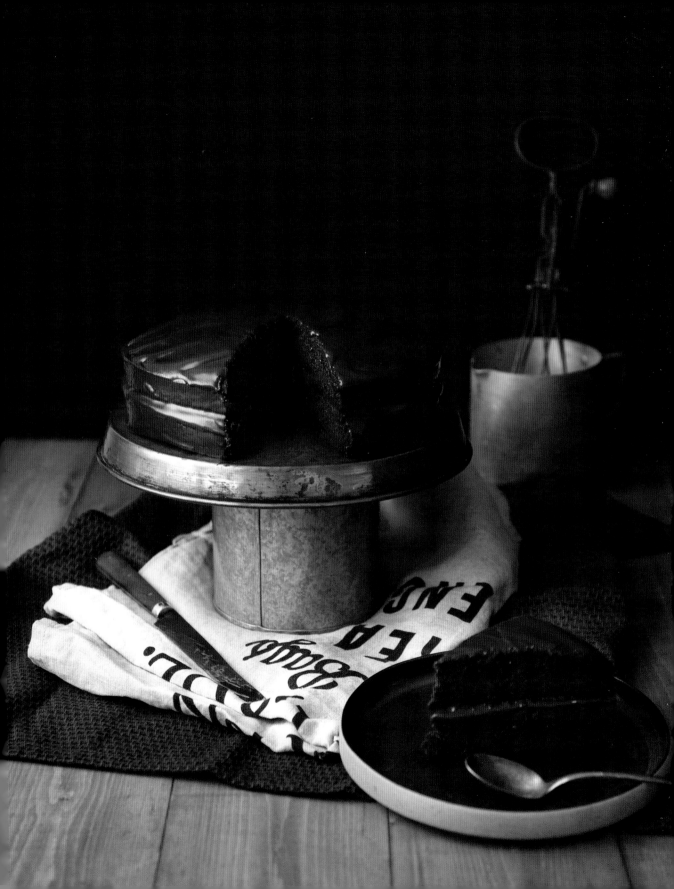

Tips for Frosting a Cake

► **NO CRUMBS:** So often, when we frost a cake, crumbs get into the frosting. To avoid this, once the cake is out of the oven and cooled down, carefully wrap it in plastic wrap and chill it in the refrigerator for 20 to 40 minutes. For best results, if you have the time, make the cake a day ahead of time, cool it on the counter, then wrap it, and put in the refrigerator until you're ready to frost. This reduces the "crumby" factor considerably.

► **CLEAN CAKE STAND:** Just prior to frosting your cake, place a sheet of parchment paper on the cake stand (or cake plate) first. Frost the cake, and then carefully slide out the parchment paper. Voila! A beautifully clean cake stand!

► **FROSTING CONSERVATION:** If you're short of frosting, only lightly frost the middle layers and reserve most of the frosting for the top and sides. The frosting that goes in the middle is really the glue that holds the cake together, so you don't need a huge amount.

► **LIKE THE PROS:** Once the cake is put together, frost the top first, then the sides. To keep the edges crisp looking, frost the top separately from the sides. It's okay if some frosting dribbles off the top of the cake to the sides, but don't purposefully smooth the frosting from the top of the cake down to the sides, because the sides will be rounded. To give the final frosting a smooth look, take a clean knife and run it around the sides, then run a clean knife flat across the top.

(Thanks to star recipe-tester Jenn Bridge for these tips!)

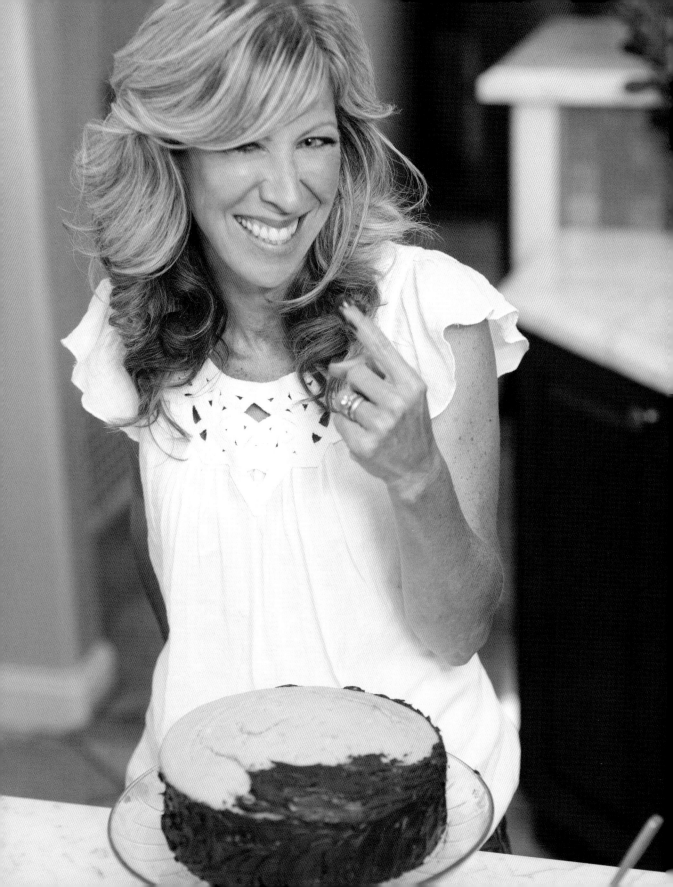

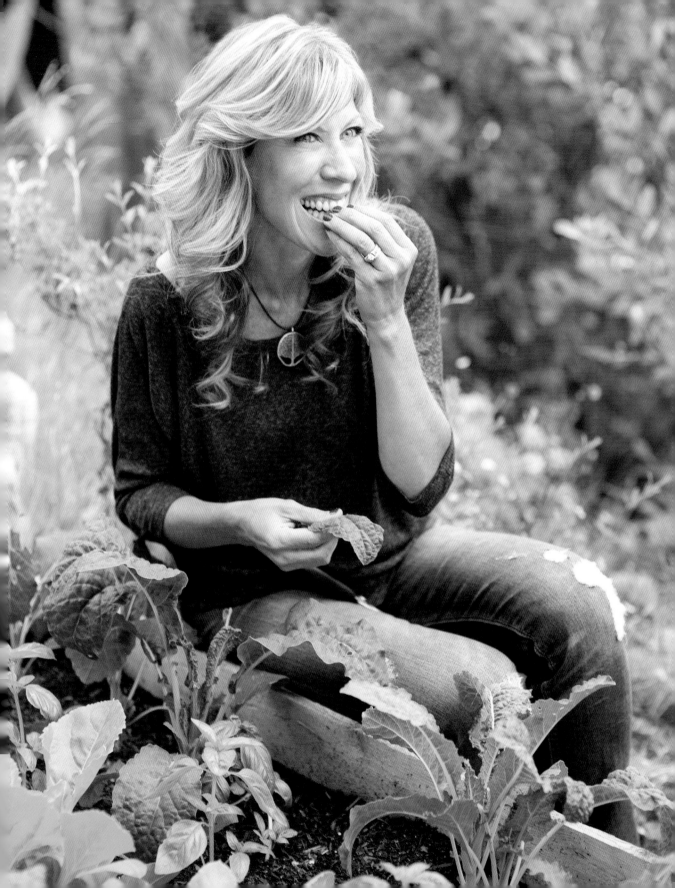

Cutting out the Middle Cow and Getting Calcium Directly from the Source

If I were to ask you to tell me the best source of calcium, you would most likely say cow's milk. You wouldn't say horse's milk, dog's milk, or even human's milk. You wouldn't say kale, collards, or bok choy. From a very young age, we have been sold the idea that cow's milk is an essential and healthful food for humans to consume, lauded for all the calcium it contains.

And while it's a fact that there is calcium in cow's milk, the question is *why*? To answer that question, we have to ask a few more:

What is calcium?
It's a mineral.

Where are minerals found?
In the ground.

Why is calcium found in the milk of cows?
Because they eat mineral-rich grass—or, rather, they're *supposed* to eat grass.

Three out of four cows bred and kept for their milk do not eat grass. They're kept on dry lots, which are essentially dirt lots devoid of pasture. To ensure that the cows' milk is rich in calcium to live up to the marketing claims, the producers supplement the cows' feed with calcium.

CHALLENGE YOUR THINKING:
Because cows aren't getting the calcium from the grass—the source of this mineral—producers supplement their feed with calcium.

CHANGE YOUR BEHAVIOR:
Skip the middle cow, and get your calcium straight from the source: green leafy vegetables.

You could supplement *your* feed with calcium. If we look at this entire process simply from the perspective of resource-use alone, we would see how very little sense—but how very much money—it all makes.

If you ever pass by cattle grazing in a pasture, you're most likely seeing "beef cattle"—not dairy cows. (You can generally determine this by knowing a little about the different "breeds" of cattle; generally, if they're bulky and stocky, they are most likely "beef cattle." If they're tall with udders noticeably swinging between their back legs, they're "dairy cows.") In most operations large and small, cows are hooked up to milking machines three times a day. If producers allowed the cows to graze freely, it would be too labor- and cost-intensive to round them up each time they had to be brought to the milking machines. So, without grass and foliage, the natural diet of this ruminant whose wild ancestors hearken back thousands of years, cows do not consume enough calcium to justify the claims made by the dairy industry.

By now, you may be asking another question: *if cows get calcium from the grass, wouldn't it make more sense for us to do the same?*

Good question! That's exactly what I'm getting at, and though I'm not suggesting we all start grazing on our front lawns, I am suggesting that we stop going *through* an animal to get a nutrient we can better obtain (and absorb) directly from the source: plant foods, particularly dark green leafy vegetables!

CALCIUM INTAKE—STRAIGHT FROM THE SOURCE

Part of the reason we are so willing to buy the myth—and the milk—is because we want to be healthy and do the right thing for our loved ones and ourselves. We're told that we need calcium (and we do) and vitamin D (and we do) and that the best source of these nutrients is cow's milk (and it isn't).

It's accurate to say we need calcium; it's inaccurate to say we need cow's milk or goat's milk or llama's milk or buffalo milk or sheep's milk. For the animals' sake and our own health, the best thing we can do is go directly to where the calcium resides—straight to the green leafy vegetables, where we also benefit from the presence of vitamins, minerals, fiber, folate, and phytonutrients.

CALCIUM-RICH GREENS:

One cup cooked collard greens contains 266 milligrams of calcium; one cup raw contains 52 milligrams.

One cup cooked turnip greens contains 197 milligrams of calcium; one cup raw contains 104 milligrams.

One cup cooked bok choy contains 158 milligrams of calcium; one cup raw contains 74 milligrams.

One cup cooked mustard greens contains 104 milligrams of calcium; one cup raw contains 58 milligrams.

One cup cooked kale contains 179 milligrams of calcium; one cup raw contains 90 milligrams.

One cup cooked broccoli contains 62 milligrams of calcium; one cup raw contains 43 milligrams.

NOTE: *Often when people think of calcium and green leafy vegetables, they tend to name spinach as a good source, but it's worth noting that the high amount of oxalates present in spinach, Swiss chard, and beet greens substantially decrease our body's ability to absorb their calcium. That doesn't mean we shouldn't eat these nutritious and delicious leafy greens, but calcium just isn't their star quality.*

Outside of greens, there are plenty of high-calcium foods, including

- Blackstrap molasses, one tablespoon of which contains 137 milligrams of calcium

- Soybeans, one cup of which contains 175 milligrams of calcium

- One cup of cooked navy beans, which contains 126 milligrams of calcium

- One quarter cup almonds, which contains 92 milligrams of calcium

- Five figs, which contain 90 milligrams of calcium

- One half cup tempeh, which contains 92 milligrams of calcium

And then, of course you have your calcium-*fortified* foods. That means that calcium is added during the processing.

- One cup calcium-fortified Total cereal contains 1,000 milligrams of calcium.

- One cup calcium-fortified Special K Plus cereal contains 600 milligrams of calcium.

- One cup fortified plant-based milk (soy, almond, rice, hemp) contains about 300 milligrams of calcium.

- One cup calcium-fortified orange juice contains about 250 milligrams of calcium, the same as a cup of cow's milk.

- One half cup firm calcium-set tofu contains 861 milligrams of calcium.

    NOTE: *The calcium content in tofu varies according to the brand and type of agent used to set the tofu. When calcium sulfate is used, the calcium content is very high. Calcium sulfate is the most common coagulant used to make firm tofu. So, just check the label of the tofu you buy to see if it's a calcium-fortified; i.e. if it's made with calcium sulfate.*

CALCIUM ABSORPTION AS IMPORTANT AS CALCIUM INTAKE

I think it's clear that calcium is abundant in plant foods, but there is a lot more to say, because intake is just one aspect of calcium status. As with all nutrients that are required from our diet, it is not simply a matter of *taking in* the nutrient. It's also a matter of *absorbing* it and *utilizing* it. Our body's ability to absorb and utilize a nutrient from a food is called *bioavailability*.

In other words, though it's helpful to know how much calcium is in certain foods, it's also necessary to know how much of that calcium we actually absorb.

Broccoli: Over 60% of the calcium in broccoli is absorbed by our bodies—so it's a very good source.

Kale: About 50% of the calcium in kale is absorbed by our bodies, so it's also a very good source.

Bok choy: Fifty-three percent is absorbed by our bodies. Very good.

Fortified beverages: The calcium used to fortify most juices and plant-based milks has a high bioavailability, ranging from 40 to 60%.

Calcium-set tofu: Calcium-fortified tofu (the tofu coagulated with calcium sulfate), has a bioavailability of over 30%.

Cow's milk: The bioavailability of cow's milk is 30%. Therefore, not only are the green leafy vegetables a better source of calcium because you're getting all the good stuff (and none of the harmful stuff) when you consume them, you also absorb a lot more of the calcium from these vegetables—50-60% in most cases versus 30% from cow's milk. You tell me what makes more sense.

INCREASING CALCIUM ABSORPTION AND DECREASING CALCIUM LOSS

Overall, it's estimated that North Americans absorb about 30% of the calcium present in food (even cow's milk has 30% bioavailability), so we want to increase absorption in as many ways as possible.

The best way to maximize absorption of calcium is to increase exposure to or intake of vitamin D. Vitamin D supplements are recommended for those who are deficient, those in certain age groups, and for people who lack exposure to the sun. This applies to everyone—not just vegans. Just as the feed of cows is supplemented with calcium, so, too is their milk fortified with vitamin D during processing. (Most plant-based milks are fortified, as well.) People with light skin would do well to expose their face and forearms to 10 to 15 minutes of warm sunlight a day. People with dark skin may require three times as much.

To determine your vitamin D levels, the Vitamin D Council has collaborated with ZRT Labs to make a discounted take-home vitamin D test kit available. Search online to purchase a kit.

In addition to taking in calcium and increasing our bodies' absorption of calcium, we also want to avoid losing that which we take in. The latter has much to do with other characteristics of our diet, namely our intake of protein and sodium, both of which contribute to loss of calcium in our bones. Plant protein contains less concentrated sulfur amino acids than animal protein, but high quantities of protein powders—including concentrated soy protein—could play a role in calcium excretion. To avoid such losses, experts recommend keeping protein intakes closer to recommendations and sodium intake under 2,300 milligrams a day and below 1,500 for people with high blood pressure, diabetes or chronic kidney disease, African-Americans, and people ages 51 and older.[44] Also, be sure to participate in weight-bearing exercises to keep your bones strong.

DAILY RECOMMENDATIONS FOR CALCIUM

How much calcium do we actually need?

In the United States, the daily recommendations are 500 milligrams for ages 1 to 3; 800 milligrams for 4 to 8 year-olds; 1,300 milligrams for adolescents 9 to 18 years; 1,000 milligrams for adults 19 to 50 years of age and increasing to 1,200 for women 51+ years of age and for men 71+ years of age.[45]

There is absolutely no dearth of calcium-rich foods available to us, and skipping the middle cow (or goat or sheep or llama or buffalo) means that we also skip the harmful saturated fat, dietary cholesterol, animal protein (casein), and lactose.

DEFYING NATURE: LACTOSE INTOLERANCE

We need to address another component of cow's milk, and that's lactose. It's important to talk about lactose in this context because it will help you walk away truly absorbing (pun intended) this information.

All mammals lactate for one purpose: to provide nourishment and sustenance for their offspring. Though breastfeeding in industrialized countries is much lower than in other parts of the world and was even discouraged when I was a babe, technically, humans can nurse for up to five years or more.

Once we're weaned, we don't need to consume even our own species' milk, and in fact, our bodies stop producing an enzyme called lactase by the time we are past the age of weaning—at about four years old. Lactase is the enzyme that enables us digest lactose, which is the sugar in the milk of mammals, including humans. So, by the time we should be weaned, our bodies don't make this enzyme anymore. Although some people around the world adapted genetically to continue consuming animal milk without discomfort, a huge percentage of the world's population suffer from "lactose intolerance," experiencing gas, bloating, abdominal cramping, and diarrhea. According to the Journal of the American Dietetic Association, approximately 75% of the world's population loses the ability to digest lactose after infancy.[46]

> **CHALLENGE YOUR THINKING:**
> Our bodies stop producing lactase, the enzyme that enables us to digest lactose, because we're not supposed to consume this milk sugar once we're weaned. Lactose intolerance is not a disorder. It's normal.

Lactose intolerance is not a *disorder*. It's *normal*! We're not *supposed* to be consuming lactose once we're weaned.

Skipping the middle cow is health- and life-enhancing for everyone, including the cows—and the goats. The goat's milk industry targets "lactose-intolerant" people, purporting it to have lower amounts of lactose than cow's milk. And it's true: goat's milk has 6% less lactose than cow's milk. 6%. Not a big difference in my book. The bottom line is cows and goats stop drinking their own mother's milk when they become adults. We should do the same.

DYING FOR CALCIUM

Before I realized that cows had to be pregnant to produce milk, I also believed that consuming animals' milk didn't contribute to suffering because the cows didn't have to be killed for us to take their milk. I believed it because that's the story we're told and because I desperately didn't want to believe that my consumption of cow's milk, cheese, and butter were harming anyone.

But I was wrong.

Because a cow's life is only as valuable as the offspring and amount of milk she is able to produce, when she is no longer profitable (i.e. when the costs to feed, medicate, and shelter her exceed the revenue derived from her milk output), she is sent to slaughter.

Cows are impregnated beginning at about 15 months young, even though they don't reach physical maturity until they are 4 years young. By the time she is five, after having endured three or four pregnancies (and the abduction of the same number of her calves), she is sold to slaughter. Cattle have a natural life expectancy of 15 or 20 years,[47] but dairy cows—all dairy cows—are sent to slaughter at about 4 to 5 years young.

CHALLENGE YOUR THINKING:
Every dairy cow is killed to be sold for her flesh when she is no longer "profitable"; i.e. when she no longer produces enough milk to justify her life. A slaughter-free animal agricultural system is simply not viable.

CHANGE YOUR BEHAVIOR:
Make calcium-rich recipes from plant foods!

Whether she is used on a small farm, organic farm, "humane" farm, "family-owned" farm, artisan farm, whatever-it's-called-farm, she is sent to slaughter when her milk production wanes.

Whether the milk is labeled organic, whole, pasteurized, unpasteurized, homogenized, raw, lactose-free, low-fat, 2%, 1%, skim, fat-free, rBST-free, or natural, she is sent to slaughter.

More than 18% of U.S. beef comes from spent dairy cows,[48] the majority of which is sold for fast-food hamburgers and supermarket retail. In the United States, of the 9.2 million cows raised for milk, approximately 50 to 70 thousand are slaughtered each week[49] or about three million each year.

Make no mistake about it. There is no retirement spa for used-up cows.

As far as I'm concerned, there is simply no ethical way to keep cows or goats (or any animal) "just for their milk." You cannot stimulate lactation without pregnancy, and to keep milk production high and consistent, you have to keep impregnating them, while keeping their offspring from drinking the milk that was made just for them. To stop the offspring from competing for what is rightfully theirs, they're sold for slaughter. To eliminate the costs of caring for "nonproductive" animals, males are killed. Perhaps a stud or two is kept for their semen, but you need only so many males for this purpose, and they are carefully selected for their genetic characteristics.

 As much as we want to distance ourselves from responsibility and culpability, there is no such thing as a slaughter-free animal agriculture system. It is not economically viable to feed, shelter, treat, and house animals for the duration of their lives and generate no profit in return.

We have no physiological requirement for cow's milk, but we do have an ethical imperative to make choices that create as little harm as possible.

So, let's just do what the cows do and go directly to plants where the calcium resides.

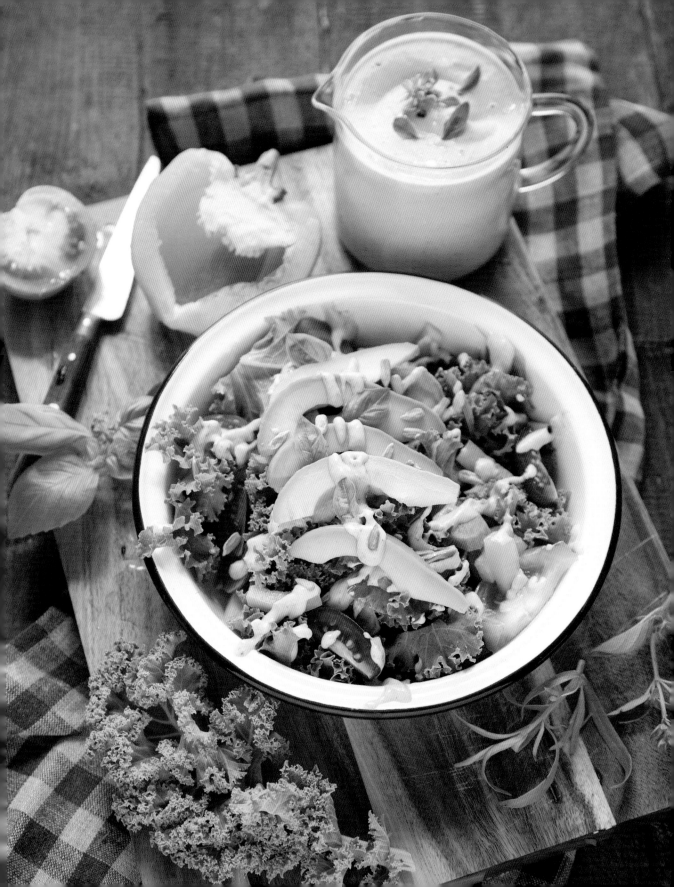

Green Goddess Dressing

YIELD 1 cup **ALLERGY** Soy-free, gluten-free, wheat-free, oil-free (if you eliminate the oil)

INGREDIENTS

1½ cups any combination of
    mixed herbs and alliums
    (parsley, chives, green onions,
    basil, tarragon, cilantro)

2 cloves garlic, peeled

¼ cup (60 g) raw tahini
    (sesame seed paste)

¼ cup (60 ml) apple cider vinegar

¼ cup (60 ml) fresh lemon juice

¼ to ½ cup (60 to 120 ml) water

2 tablespoons agave nectar or
    maple syrup

¼ cup (60 ml) olive oil

½ teaspoon salt

½ teaspoon black pepper

¼ teaspoon red pepper flakes
    (optional)

PER SERVING (2 TABLESPOONS):
Calories: 127, **Protein:** 1.8 g, **Fat:** 10.5 g,
Carbohydrates: 7.6 g, **Fiber:** 1.2 g,
Cholesterol: 0 mg

Dedication

From: Elaine Johnson
To: My beautiful daughter,
Persephone Rose

Enjoy this delicious homemade version of the popular commercial dressing, believed to be a San Francisco invention from 1923. Play with your own herb combinations and make it more or less garlicky.

DIRECTIONS

- In a food processor or blender (high-speed or regular), add the fresh herbs, and mince them up. Add the garlic cloves to help them along.
- Next, add the tahini, vinegar, lemon juice, ¼ cup of water, agave nectar or maple syrup, olive oil, herbs, salt, pepper, and pepper flakes (if using).
- Blend well (at least one minute) until the dressing is emulsified and very green. Check thickness, and add the remaining ¼ cup of water (or more) if the dressing is not thin enough to pour.
- This dressing will keep well in the refrigerator for several days, though it may become discolored over time.

Suggestion for Serving

Pair with your favorite salad greens; my favorite are arugula (rocket) or coarsely chopped curly or lacinato kale. Massage the kale with your hands for about 5 minutes to tenderize the leaves and make them less bitter. Add tomatoes, avocados, carrots, bell peppers, sunflower seeds, and other favorite raw veggies, nuts, and seeds.

FOR YOUR MODIFICATION

I've left out the oil with great results. Feel free to do the same.

Broccoli Slaw

YIELD 4 cups **ALLERGY** Soy-free, wheat-free, gluten-free

INGREDIENTS

2 cups (200 g) shredded broccoli
stems (3 to 4 large stems)

1 cup (90 g) shredded carrots
(2 to 3 medium carrots)

½ cup (50 g) shredded fennel
bulbs (1 medium bulb)

1 red bell pepper, cut in thin
2-inch julienne

¼ to ½ cup (10 g to 20 g)
chopped cilantro or parsley

2 tablespoons chopped mint leaves

½ to 1 serrano chile, minced (and
seeded if you want less heat)

3 to 4 tablespoons seasoned
rice vinegar

1½ to 2 tablespoons toasted
sesame oil

1 teaspoon Dijon mustard

2 teaspoons minced or grated
fresh ginger

1 medium garlic clove, minced

Salt, to taste

2 tablespoons black sesame
seeds (optional)

PER SERVING (1 CUP):
Calories: 134, **Protein:** 3.2 g, **Fat:** 9 g,
Carbohydrates: 10 g, **Fiber:** 4 g,
Cholesterol: 0 mg

Turn to this recipe when you cook with broccoli and don't want to simply discard the nutritious and delicious thick stems!

DIRECTIONS

◗ In a large bowl, combine the shredded broccoli, shredded carrots, shredded fennel, julienned bell pepper, cilantro or parsley, mint, and chile, and toss together until well combined.

◗ In a separate bowl, whisk together the vinegar, sesame oil, mustard, ginger, garlic, and salt, to taste.

◗ Pour the dressing into the bowl with the shredded vegetable mixture, and toss to thoroughly combine. Serve right away, or refrigerate until ready to serve. It will keep well in the refrigerator for 2 days. More than that, and it will lose its crunch. Alternatively, you may refrigerate the vegetables separate from the dressing, and only toss them together before you're ready to serve, at which point you can add a sprinkling of the sesame seeds to each serving.

FOR YOUR EDIFICATION

The easiest way to shred the broccoli stems is to cut off the florets (and use for another recipe or store in fridge for future use), cut off the tough bottom tip, then rinse and pat dry. Using a standard vegetable peeler, peel away the skin as you would a carrot. (I recommend discarding the top layer you peel away, as it's the toughest layer.) You may want to cut the shreds in half before tossing them into your bowl, but it depends on how long and wide they are.

Dedication

From: Lindsay Hazelett-Cordner
To: Our beloved companion,
Miss Mackey

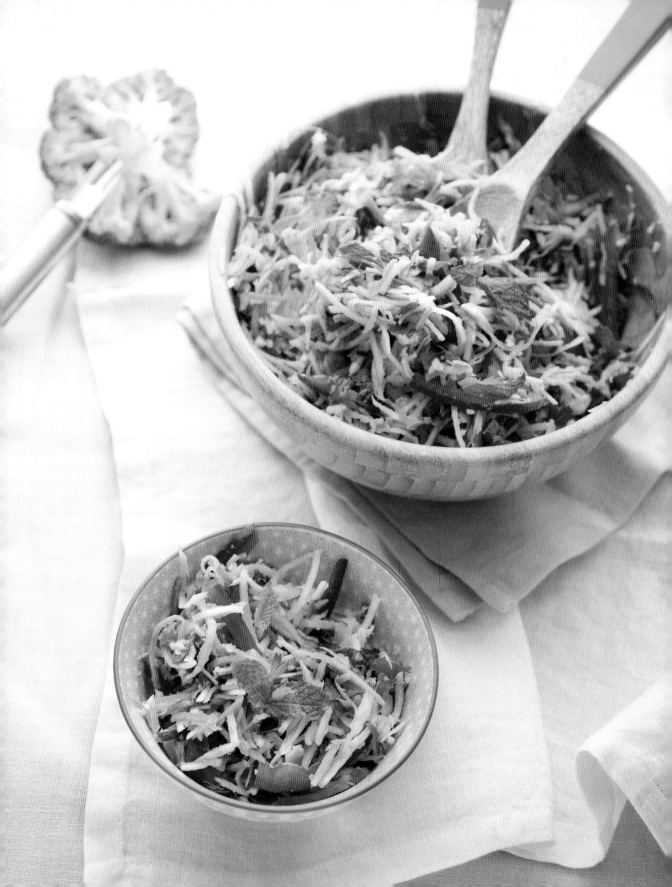

Hazlenut Milk

Soy Milk

Rice Milk

Almond Milk

Plant-Based Milks: Ancient Beverages

You're at the beginning of your third week of the Challenge, and surely, by now you've seen all the plant-based milks on the market. I imagine you've even bought one or two. Plant-based milks have no saturated fat, no cholesterol, no lactose, and no casein; have been around for centuries; and are delicious, nutritious, and widely available. Understanding their history, as well as how we became so dependent on animal milk, will help ground you in your new habit.

> **CHALLENGE YOUR THINKING:**
> Animal-based milks became the imposter, the "alternative," the substitute for what is indisputably the most natural, nutrient-rich substance for humans to consume in our developing years: human milk.

People tend to refer to plant-based milks as "alternatives to" or "substitutes for" animal-based milks, and the dairy industry rather scathingly calls them "imitation milks." In fact, the National Milk Producers Federation has been trying for years to make it illegal for nondairy milk companies to use the word "milk," claiming they have proprietary ownership of that word.[50] Just try telling a lactating mother she has to call her milk "breast beverage"!

The words "alternative" and "substitute" imply that the thing they are being measured against is superior—that you choose the "substitute" when you can't get the "real thing." By that definition, when you examine our history and physiology, it's clear that cow's and other non-human-animal milks displaced human milk. In other words, animal milk is the imposter, the "substitute," and the "alternative" to what is indisputably the most natural, nutrient-rich substance for humans to consume in our developing years: human milk.

The only reason female mammals lactate is to feed their young. The milk their bodies produce is meant for the baby who has been growing inside of them. Lactation is stimulated by pregnancy—for *all* mammals. (The word literally refers to the milk-producing mammary glands all mammals share.) Depending on the species of animal, at a certain age, infants are weaned; that is, they move from mother's milk to solid food to get their nutrients. This is the natural progression of things. However, in the case of humans:

after we're weaned, we're sold the idea that we should then switch to the milk of another animal—even though the offspring of that other animal—whether they're calves, kids, or lambs—stop drinking their mother's milk once they're weaned and developing into adults.

Just as other species don't drink their own species milk into adulthood, neither do we. At the very idea of consuming our own human milk or any foods derived from it (ice cream, cheese, sour cream), people wrinkle up their noses in disgust. In fact, I see similar sneers at the suggestion that humans drink rat's milk or cat's milk or dog's milk. Cow's milk, goat's milk, and sheep's milk? No problem. But dog's milk? "That's just disgusting," folks think.

Perhaps we have to ask ourselves why we reject consuming the lactation fluid of some species but accept consuming that of another. After all, rat, cat, and dog milk is very nutritious. Why haven't we tried them?

Could it be because we recognize—instinctively and without marketing manipulation—that rat's milk is made for baby rats, cat's milk is made for kittens, and dog's milk is made for puppies? Could it be because we concede that animal's milk is indeed very nutritious—for the offspring of the respective species and even then only up until a certain age?

And, because a mammal cannot lactate without being pregnant (and subsequently giving birth), it's important to point out that the offspring of a dairy cow (or goat or sheep) is merely incidental; he or she is simply the consequence of a pregnancy that is required to keep the animal lactating. Every year, almost 800,000 male calves born to dairy cows in the U.S. are slaughtered and sold as "veal"—all for a product that is definitely not necessary for humans to consume.

CHALLENGE YOUR THINKING:
Cow's milk was chosen because of the nature of the animals—not because of the quality of the milk. Humans have no more nutritional requirements for cow's milk than they do for rat's milk.

CHALLENGE YOUR THINKING:
The offspring of a dairy cow is merely incidental; he or she is simply the consequence of a pregnancy that is required to keep the animal lactating.

The situation is similar for dairy goats, though they have a shorter gestation period—about five months. They are milked for seven to eight months, re-seminated, and milked another two to three months. Males are unwanted and sold to slaughter, and goat pregnancies are doubly problematic, because twin births are common, resulting in more unwanted lives and thus more slaughter.

By foregoing animal milk, we turn to plant-based milks, which have been around for centuries and which vary according to where you are in the world. Though water is really the only beverage we have a physiological need for (beyond mother's milk when we're young), it is certainly convenient and tasty to be able to make creamy, nutrient-rich milk from nuts (almonds, hazelnuts, peanuts, and cashews), grains (oats and rice), legumes (soybeans and peanuts), and seeds (coconut, hemp, and sunflower).

Whether your decision to wean off animal milk is based on your compassion or your health or both, there are several facts to consider when choosing which plant-based milk is right for you:

- All of these milks will taste different to you if you compare them to what you've always known. This is why I don't recommend doing a side-by-side comparison of the cow's milk you've been drinking for decades and the almond milk you've never tried. Give your taste buds a chance to adjust and resist the temptation to judge the new milks as "inferior" just because they're unfamiliar to you.

- Variety in our diets is ideal for a number of reasons, not the least of which is allergy-avoidance. Too much of one thing can create an allergy, so don't just drink one type of milk—vary them.

- Different types and brands of milk vary in terms of taste and texture, so if you don't like one, don't throw the baby out with the bathwater and reject the whole lot. Try another.

- All of the plant-based milks are interchangeable (with the exception of coconut milk that comes in a can, which is not drunk as a beverage but rather is used to make Asian curries or for baking). However, So Delicious has a coconut milk *beverage* that is delicious.

- Some milks are creamier than others; the thinnest of the bunch is rice milk, so it's the one I tend not to use when I need a thick milk. Oat, almond, and soy are the thickest.

- As with cow's milk, plant-based milks are fortified with calcium, B_{12}, and vitamin D. Check the package to be sure.

- Most plant milks come in plain, vanilla, and chocolate—and some are unsweetened. Many brands also have special flavors such as hazelnut, mocha, and "nogs," which are very popular in the winter holidays.

- Many plant-based creamers are available, too!

Find plant-based milks either in the refrigerated section of the grocery store or on the shelf, packaged in aseptic cardboard boxes that don't require refrigeration until they're opened.

One more thing to keep in mind: because of clever marketing language, many people believe they're drinking low-fat cow's milk when they choose 1% and 2% versions. Although it's true that only 2% of the total *volume* of "2% milk" is fat (milk is mostly water), in reality, relative to total calories, the true percentage of fat in "2% cow's milk" is 35%; in "1% cow's milk", it's 20% fat.

> **CHALLENGE YOUR THINKING:** The true percentage of fat in "2% cow's milk" is 35%; in "1% cow's milk," it's 20% fat.

PLANT MILKS

Soy Milk

The most known of the bunch, soy milk originated in China thousands of years ago and was used long before we have written records to document the precise "day of discovery." You can certainly buy a soy milk maker and create your own milk at home by boiling and straining soybeans. It's simple but time-consuming. However, many commercial brands and varieties are available—including unsweetened, vanilla, plain, chocolate, and a thicker "creamer" that comes in many different flavors that people enjoy adding to their coffee or tea.

Almond Milk

Used widely in the Middle Ages in regions stretching from the Iberian Peninsula to East Asia, almond milk has always been valued for its protein content and for its ability to be preserved better than animal-based milk, which went bad if not used in a short amount of time. Almond milk is easy to make at home (see page 207 for recipe).

Rice Milk

Most commercial brands of rice milk are made from brown rice, and of course, there is a variety of flavors to choose from: plain, vanilla, chocolate, and unsweetened.

Coconut Milk

Coconut milk is what we typically call the sweet, thick, white liquid derived from the meat of a mature coconut and, with the exception of a coconut-milk-based beverage made by Turtle Mountain Foods, is often used for cooking (such as for making Thai curries) and not for drinking. Different from *either* of these, the juice of the young coconut is coconut water and drunk as a beverage. It's naturally fat-free and low in calories with high nutrition content. You'll often see coconut water served right in the coconut itself with a straw in restaurants specializing in Thai, Burmese, and Vietnamese cuisines).

>   **NOTE:** *If you love the coconut flavor but don't want the fat that is part of canned coconut milk, add a few drops of coconut extract to your favorite plant-based milk.*

Hemp Milk

Hemp milk is made from soaked hemp seeds, yielding a creamy, nutty-tasting beverage. Aside from healthful vitamins and minerals, hemp milk also boasts a high amount of essential fatty acids and poses no allergic threat.

Other Plant Milks

Other commercial plant milks include cashew, hazelnut, oat, peanut, and sunflower, and they're all delicious. Of course, you can also make any of these at home, and aside from recipes I have in previous books, you can find recipes and guidance online.

Whether you make your own or buy your favorite commercial version, you can congratulate yourself for finally being weaned! It's one of the first signs that we're growing up—healthy and strong.

Homemade Almond Milk

YIELD Makes 4 cups **ALLERGY** Soy-free, oil-free, gluten-free, wheat-free

INGREDIENTS

1 cup (170 g) of raw almonds

3 cups (720 ml) water for soaking the almonds

4 cups (960 ml) water for blending the almonds

PER SERVING (1 CUP):
Calories: 35.0, **Protein:** 1.3 g, **Fat:** 3.0 g, **Carbohydrates:** 1.3 g, **Fiber:** 0.8 g, **Cholesterol:** 0 mg

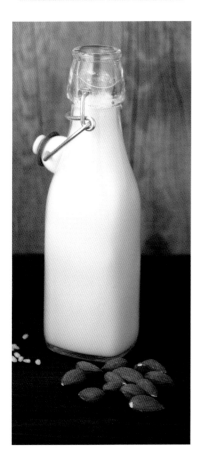

Although there are some wonderful commercial brands available, there's truly nothing like homemade, and you need no special equipment. For coffee drinkers, this is an ideal creamer and froths up beautifully when making lattes.

DIRECTIONS

- Soak the almonds (with the skins on) in the three cups of water for 8 to 10 hours, or up to two days. (Refrigerate if soaking over 8 hours.)
- Drain and rinse the almonds and place them in a high-powered blender with the four cups of water. Blend well until the mixture is white and creamy and there are no visible particles of almond in the liquid, 3 to 4 minutes on high.
- Strain through a nut milk bag or fine cheesecloth, squeezing as much milk out of the pulp as possible. The milk will keep in the refrigerator for 4 days and is fantastic on cereal or in coffee, tea, smoothies, and oatmeal.

FOR YOUR EDIFICATION

The pulp can be dried in a 200°F oven until crumbly and processed into a powder in a food processer. It can then be used as breading for tofu or tempeh, or added into muffins or cookies.

FOR YOUR INFORMATION

Once you blend the water and almonds, you will have a thick milk, but you still must strain out the pulp, or your milk will be bitter.

Demystifying Tofu: It's Just a Bean!

Having talked about plant milks, including soy milk, it makes sense to spend some time addressing one of the most popular foods made from a plant-based milk: tofu. Hopefully, by this time in *The 30-Day Vegan Challenge*, you're experimenting with new foods and exploring new vegetables, fruits, and grains. You're probably aware that tofu is an option, and maybe you've ordered it in restaurants but are intimidated by the idea of cooking it yourself. Perhaps you've tried tofu but didn't like it. If so, I encourage you to try it again. Many who don't like tofu tend to have a problem with the texture, but it's important to understand that not all tofu is created equally. There is a huge variety of brands and many different textures.

Although the public tends to associate tofu with vegans and vegetarians, as if it's reserved only for these groups, eating tofu is certainly not a prerequisite to being vegan, but if you've been holding off preparing it yourself for one reason or another, I want to try to demystify this wonderful albeit misunderstood food!

CHALLENGE YOUR THINKING: Casein, the protein in animal milk, is considered a cancer-causing substance; i.e. a carcinogen, by the researchers who organized the largest epidemiological study ever conducted on the relationship between food and health/disease. 80%-87% of the proteins in cow's milk are proteins, and in cheese, it's even more concentrated.

An ancient food, tofu originated in China about 2,000 years ago. While the details of its discovery are uncertain, legend has it that it was discovered by accident when a Chinese cook added nigari seaweed to a pot of soy milk, causing it to curdle, and the result was tofu. Tofu was introduced into Japan in the 8th century, where it was known as "okabe" until the 15th century, though it didn't gain widespread popularity in Japan until the 17th century.

Tofu's rise in the West mirrored the increasing interest in healthier foods. First gaining attention during the 1960s, tofu has been skyrocketing in popularity ever since research began to reveal the many significant benefits of this delicious legume-based food.

DEMYSTIFYING THE BIG WHITE BLOB

Tofu is produced in much the same way as cheese. First, you start with milk. In the case of dairy-based cheese, that milk is from a pregnant female, but the origins of tofu are much more simple, humane, and healthful. You start with a soybean and make milk by soaking, grinding, boiling, and straining dried soybeans.

Once you have your soy milk, next you add a coagulant. When you *coagulate* something, you cause it to *curdle*. In other words, you transform it from a liquid into a soft semisolid or solid mass. Most of us have seen curdling when cow's milk starts to go off and you see little semi-solid white lumps floating around. Those are curds. That particular process of curdling indicates that the milk is spoiling—that it's turning *sour*.

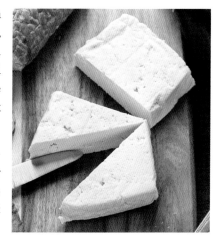

But, there are ways to sour milk intentionally. You do this by adding an agent that will produce the souring effect, such as vinegar or lemon juice. Just squeeze some lemon juice or vinegar into nondairy milk (about 1 tablespoon per 1 cup), and you have what is considered "buttermilk."

The commercial tofu industry, however, uses other coagulants to curdle their milk, and we'll get to those in a moment. First, for the purposes of comparison, let's look at what is used to curdle cow's milk for the making of dairy-based cheese: rennet. Rennet is essentially a bunch of enzymes produced in the stomach of mammals to help the respective offspring digest his or her mother's milk. One of these enzymes causes the milk to coagulate—to *curdle* or separate into solids (*curds*) and liquid (*whey*).

What's actually happening is that the milk proteins, called caseins, are tangling up into solid masses or *curds*. What remains are whey proteins. In cow's milk, 80%-87% of these proteins are caseins. According to the results of the largest and longest research project ever conducted on the relationship between food and health (The China Study), casein is the *number one carcinogen* (i.e. cancer-causing substance) that people encounter on a daily basis.[51] Considering how much cow's milk and dairy-based cheese people are consuming, these findings should compel us to sit up and take notice.

Though vegetarian rennet is sometimes used in the production of kosher cheeses, nearly all of them are produced with either microbial rennet or genetically modified rennet. Microbial rennet is produced by using certain fermented molds that apparently results in a slightly bitter-tasting cheese, which is unfavorable to many.

However, with the development of genetic engineering, scientists started using calf genes to modify bacteria, fungus, or yeast to make them produce chymosin, one of the first artificially produced enzymes to be registered and allowed by the FDA in the USA. In 1999, about 60% of U.S. hard cheese was made with genetically engineered chymosin. And, people turn their noses up at tofu! If you're eating animal-based cheese, either you're consuming enzymes extracted from dead baby calves, or you're consuming genetically engineered enzymes originated from the genes of dead calves.

If you eat tofu, you're consuming the milk from soaked beans and one of two types of coagulants.

SALT COAGULANTS: An example of a salt-based coagulant is calcium sulfate, which is essentially tasteless. Tofu that's made with calcium sulfate is obviously rich in calcium. Other salt coagulants used are nigari salts, such as magnesium chloride and calcium chloride. Calcium chloride is a common coagulant for tofu in North America. You'll recognize this coagulant on the list of ingredients, because it will most likely say *nigari*.

ACID COAGULANTS: Although it sounds scary, glucono delta-lactone (GDL) is a naturally occurring organic acid, and is used as the coagulant for silken tofu producing a very fine-textured tofu that is almost custard-like.

Tofu producers may choose to use one or more of these coagulants, as they each play a role in producing a desired texture in the finished tofu. So, when you notice a different taste or texture in tofu depending on the brand, a lot of this depends on the coagulant used.

Once you have your curds, you press them. The curds are processed differently depending on the form of tofu being made. For silken/soft tofu, the soy milk is curdled directly in the tofu's selling package. For standard firm Asian tofu, the soy curd is cut, strained of excess liquid using muslin, and then lightly pressed to produce a soft cake. Firmer tofu is further pressed to remove even more liquid.

TEXTURE VARIETIES

People's heads tend to spin as they scan the shelves of silken, soft, medium, firm, extra firm, and super firm tofu. What about these varying textures and when do you use which one?

SOFT/SILKEN

The texture of soft and silken tofu is similar to that of very fine custard. You use this type of tofu when you want to make something creamy, such as mousses, pie fillings, and puddings. You can also use it for salad dressings and sauces, and silken tofu also works great in baked goods instead of using chicken's eggs. See Day 14: Baking Without Eggs (It's Better!).

In the grocery store, you'll find silken tofu in an aseptic cardboard (vacuum-packed) box most likely in the Asian foods aisle—*not* in the refrigerated case with the fresh tofu. *Mori-nu* is the most common brand of this type, and it can be stored in your cupboard for up to a year—unless you open it. Then it needs refrigeration.

It can start to get confusing when you look at the little box of silken tofu and notice that—even though it says "silken," it will also say "soft," "firm," or "extra firm." These are just degrees within the texture of silken tofu itself. But, heed my warning: even if it says "extra firm" on the box, this is not the type of tofu you can grill or stir-fry; it's much too soft and crumbly for such a purpose. Recipes will typically specify which variation of silken is called for, but "silken firm" is a good middle-of-the-road bet when you're not sure.

> **NOTE:** *"Soft" tofu is similar to silken and found in water-filled tubs in the refrigerated case of the grocery store.*

FIRM/EXTRA FIRM TOFU

Choosing the texture that is appropriate for the dish you're making is the key to enjoying tofu. It needs to satisfy the mouthfeel you're aiming for, whether it's creaminess or chewiness.

SUPER FIRM TOFU

Yes, there's even super firm, which is—well—super firm! The brand that originated this texture is Wildwood, and while they offer *regular* firm and *extra* firm, they also make *super* firm tofu, which absolutely satisfies the desire for a hearty, dense texture. Although it is carried by major national grocery store chains throughout the U.S., it's also worth noting that as of this writing, Trader Joe's private-labels Wildwood's super firm tofu under the Trader Joe's brand, and so it might be easier to find if you have a TJ's near you.

Here are some ways to use firm and super firm tofu:

- ▶ Cut the tofu into cubes or simply crumble it up; add it to your favorite green salad, and toss.
- ▶ Crumble it, add it to a sauté pan, and add taco seasonings. Cook, and fill soft or hard taco shells.
- ▶ Crumble it up; add it to a sauté pan, along with salt, cumin, and turmeric for a tofu scramble. (See page 117 for Tofu, Mushroom, and Sausage Scramble.)
- ▶ Cube or slice it, and add it to a vegetable stir-fry.
- ▶ Slice it up, then grill, broil, or bake it.

Delicious as firm and super firm tofu is, there's a way to transform it to make it even better—in my opinion. You freeze it.

FREEZING TOFU

You've probably heard of "pressing tofu." You wrap a block of tofu in a towel, press something heavy on it, and allow some time (about 20 minutes) for the water to come out of the tofu and into the towel. Pressing out water means you create room for another marinade to soak in, but you'll never get as much water out of tofu pressing it as you would freezing it. Besides, freezing tofu will change your life! Well, it will at least change your experience and perception—as well as the texture—of tofu.

This procedure does not apply to silken tofu—only firm: regular firm, extra firm, and super firm. You will find all of these in the refrigerated section of the grocery store, and each of them will be either water-packed in a tub or water-packed in a vacuum-sealed package. Upon arriving home with your tofu, put it directly in the freezer. Do not open it. Do not transfer it to another container. Nothing. Simply put it in the freezer unopened. To get the best results for our purposes, let it freeze for a minimum of 24 hours (but you can leave tofu in the freezer for several months). I always buy more than I need so I have frozen tofu at all times!

When it comes time to use it (and you're planning in advance as recommended in Day 7, right?), take it out of the freezer, place it on a plate or towel, and thaw it on a towel on the counter for about four or five hours. (It thaws faster on the counter than in the refrigerator).

Now, for the life-altering (or at least tofu-altering) moment! Make sure the tofu is completely thawed (squeeze the center to be sure), and open the package. Holding the block of tofu over the sink, squeeze! As with a sponge, water will come gushing out of the tofu like a waterfall.

So what?

Because tofu—a water-based food—is so porous, by releasing all that water, you have not only dried it out somewhat, you have also created thousands of empty little pores (you can easily see them). That means you have all this room now for another liquid—such as a marinade—to soak into the tofu. That means a lot more flavor. Also, by freezing it, thawing it, and squeezing out the water, you've also altered the texture and mouth-feel of the tofu. Although I praise the super firm tofu for its hearty texture, thawed tofu is not only heartier, it's also chewier, and that is exactly the kind of texture so many of us associate with a very satisfying mouthfeel.

You can do everything to thawed tofu that you can do to tofu you didn't freeze and thaw (see ideas above). You can grill it, bake it, marinate it, sauté it, cut it up and add to a green salad, or crumble or cube it and add it to a pasta sauce or chili, or crumble and salt it to use it as feta on a Greek salad. Thawed tofu is more delicate than regular tofu, though, and it can fall apart easily. If you are going to try to keep it in tact by slicing or cubing it, you'll just want to handle it more carefully. If you're going to crumble it up, it doesn't matter how you handle it.

The more you use tofu, the more comfortable you become, and the more you understand what textures and brands work best for your purposes. Certainly, you can just use whatever type of tofu a recipe calls for, but to really learn the nuances between all the different types of tofu, the secret is first thinking about what your ultimate goal is.

For instance,

- If you want hearty tofu steaks that you marinate with BBQ sauce and throw on the grill, the firmest tofu you can find is best (extra or super firm).

- If you're making a tofu scramble (see recipe on page 117) you will want to use extra firm or super firm tofu. You don't want it to be super chewy (so you don't want to use frozen/thawed tofu), and you don't want it to by silky smooth (so you wouldn't want to use silken).

You want it to have the movement and texture we associate with scrambled chicken's eggs, which is why you'd want firm or extra firm. (I find that a combination of extra and super works really well, but if you can't find super firm, extra firm on its own is just fine.)

- If you're making a tofu "egg" salad (like my Better Than Egg Salad in *The Vegan Table),* you want it textured like hardboiled eggs, such as from extra firm or super firm tofu.

- If you are sautéing tofu as part of a stir-fry, you want to use extra firm tofu or super firm tofu to hold up to the spatula abuse the tofu will take during the sautéing process. (Frozen/thawed is great for a stir-fry, as well.)

- Extra or super firm tofu is also best for Thai curry.

- For tofu ricotta, a firm or extra firm tofu is ideal.

DON'T FEAR THE BEAN

The soybean was once the darling of health food proponents, but lately there has been quite a backlash against this innocent bean, and I wanted to take a moment to address this. As I said above, if you don't like foods made from soybeans or the beans themselves, you don't have to eat them. If you have an allergy to soybeans, of course, you shouldn't eat them. But, the way a few individuals have been spreading their anti-soy rhetoric, you'd think the soybean was threatening the very survival of the human species. Soy naysayers have claimed that soy causes thyroid problems, birth defects, male reproductive problems, nutritional deficiencies, certain cancers, and cognitive dysfunction. In summary, ***the negative claims about soy do not hold up in peer-reviewed studies (where they even exist). The overwhelming scientific research on soy is positive and concludes that soy is either neutral or is beneficial—not harmful.***

The other accusation leveled at soy is that it is responsible for the destruction of the rainforests in South America and that as a genetically modified crop it should be avoided. Actually, both of these statements are partially true—but for soybeans fed to livestock, not the soybeans being grown for tofu or soy milk. The majority of soybeans grown in the world are fed to livestock, who are then turned into meat; the destruction is being caused by the meat industry—not the makers of tofu! I recommend to always buy organic soy foods, most of which are from beans grown in the United States. (You can find out yourself by contacting the company or by looking at the label). And, currently, foods labeled "USDA-certified organic" must also be free of genetically modified organisms (GMO). The point is: tofu is not responsible for the devastating rainforest loss; animal agriculture is.

From a broader perspective, let's remember:

1. Soy is neither miracle food nor is it poison. We're talking about a bean. It's not a toxin. It's not a chemical. It's not a weapon. It's also not a panacea. It's a bean, a legume, a plant food that—like all other plant foods—contains health-promoting properties.

2. Eat foods—all foods, including soybean-based foods—in their whole state. One of the criticisms about soy is that it is processed and that it shows up in so many processed foods such as energy bars, cookies, and vegan meats. It's true that concentrated soy protein—often appearing as "soy protein isolate" on labels—is processed, but that's not characteristic of the whole soybean. Extracting a single beneficial component from a food, sticking it in a product, and labeling that product "healthy" is certainly problematic. The complexity in whole plant foods extends far beyond what we can replicate in a lab, and the health benefits of these whole foods stem from the combination of all of their components eaten at once in their *whole* state.

In other words, the problem isn't *soy*. The problem is heavily *processed food*. There's a big difference between eating processed foods made with soy protein isolate and eating whole or minimally processed soy foods, such as the soybeans themselves, soybean sprouts, edamame, tempeh, miso, tofu, and soy milk. Yuba, essentially the skin of steamed soy milk, can also be enjoyed in a whole foods diet, as can be tamari soy sauce as a condiment.

Does mean we should never eat soy cheese on our pizza, vegan hot dogs at a baseball game, or energy bars on a hike? In my opinion, no. I don't think it's realistic or necessary to make our goal "never eat processed foods." However, I do recommend that we base our diets on whole foods and eat *highly* processed foods (those so far from their natural state that the complexity of their nutrition has been lost) in smaller amounts.

I make this distinction between "processed" and "highly processed" foods, because there is a very wide range when it comes to "processed foods." For instance, blueberries plucked off their vines and frozen, apples picked from their trees and turned into applesauce, garbanzo beans cooked and mashed to make hummus, and peanuts ground down into butter—are all processed foods. But, is there something inherently wrong with frozen berries, applesauce, hummus, or peanut butter? No! If you blend a fruit smoothie, can some beans, or dehydrate kale, you're *processing* the foods from their original state to a different one. But, there's nothing wrong with blended fruit, canned beans, and dehydrated kale chips. Eating foods in their different states brings pleasure and variety to our lives.

We can certainly exercise our right to avoid highly processed foods, but scapegoating one component of these products (soy isolate protein) and thus demonizing the original food (soybean) makes no sense.

In addition to the Tofu Cacciatore on page 215, try the Tofu, Mushroom, and Sausage Scramble on page 117.

Tofu Cacciatore

YIELD 2 servings **ALLERGY** Gluten-free, wheat-free

INGREDIENTS

1 pound extra firm tofu, frozen
and thawed

3 tablespoons olive oil, divided

½ teaspoon salt, divided

¼ teaspoon freshly ground
pepper, plus more to taste

3 carrots, cut into thin slices

1 small yellow onion, cut into
thin slices

1 large red bell pepper, cut into
thin slices

3 garlic cloves, finely chopped

½ cup (120 ml) dry white wine

1 25-ounce jar tomato sauce
(about 3 cups or 800 ml)

3 tablespoons drained capers

1½ teaspoons dried oregano leaves

⅛ to ¼ teaspoon red pepper flakes

¼ cup (57 g) coarsely chopped
fresh basil leaves (optional)

Salt and pepper, to taste

PER SERVING
Calories: 611.0, **Protein:** 31.0 g, **Fat:** 33.5 g,
Carbohydrates: 43.6 g, **Fiber:** 13.1 g,
Cholesterol: 0 mg

This Cacciatore is much healthier, much cleaner, and much more compassionate than the version made with chicken. The trick is using tofu that has been frozen and thawed; it yields an incredibly satisfying chewy texture. (See the earlier part of this chapter for directions on freezing and thawing tofu.)

Note: *Be sure to take your tofu out of the freezer and have it thawed by the time you're ready to cook. Also if you plan on serving this with rice or pasta, you'll want to start cooking those as you start preparing this dish.*

DIRECTIONS

◯ Holding the tofu over the sink or a bowl, gently squeeze out all of the water. Transfer the block of tofu to a cutting board and cut into 1½-inch-long slices.

◯ Sprinkle the tofu pieces with ¼ teaspoon of each salt and pepper. Gently toss to combine.

◯ In a large heavy sauté pan, heat 2 tablespoons of the oil over a medium-high flame. Add the tofu pieces to the pan and sauté just until golden brown and crispy, about 5 to 7 minutes per side. Transfer the tofu slices to a plate, and set aside.

◯ Add the carrot slices, onion, bell pepper, and garlic to the same pan, along with the remaining tablespoon of olive oil. Sauté over medium heat until the vegetables are tender but still crispy, about 5 minutes. Take care not to over-cook the peppers and carrots, or they'll be too soft. Season with a pinch of salt and pepper.

◯ Add the wine and simmer until reduced by half, about 5 minutes. Add the tomato sauce, capers, oregano, and red pepper flakes. Return the tofu to the pan and turn them to coat in the sauce. Bring the sauce to a simmer, turning the heat down to medium-low. Continue simmering until the tofu and veggies are heated through, about 5 minutes.

◯ Serve on its own as a main dish, along with salad and veggies on the side or over spaghetti, penne pasta, or even brown rice. Top with chopped basil, and sprinkle with additional salt and pepper, if desired.

Putting to Rest the Great Protein Myth

If I had a nickel for every time someone asked me, "Where do you get your protein?" I would be a very wealthy vegan—and so would every other vegan, because it's the most commonly asked question.

I certainly applaud people for asking questions about health and nutrition, but we need to get away from the idea that vegans have to eat one way and nonvegans have to eat another way. The fact is *we all* need to make sure we're getting the nutrients we require not only to be healthy but also to thrive. Despite all the advanced medical training and technology in "developed" nations, millions of people are suffering and dying from what are mostly *preventable* diseases. There is a lot we can do to improve our health, so certainly *everyone* should be asking questions about how to do better—not just once you consider going vegan.

When it comes to protein, the idea that we can't get enough on a vegan diet is simply not true, as emphasized by the American Dietetic Association's (ADA) position paper on vegetarianism:

> *Plant protein can meet requirements when a variety of plant foods are consumed and energy needs are met.*

Breaking this down, what does it mean to consume a "variety of plant foods" and meet your energy needs? The first one is self-explanatory. The idea is to enjoy a variety of plant foods throughout the day: vegetables, fruits, grains, nuts, seeds, and legumes. Aside from meeting your protein needs, you will also be taking in a number other essential and healthful vitamins, minerals, and phytochemicals. Variety is the key.

As far as meeting energy needs, that is just a different way of saying you need to take in the adequate number of calories for your body type, weight, and lifestyle, and this pertains to vegans and nonvegans. I think this is vital to understanding the transition that takes place from eating an animal-based diet to a plant-based diet. Because of the nutrient profile of animal products versus plant foods, when you become vegan, you very naturally consume fewer calories because plants are much less calorie dense than animal flesh and fluids. (Read more about this on Day 27: Understanding Weight Loss.)

This is not necessarily a bad thing. Many, many people are consuming far more calories than they're expending each day, so they would do well to reduce their caloric intake. And, since they're consuming so many calories—the majority of which are from animal products—they're also far exceeding their protein needs. And that is not necessarily a *good* thing. So, when they switch to a plant-based diet and consume fewer calories and thus less (animal-based) protein, they mistakenly perceive that as a negative thing. After all, we live in a society where "more" is better.

What I suggest is that we keep things in perspective and understand that everything is relative. Consuming fewer calories and thus less protein when you become vegan is natural and—if weight loss is something you strive for—even optimal. Consuming no animal protein is also optimal, as we have no nutritional need for it. Now, in terms of specific ways in which people would *not* actually meet their protein needs, we see it only in a few scenarios; again, this is the case whether you're vegan or not.

1. You stop eating. People who suffer from anorexia, depression, extreme poverty, severe illness, or extreme dieting don't meet their energy needs, because they're not eating! If they're not eating, they aren't getting enough protein—or other macronutrients and micronutrients.

2. You are an endurance athlete and do not increase your caloric intake. When you increase your calorie expenditure to the degree that endurance athletes do, you absolutely must also increase your calorie intake to be sure you're getting all of your nutrients, including protein.

Assuming you're taking in adequate calories, not eating low-protein/low-nutrient foods such as potato chips all day, and you're not eating a fruit-only diet, the risk of protein deficiency is a nonissue.

The simple truth is that people in developed countries tend not to suffer from diseases of deficiency, but rather diseases of excess. In fact, most people have never even met anyone with serious protein deficiency; they may have seen images from hunger organizations who show children with thinning hair and distended (swollen) bellies. *They* have protein deficiency because they're not getting enough *food*. There is even a scientific term for this; it's called kwashiorkor. It's a disease we see in countries where rampant poverty prevents people from consuming the calories and nutrients they need to survive or thrive. In industrialized nations, we do not have kwashiorkor wards in hospitals; we do not know any kwashiorkor specialists, and we probably do not have any friends—vegan or not—with kwashiorkor. But what we do have are diseases linked to our excess intake of animal protein: cancer, gout, and kidney problems such as kidney stones.[52]

The problem isn't that vegans "can't get enough protein"; the problem is that most people are consuming way more protein than they need—particularly from animal sources, and that's neither necessary nor healthful.

COMPLEMENTING YOUR PROTEIN

Regarding protein and a plant-based diet, The American Dietetic Association states:

Research indicates that an assortment of plant foods eaten over the course of a day can provide all essential amino acids; thus complementary proteins do not need to be consumed at the same meal.

One of the biggest myths about protein is that vegans (and vegetarians) have to "complement" our protein at each meal; i.e. that is, we have to *combine* certain foods to get a *complete* protein. Unfortunately, this myth started with a book whose intention was to inspire a plant-based diet. The premise of Frances Moore Lappé's 1971 book, *Diet for a Small Planet* was that we could feed a hungry world by feeding everyone a plant-based diet, eliminating the intensive, wasteful resources of animal-based agriculture. With the intention of making sure people did this healthfully, she popularized the idea of "complementary proteins."

Her recommendations were based on the fact that protein is made up of amino acids—every type of protein, whether animal- or plant-based. The body can produce *some* amino acids, and those that it cannot are considered "essential"; i.e. we must get them from food. Plant proteins have all of the essential amino acids; some foods simply have higher amounts of certain amino acids than others do. For instance, beans are lower in methionine, and grains are lower in lysine, and so the idea that became perpetuated was that we would have to consume beans and grains in one meal to get *all* the amino acids—to get a "complete protein."

We've known for decades this isn't necessary, and yet the myth persists. As long as we're eating a variety of foods throughout the day, our bodies are smart enough to assimilate and store the amino acids we need.

HOW MUCH PROTEIN DO WE NEED?

Taking into account our various body sizes and activity levels, you can calculate for yourself your optimum intake. *Current guidelines recommend that adults eat 0.36 grams of protein per day for every pound of healthy body weight.*[53] Infants, children, competitive athletes, pregnant, and nursing women require more protein. Infants, children, competitive athletes, and pregnant and nursing women require more protein. (See Day 23 for specifics.) If you want to be even more precise, many experts suggest adding 10 percent to these recommendations for vegans, since the digestibility of protein in plant foods is slightly reduced.

PROTEIN IN PLANT FOODS

Though we've all been indoctrinated to believe that meat, dairy, and eggs are the only sources of protein, the fact is that protein is plentiful in plants. Certainly, some plants contain more protein than others do, but many grains and vegetables contribute a significant amount of protein to our diets. Unfortunately, we're never taught that broccoli, oatmeal, and carrots have protein, but just think for a moment about the largest, strongest land animals on the planet: giraffes, elephants, bulls, and bison. They're all vegetarian animals, and they get plenty of protein—from the plants.

Just a glance at the chart below demonstrates how easy it is to consume a healthful amount of protein each day. So next time someone says to you, "You're as strong as an ox," you can say, "Well, of course I am. I get my protein from the plants—just like the ox!"

Plant-Based Food	Protein in grams
Protein shakes (soy, rice, hemp, pea)	amount varies; check label
1 cup of firm tofu	40 g
1 cup of cooked tempeh	30 g
1 cup of cooked soybeans	29 g
1 cup of cooked lentils	18 g
1 cup of cooked pinto beans	15 g
1 cup of cooked black beans	15 g
1 cup of cooked chickpeas	15 g
3 slices veggie deli slices	14 g
¼ cup sunflower seeds	8 g
¼ cup almonds	7.4 g
8 ounces nondairy milk	5–10 g
6-ounce container soy yogurt	5–7 g
1 cup cooked corn	5.4 g
1 cup quinoa	8 g
2 tablespoons peanut butter	8 g
1 cup cooked broccoli	8 g
1 cup cooked brown rice	8 g
1 cup cooked oatmeal	7 g
1 bagel	7 g
1 medium baked potato	4.5 g
½ ounce walnuts (7 halves)	4.3 g
1 cup chopped cooked kale	2.5 g
1 cup raw spinach	1.6 g
1 medium raw carrot	0.7 g

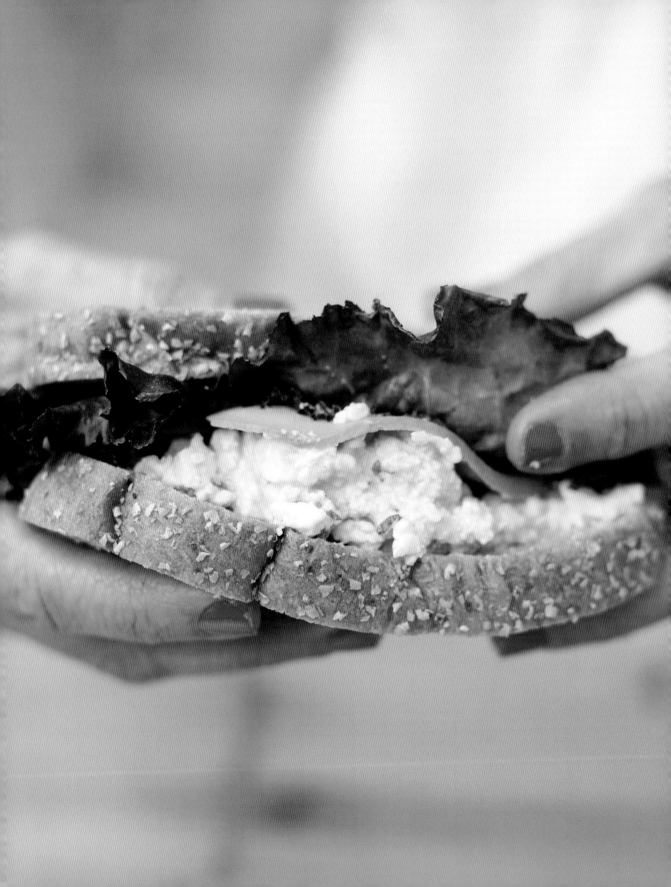

Strong Like Popeye:
Increasing Your Iron Absorption

Popeye ate spinach. Popeye was strong. Wimpy ate burgers. Wimpy was... wimpy. Popeye was onto something. Plant-based iron—not burgers—makes you strong.

Despite the pervasiveness of this muscled pop culture icon, I continue to meet people who claim to have become anemic (i.e. iron-deficient) after becoming vegetarian or vegan based on feeling fatigued. Having self-diagnosed, most of these people never actually had their iron levels checked by a doctor; they just assumed they were anemic because they were tired and because friends told them their lack of eating meat was the cause.

> **CHALLENGE YOUR THINKING:**
> Popeye ate spinach. Popeye was strong. Wimpy ate burgers. Wimpy was wimpy. Plant-based iron makes you strong—not burgers!

Having said that, iron deficiency is the most common nutrient deficiency in the United States; the typical North American diet provides only 5 to 6 mg of iron for every 1,000 calories consumed. Worldwide, it's the most prevalent nutritional deficiency, and the most susceptible are menstruating women (women of childbearing age), pregnant and lactating women, teenagers, and children aged six months to four years. This is true for vegetarians, vegans, and nonvegetarians.[54]

INCREASING ABSORPTION

Studies show little difference in the incidence of iron deficiency between vegans and nonvegetarians in developed countries. In fact, the amount of iron in vegan diets tends to be higher than or at least equal to, that in nonvegetarians diets. Why? Because almost everything that crosses a vegan's lips contains iron: beans, nuts, seeds, grains, vegetables, and fruits.

There are two different types of iron in foods: *heme* iron and *nonheme* iron. Heme iron is found in animal products; nonheme iron is found in both plant foods and animal products. After being absorbed and reaching our cells for building hemoglobin and other purposes, *our body doesn't care whether the iron was originally heme or nonheme*. So, when people assert that our bodies need *heme* iron from meat, it's simply not true. The body needs to *absorb* iron, but it ultimately doesn't matter where it originated.

CHALLENGE YOUR THINKING:
The body needs to absorb iron, but it doesn't care whether the original source of the iron was heme (animal-based) or non heme (animal- and plant-based).

CHANGE YOUR BEHAVIOR:
Eat foods rich in iron, eat foods that increase iron absorption, and when eating iron-rich foods, avoid eating them with foods that decrease iron absorption.

Dietary factors most certainly influence our body's ability to absorb iron, and it's these dietary factors we want to increase. Vegans tend to be ahead of the game because of the amount of plant foods they eat—particularly those rich in vitamin C. This is an important vitamin for many reasons, not the least of which is its ability to increase our absorption of iron; in other words, vitamin C increases the iron's *bioavailability* (our body's ability to absorb and use nutrients). Furthermore, if you cook vitamin C containing foods, such as tomatoes or lemon juice, in cast iron cookware, that also increases the iron's bioavailability.

Eating vitamin C-rich foods at the same time we eat iron-rich foods is one of the best things we can do. Fruits and vegetables are our main sources of vitamin C, with the richest being tomatoes, citrus fruits (oranges, tangerines, and grapefruit), strawberries, kiwi, papaya, green vegetables (broccoli, kale, collard greens, Swiss chard, and brussels sprouts), bell peppers (all colors), and cauliflower.

And what are some delicious ways to pair iron-rich and vitamin C-rich foods?

► Make a bean or lentil salad that includes lemon juice, chopped chard, and chopped bell peppers. Add a little seasoned rice vinegar or balsamic vinegar and some salt, and it's perfect and delicious.

► Make a kale salad and toss with a drizzle of olive oil, salt, and white beans and barley, plus slices of oranges or tomatoes!

► Bake a potato and top with sautéed onions and peppers!

There is no shortage of iron in plant foods, but some contain higher amounts than others do.

Food	Iron Content
Fortified cereals	amount varies; check label
1 can white beans	40 mg
1 cup cooked lentils	30 mg
1 cup cooked barley	29 mg
1 cup of cooked lentils	18 mg
1 cup cooked chickpeas	15 mg
1 cup cooked pinto beans	15 mg
1 tablespoon blackstrap molasses	15 mg
1 medium baked potato	14 mg
¾ cup cup cooked oatmeal	8 mg
½ cup firm tofu (brands vary; check label)	7.4 mg
½ cup cooked quinoa	5–10 mg
1 cup cooked mushrooms	5–7 mg
1 ounce pumpkin seeds	5.4 mg
3½ cups of raw broccoli	8 mg
12 dried apricots	8 mg

HOW MUCH IRON DO WE NEED?

There are some variations for babies, toddlers, and seniors, but the daily recommendation for the U.S. and Canada is 8 milligrams for adult men; 18 milligrams for adult menstruating women, and 27 milligrams for pregnant women. Neither should exceed 45 milligrams a day, as too much iron can cause hemochromatosis (iron overload), a serious disease.[55]

THINGS THAT DECREASE ABSORPTION

Just as there are things we want to do to increase absorption, there are things we want to do to avoid *decreasing* absorption. When we consume calcium supplements, coffee, or tea at the same time we eat iron-rich foods, we inhibit iron absorption. So, just avoid these things when eating iron-rich foods if you want to increase your iron absorption. The bioavailability of iron can be reduced by up to 60% by the tannins in black or green teas.

Also, there are foods that are high both in iron and in phytates that prevent absorption. These iron-rich foods include wheat bran, whole grains, and legumes. Soaking, sprouting, leavening, and fermentation of whole grains render the iron more bioavailable by degrading the phytates. While eating whole grains is desirable, we should not be sprinkling wheat bran over our food.

Finally, the other thing to consider is that vegans have a considerable advantage in the iron department not only because they eat more iron and vitamin C-rich plant foods but also because they don't eat dairy. Cow's milk—both the liquid stuff and products made from it—are poor sources of iron. They displace iron-rich foods from the diet, and the presence of cow's milk or cheese in the diet has been shown to decrease the absorption of iron from a meal by as much as 50%.[56]

WHAT TO DO IF YOUR IRON STORES ARE LOW?

Many people assume they have anemia just because they're tired, but they might be tired for a number of other reasons, such as not eating enough calories, eating too many high-sugar foods, and possibly not getting enough sleep. This doesn't mean that iron-deficiency is not real for some people, but if you're concerned, don't self-diagnose. Check with your doctor and get your iron tested.

Having said that, it's also important to understand a few things your iron status means. There are three stages of actual iron deficiency:

- The first is just iron depletion—it means your stores are low, but it doesn't affect how you feel.

- The second is iron deficiency, and you may feel tired and a sensitivity to cold.

- The third is iron deficiency anemia, and your blood hemoglobin is below the normal range. You are likely to feel exhaustion, irritability, lethargy, and headaches. Your skin may also appear pale.

If you are suffering from the symptoms of iron-deficiency, have your doctor measure your iron status. If your doctor thinks your iron stores are too low, he or she may suggest that you eat meat (which is unnecessary) or that you take an iron supplement. You might want to talk to him or her about first increasing your vitamin C intake by taking 100 milligrams of vitamin C with meals (or increasing intake of vitamin C-rich foods by 100 milligrams) twice a day for 60 days and refraining from tea and coffee during meals. If this doesn't work, then—under your doctor's guidance—you may want to take iron supplements.

Remember, there is a prevalence of iron deficiency in nonvegetarians, and though ideally, their doctors should encourage them to eat *less* meat and *more* vitamin C-rich plant foods, they usually just recommend iron supplements. They don't tell their iron-deficient meat-eating patients to eat *more* meat.

IS LOW IRON A BAD THING?

Although there is little difference in the incidence of iron deficiency between vegetarians and nonvegetarians, vegans and vegetarians do often have iron stores on the low end of the normal range. *However,* this doesn't seem to pose a problem. For those in generally good health and with abundant food available, iron stores at the low end of the normal range is just not a problem. In fact, there are a few potential upsides:

1. Low iron stores are associated with higher glucose tolerance and therefore could prevent diabetes.[57]

2. High iron stores have been linked to cancer and cardiovascular disease because of increased evidence of free radical damage. Having lower iron stores seems to protect cells from free radical damage.[58]

Consuming too much iron, particularly if you're taking a lot of it in supplement form, can be a problem. Too high an iron level can lead to zinc and copper deficiency and can cause iron overload. (Excess iron is not easily eliminated from the body.) This is one of the reasons many experts recommend getting iron from the diet rather than from multivitamins.

Skipping the Middle Fish: Getting Our Omega-3s Directly from the Source

Another nutrient—like protein and calcium—that has been touted as strictly animal-based is Omega-3 fatty acids. Fish oil supplements are flying off the shelves, and fish is routinely recommended as the best source of omega-3 fatty acids. Not only is this doing serious damage to the oceans and killing millions of marine animals each year, people are consuming mercury, other heavy metals, and a variety of environmental contaminants (PCB's DDT, dioxins, etc.).

CHALLENGE YOUR THINKING:
We absolutely do not need to eat fish to take in the healthful EPA and DHA fats. Even fish don't make these fats; they consume them through the omega-3 rich algae and phytoplankton.

CHANGE YOUR BEHAVIOR:
Do what the fish do and go to the plants for your omega-3 fatty acids.

So, if we're to take the experts' advice and get our omega-3 fatty acids from fish, we do so at the cost of damaging the oceans, killing millions of marine animals, and consuming heavy metals and other toxic chemicals—not to mention consuming unhealthful saturated fat and dietary cholesterol.

Well, that doesn't sound so good.

And so, we're offered another solution: eat farmed-raised salmon. Having pretty much wiped out the wild salmon population on the East Coast and having almost succeeded in doing the same on the West Coast, 90 percent of the salmon eaten in the United States are—in fact—raised on aquatic farms.[59] Of course, as with all animal factory systems, the fish are kept in intensive confinement where they absorb and consume antibiotics and pesticides, along with over 100 other pollutants.

Moreover, they're fed a cheap diet of what's called "fish meal," which is comprised mostly of wild-caught fish; in other words, farm-raising fish contributes to even more animals taken from the ocean. And of course both wild and farmed fish are still contaminated with heavy metals (farmed fish are, after all, eating the mercury-laden wild-caught fish), and they contain unhealthful saturated fat and dietary cholesterol.

It seems to me we have *another* option—a better option for everyone involved—for obtaining essential fatty acids. We can stop going *through* the fish to get to the nutrients that the fish get from eating plants.

Most everyone these days can tell you that they know it's important to eat omega-3 fatty acids or what they've been told are "healthful fats" or "fish fat," but not many could tell you why these fats are important or where they originate.

Omega-3 fatty acids—such as EPA and DHA—are absolutely essential for optimal health. Think reduced inflammation when you think of omega-3 fats. When you reduce inflammation—all throughout the body—blood flows beautifully and easily, keeping the various organs functioning optimally. Where there's inflammation, blood flow is hindered. So, since omega-3 fats help reduce inflammation, they help reduce the risk of atherosclerosis (heart disease and stroke); they reduce joint pain—such as that associated with arthritis. And because they concentrate in the brain, they are very important for cognitive and behavioral function—which means improved brain memory and performance (including protecting us from diseases such as Alzheimer's) as well as reducing depression and fatigue.

So, it's VERY important to consume omega-3s. But, we don't need fish to do this.

In fact, fish don't even make EPA and DHA; these special omega-3 fatty acids are made by algae and phytoplankton—*not fish*. Salmon are carnivorous—they eat other sea animals, namely zooplankton, herring, and krill. Krill, small shrimp-like animals, in turn, eat phytoplankton and algae. Algae are composed of high-quality healthful fats (among other healthful nutrients such as carotenoids). In other words, the *algae*—not the fish—provide the nutrients. The fish take in these fats from plants, and we can do the same thing.

For the sake of our health, the fish's lives, and the health of the ocean, we need to eliminate the middle fish and go directly to the source of the nutrients. We need to:

▶ Consume plant foods rich in omega-3s.

▶ Increase our *absorption* of these fats and the *conversion* of these dietary fats into usable DHA (I'll get back to this).

▶ Decrease our consumption of omega-6s. Though you've most likely heard of omega-3s through media sound bites, you may not have heard as much about omega-6s, but you can't really talk about one without talking about the other.

LET'S TACKLE THE FIRST ONE FIRST: CONSUME OMEGA-3-RICH PLANT FOODS

Flaxseeds, chia seeds, and hemp seeds are rich sources of omega-3 fatty acids, and they're widely available in stores today—or online. Flaxseeds need to be ground first, and I recommend buying them whole and then grinding them at home using a coffee or seed grinder. (Otherwise, you don't know if they've been stored properly and for how long at the store.) Or, use a blender to grind two cups or more. Store them in a container in the freezer or refrigerator. Whole, unground seeds can remain in the cupboard.

> **NOTE:** *In terms of nutrition, both brown and golden flaxseeds are essentially the same, so choose what is most readily available and most affordable.*

Ground flaxseeds are only one option and can be added to your oatmeal, breakfast shakes and smoothies, morning cereal, green or grain salads, or soup and stews. Hemp seeds and walnuts can also be easily added to your favorite foods.

- ground flaxseeds (1 tablespoon [7 g] per day)
- chia seeds (1 tablespoon [11 g] per day
- shelled hemp seeds (3 tablespoons [21 g] per day)
- walnuts (about 14 halves [1 ounce] per day)
- flax oil (1 teaspoon [5 ml] daily)

> **NOTE:** *Although you can bake with flaxseeds (ground or not), you don't want to cook with flax oil. Either take your daily teaspoon of oil directly from a spoon, or use it to make a salad dressing. If you like the taste, you can also add it to oatmeal, soup, or a smoothie. (See Day 14 for more on baking with ground flaxseeds.)*

SECOND, WE NEED TO INCREASE OUR ABSORPTION AND CONVERSION OF OMEGA-3S INTO A FORM OUR BODIES CAN USE. THIS FORM IS CALLED DHA.

Consuming a daily dose of omega-3 fatty acids is important, but so is increasing the absorption of these fats. Omega-3 fatty acid is also known as alpha-linolenic acid—or ALA—and it's one of the two main *essential fatty acids* (often abbreviated as *EFAs*). The other is omega-6 fatty acid, also known as linoleic acid—or LA.

> **NOTE:** *When a nutrient is "essential," it means our bodies can't manufacture it, so it's essential that we get it from our diet.*

THIRD, DECREASE OUR CONSUMPTION OF OMEGA-6S

Now I know you've heard of *saturated* fats and *monounsaturated* fats. Both omega-6s and omega-3s are *polyunsaturated* fats, and it is indeed essential that we take in enough of these fats, but we also want to obtain a balance between the two. The problem is that many people do not get sufficient omega-3s, but they are taking in too many of the omega-6s. This is because they're cooking with such commercial oils as corn, sunflower, safflower, and vegetable (often just a combination of these other oils). In addition, they're eating many packaged foods, which contain high amounts of shelf-stable omega-6 fats. What's more, they're also consuming omega-6 fats by way of arachidonic acid, which is in meat, dairy, and eggs.

So, one solution to finding this balance is to eat fewer omega-6-rich oils. Great. Done. You're all set! You're going to be

> ► taking in more omega-3s

and

> ► taking in fewer omega-6s

But, now you want to improve your body's ability to convert these omega-3s into a form your body can use, namely into EPA and DHA. So, how do we do this? And does everyone's body convert these fats equally well?

First, let me say that EPA and DHA originate primarily in sea vegetables, such as in the algae I mentioned above. So, one thing we can do is go straight to a DHA supplement and not even rely on our bodies to convert the EPA. And, where is this DHA sourced from? Not fish. Remember where the fish get DHA? From algae! That's correct. We can get DHA supplements sourced from algae. By doing so, we skip the heavy metals, saturated fat, dietary cholesterol, and pollutants and get only the good stuff.

Now, does *everyone* have to take a DHA supplement? Not necessarily. Most people's bodies are able to efficiently and effectively convert omega-3 fatty acids into DHA, but some aren't, and they may be more inclined toward allergies and depression. In addition, people with diabetes tend not to efficiently convert ALAs into EPA and DHA, and the consumption of excessive saturated fat, dietary cholesterol, and trans fat in the diet hinder this conversion. Finally, the rate of this conversion slows down, as we get older, so that's something to consider, as well.

So, in terms of what experts recommend based on the evidence available:

> ► If you are over 65, you might want to consider taking a DHA supplement.

> ► If you have diabetes, you might want to consider taking a DHA supplement.

> ► If you're pregnant or lactating, you'll want a DHA supplement. This is especially important because the rate of conversion from omega-3s to DHA is also limited in infants.

- ▶ If you've been suffering from depression, Attention Deficit Hyperactivity Disorder, allergies, Alzheimer's disease, or schizophrenia, studies indicate that stores will increase after several months of taking DHA directly.

- ▶ If you've been consuming many saturated fats and trans fats, bring those down, and take a direct DHA for a few months while getting into the habit of consuming flaxseeds or flax oil.

If you're not in any of these groups—and that's most of us—the conversion to from omega-3 fatty acids into DHA tends to happen naturally with no trouble, and you can absorb essential fatty acids through the foods I named above.

Although I'm not in any of these groups and feel confident about my conversion, I also really like the insurance of periodically taking a DHA supplement. I may take the supplement for three months on and three months off, while consuming ground flaxseeds daily (and eating very few omega-6s), because I just like to be sure. See recommended DHA supplements in Resources for You.

B$_{12}$: A Bacteria-Based (Not Meat-Based) Vitamin

Before you started The 30-Day Vegan Challenge, you might have been concerned about vitamin B$_{12}$ intake, assuming B$_{12}$ is an animal-based vitamin that you can get only from meat and animal products. Like all other nutrients, B$_{12}$ is not animal-based, but it's not plant-based either—bacteria synthesize it. B$_{12}$ is found on bacteria and fungi, microscopic organisms that reside in the soil. We used to consume B$_{12}$ from the ground when we ate some soil along with our vegetables, but now that our modern practices dictate that we scrub our veggies clean because we're (justifiably) concerned about pesticides and toxins, we eat less soil and cannot rely on B$_{12}$ from that source.

Vitamin B$_{12}$, also called cobalamin, is a water-soluble vitamin that plays a huge role in maintaining a healthy digestive system and protecting the nervous system. Without vitamin B$_{12}$, very serious and irreversible damage may occur, resulting in heart disease, blindness, or dementia. Symptoms of what's considered *overt* B$_{12}$ deficiency include chronic fatigue, numbness or tingling in the hands or feet, loss of appetite, loss of menstruation, nausea, and tongue soreness. Symptoms in the neurological system are one of the biggest concerns, and nerve damage can be irreversible if not caught early enough.

CHALLENGE YOUR THINKING: Research indicates that B$_{12}$ function cannot be restored to optimal levels by adding small amounts of animal products into the diet, despite professionals and lay people making these recommendations. Increasing B$_{12}$ through regular supplementation will be the most effective step to maximizing your B$_{12}$ status, whether you're vegan or not.

CHANGE YOUR BEHAVIOR: To ensure optimum intake and absorption, take a daily multivitamin that contains B$_{12}$, along with 1,000 mcg of a separate B$_{12}$ supplement twice a week.

Aside from *overt* B_{12} deficiency, there is also *mild* B_{12} deficiency, which is harder to detect but still serious. One of the numbers I suggested you look at early on (see Chapter 4 Know Your Numbers) is your homocysteine level. Just as lowering your cholesterol helps to prevent heart disease and strokes, so does lowering your homocysteine level, and B_{12} helps do this. In fact, studies show that vegans who don't supplement their diet with vitamin B_{12} have high homocysteine levels, which can contribute to heart disease.[60]

HOW MUCH IS NEEDED?

One of the things that's so remarkable about this essential vitamin is how little of it our bodies require; it's such a small amount that it's actually measured in micrograms. Some new vegans erroneously conclude that because our B_{12} intake requirement is so small and because our body stores it for years, we don't need to worry about B_{12}. Although it *is* true that at the time they become vegan some people have enough B_{12} stored in their livers to prevent overt B_{12} deficiency for a number of years, it is also true that these stores cannot prevent mild B_{12} deficiency; i.e. elevated homocysteine levels, and thus putting us at risk for heart disease.

One of the benefits of our modern era is that we can prevent nutrient deficiencies that once plagued our forebears simply by taking advantage of fortified foods and supplements. I'm not suggesting we use supplements as a *replacement* for eating healthfully but merely as insurance. By consciously ensuring adequate intake of B_{12} and striving for optimum nutrition via the other suggestions outlined in this book, vegans can be shining models of health that everyone will be inspired to emulate. So how much is needed to acquire this?

The U.S. Daily Recommended Intake for vitamin B_{12} is 2.6 micrograms (mcg) per day, but research suggests an optimal range is closer to 5 to 10 mcg per day. This is still not a problem, because single B_{12} supplements as well as multivitamins tend to provide large amounts of vitamin B_{12}, well above even these higher recommendations. This extra amount is nontoxic (as a water-soluble vitamin, unused B_{12} is excreted from the body), but desirable to ensure that everyone is getting an adequate supply to the tissues. It also means you can take the supplement less frequently.

If a chewable multivitamin has 10 mcg/µg or more of B_{12} (as cyanocobalamin), and is taken daily, that should be sufficient. (Chewables tend to be better absorbed.) But if you want to be certain you're getting optimal amounts of vitamin B_{12}, you can take 1,000 mcg/µg twice a week along with your daily multivitamin.

The only time you may need additional supplementation is if you're truly deficient or if you haven't had a regular, reliable source for a while, in which case experts recommend increasing the amount of B_{12} to 2,000 mcg once a day for two weeks, then proceeding with regular recommendations. (If you have a true deficiency due to lack of absorption, you can determine and treat this with your health professional.)

Individual B_{12} supplements come in tablets, sublinguals (that dissolve under your tongue), lozenges (that also dissolve in your mouth), and liquid drops. According to research, sublingual tablets and liquid drops may provide the most rapid response, especially if you're looking to bump stores up right away.

It's also worth saying that B_{12} function cannot be restored to optimal levels by adding small amounts of animal products into the diet, despite professionals and lay people making these recommendations. Increasing B_{12} through regular supplementation will be the most effective step to maximizing your B_{12} status, whether you're vegan or not.

Recommended Dietary Allowance (RDAs) for Vitamin B_{12}*

Age	Male	Female
Birth to 6 months*	0.4 mcg	0.4 mcg
7–12 months*	0.5 mcg	0.5 mcg
1–3 years	0.9 mcg	0.9 mcg
4–8 years	1.2 mcg	1.2 mcg
9–13 years	1.8 mcg	1.8 mcg
14+ years	2.4 mcg	2.4 mcg

See page 241 for daily values for pregnant and lactating women.

B_{12} IN FOOD

Some foods such as seaweed, mushrooms, tempeh, miso, tamari, and spirulina have been lauded as good food sources of B_{12}, but this was based largely on faulty testing methods. Though they may contain some amounts of B_{12}, they're not providing reliable or consistent amounts. Although these foods are nutritious for a variety of other reasons, they may not be reliable B_{12} sources.

However, many foods are *fortified* with B_{12}, including nondairy milks, vegan meats, breakfast cereals, and one type of nutritional yeast, called "Vegetarian Support Formula" made by Red Star, which grows on B_{12}-fortified molasses. (It's not a live yeast like that used to make bread.) It has a wonderful cheesy flavor (great for popcorn!) and makes delicious cheese sauces. Though it's a delicious addition to any repertoire, it's not recommended that even the fortified version be *relied* upon as the sole source of B_{12} in your diet (various factors may diminish its efficacy.) Again, it doesn't mean nutritional yeast can't or shouldn't be part of your diet; it just means it's not a *reliable* source of B_{12}.

Fortified Foods	B_{12} mcg per serving
Yves Veggie Cuisine Slices, 4 slices	1.2-1.5
Yves Veggie Ground Round, ⅓ cup	1.4
Yves Veggie Wieners or Jumbo Dogs, 1	0.7-1.5
Red Star Nutritional Yeast Flakes	8
Nondairy Milks	3
Fortified Raisin Bran or Kelloggs Cornflakes, ¾ cup	1.5
Product 19 Cereal, ¾ cup	6
Fortified Grapenuts Cereal, ¼ cup	1.5
Nutrigrain Cereal, ⅔ cup	1.5
Total Cereal, 1 cup	6.2

From Table 7.2 in Becoming Vegan

But because I center my diet on whole foods and don't necessarily eat fortified foods regularly, I just find it easier to simply take a supplement every day and enjoy the foods listed above for other reasons (texture, flavor, and convenience)—not for their contribution to my B_{12} status.

AVOIDING DEFICIENCY AND INCREASING ABSORPTION

Keep in mind that B_{12} deficiency isn't an issue only for vegans to think about; it's also typically due to inadequate *absorption* rather than simply inadequate *intake*. Because the over-50 crowd tends to lack the ability to properly absorb vitamin B_{12}, the Food and Nutrition Board recommends that *everyone* (not just vegans) over age 50 should "meet their RDA mainly by consuming foods fortified with B_{12} or a B_{12}-containing supplement."

People with digestive or malabsorption diseases, such as pernicious anemia or even celiac sprue; chronic kidney failure; B_{12} metabolism defects; or cyanide metabolism defects may also experience inadequate absorption and should consult a health professional to make sure their B_{12} intake and absorption is adequate. In fact, everyone can get their B_{12} levels checked by requesting a test from their doctor. To get the most accurate B_{12} reading possible, a urine MMA test is recommended.

So, I hope that clears things up a bit and that you feel empowered to get what you need to acquire optimal wellness.

Keeping Things Moving with Fiber: Only in Plants, Never in Animals

At this stage, you're no doubt already experiencing the benefits of a fiber-rich diet, which may mean more skipping to the loo, but rest assured these changes are contributing to a lighter and healthier you.

Although our bodies don't digest fiber, it's essential for optimal health, related to treatment and prevention of diabetes, colorectal cancer, gastrointestinal disorders, high cholesterol, heart disease, and obesity. High-fiber foods help move waste through the digestive tract faster and easier, so possibly harmful substances don't have as much contact with the gastrointestinal tract. Fiber-rich diets are also associated with weight loss, because the fiber helps create a feeling of fullness, helping to shut down appetite and preventing us from over-eating.

Everyone knows they should be consuming more fiber, but unfortunately, they tend to do so by going to the pharmacy and buying huge vats of Metamucil and other supplements rather than increasing their consumption of plants and reducing their consumption of animal products. Metamucil *will add* more insoluble fiber to your diet (it is, after all, simply psyllium husks, which you can buy in a natural food store for much less money and without all the sugars added to commercial products), but it's just not the way to achieve optimal health—not in the long-term.

Keeping your animal-based diet the same and just taking some Metamucil—or even psyllium husks—isn't going to give you all the

CHALLENGE YOUR THINKING:
Isolating one healthful component of food does not a healthful diet make.

CHANGE YOUR BEHAVIOR:
Consuming a variety of different plant foods guarantees an optimal intake of fiber—both soluble and insoluble.

added benefits from the plant foods. Isolating one healthful component of food does not a healthful diet make. Unfortunately, I think this has become the norm for people. They think they can continue eating low-nutrient foods, high amounts of animal products, but take a few supplements, concentrated fiber, and calcium tablets, and they'll get by well enough.

TWO DIFFERENT FIBERS

The two different types of fiber are equally important, and most foods provide a mixture of both. Taking in a variety of different plant foods guarantees an optimal intake of fiber—both soluble and insoluble. It's not as if you have to declare, "Today I've had a lot of soluble fiber, so now I need more insoluble fiber." But, it's worth talking about the difference between the two. The two different types are equally important, and most foods provide a mixture of both.

Soluble fiber dissolves in water and is found in a variety of fruits, vegetables, legumes, and grains. It cuts cholesterol, adds to your feeling of fullness, and slows the release of sugars from food into the blood. These actions reduce your risk for health problems including heart disease, obesity, and diabetes. Think about how oatmeal or ground flaxseeds get gooey in water; in your body, toxins and cholesterol quite literally attach to these sticky substances and get moved out of the body. Good sources of soluble fiber are oats, oat bran, oatmeal, apples, citrus fruits, strawberries, beans, barley, rye flour, potatoes, raw cabbage, and pasta.

Insoluble fiber: As you may have guessed, insoluble fiber does not dissolve in water and is found in grain brans, fruit pulp, and the skins and peels of vegetables and fruits. It is the type of fiber most strongly linked to cancer protection and improved waste removal. Think about the toughness of apple skins or the rigidity of sesame or sunflower seeds. Acting as a natural laxative, they help give stool the bulk it needs to move quickly out of the gastrointestinal tract, speeding the passage of food removal and thus contributing to a reduced risk of colon cancer.

Good sources of insoluble fiber are whole grains, whole-wheat products, cereals made from bran or shredded wheat, raw crunchy vegetables, fruits, barley, nuts, seeds, grains, whole-wheat pasta, and rye berries.

You may have noticed there are no animal products listed. That's because there is NO fiber outside of plants. There is NO fiber in meat, dairy, or eggs. None. Fiber exists only in plant foods. Fiber does not exist in any animal products whatsoever, and that includes meat, dairy, cheese, liquid milk, and eggs. The only fiber in animals is what's in their digestive tract because they eat plants. Vegans tend to consume an abundance of fiber (just ask them how frequently they skip to the loo), but on average, meat-eaters tend to eat less than what is optimal.

> **CHALLENGE YOUR THINING:**
> Fiber exists only in plants.
> There is no fiber in meat, dairy,
> or eggs. Zero. Zilch. Zip.

HOW MUCH DO WE NEED?

Fiber is a good example of a nutrient that nonvegans tend to be deficient in. Most Americans consume *far less* fiber than is recommended.

The recommendation from the World Health Organization is 27 to 40 grams per day for most adults. The recommendation from the USDA is 25 grams per day for women and 38 grams per day for men. (The recommended intakes for children range from 12 to 25 grams per day.) However, according to recent USDA surveys, the average intake of dietary fiber by women 19 to 50 years of age is about 12 grams. Intake by men of the same age is about 17 grams.

On the other hand, vegans consume an average of 40 to 50 grams of fiber per day. The rural Chinese—eating many more vegetables and grains—take in upwards of 77 grams of fiber daily.[61] In fact, it's this high intake of fiber that is thought to contribute to the many health benefits of plant-centered diets.

Here's what the American Dietetic Association says:

> *Incidence of lung and colorectal cancer is lower in vegetarians than in nonvegetarians. Reduced colorectal cancer risk is associated with increased consumption of fiber, vegetables, and fruit. The environment of the colon differs notably in vegetarians compared with nonvegetarians in ways that could favorably affect colon cancer risk.*

COOKED VERSUS RAW

There are many opinions about whether it's better to eat more cooked veggies or more raw veggies, and I'd like to add mine: eat *both*. A combination of raw and cooked fruits and vegetables makes for a healthful, varied diet—full of all the nutrients we need and can best absorb.

How much raw should we eat in proportion to cooked? Because people do tend to eat fewer raw fruits and vegetables than cooked (and overcooked), it would behoove them to increase their consumption of green salads, fruits, and raw veggies. 75% raw and 25% cooked is a good ratio in the warm months, but it might change to about 50/50 in the wintertime, and that's fine. The main thing is to take in a variety of raw and cooked foods.

> **CHANGE YOUR BEHAVIOR:**
> Increase your raw food consumption to eat about 75% raw and 25% cooked in the warmer months and 50/50 in the colder months.

FIBER FROM FOODS—NOT SUPPLEMENTS

The prevalence of our low-fiber diets is mirrored in the popularity of over-the-counter digestive aids, laxatives, fiber supplements, and concentrated bran. Instead of increasing healthful plant foods, people tend to continue consuming their regular diet of fiber-less meat, dairy, and eggs and then rely on aids to treat the symptoms. Coping with daily constipation may be uncomfortable, but it may be a step on the road to a much more serious problem. Prevention—*not* band-aids—is what's called for.

And, it doesn't take much. A group of researchers recently reviewed a number of studies and concluded that if Americans ate an additional 10 grams of fiber a day *from food sources*, "about a third of all colorectal cancer cases in the U.S. could be avoided."[62]

That's a significant risk reduction for a small change, and hopefully, you're already seeing how easy it is to add 10 grams of fiber to your daily repertoire, which you're most likely already doing just by taking this Challenge.

- ▶ That one cup of kidney beans you're now eating for lunch gives you 13 grams.
- ▶ The one tablespoon of ground flaxseeds you're now adding to your morning smoothie or oatmeal yields nearly 7 grams. One cup of oatmeal alone will give you 12!
- ▶ A mid-day snack of raspberries (8 grams in one cup) and an apple (5 grams for a medium fruit) will give you another 13.

Remember, this additional fiber has to come from *food* not supplements—and not concentrated bran fiber. As discussed in our sidebar on supplements (page 250), you cannot extract something beneficial from the whole package and expect it to work the same way the whole package works. The key is to consume the fiber via the whole food. When your diet is based on whole foods, there is no need to consume fiber as a supplement.

DEALING WITH ALL THAT FIBER!

Because there is no fiber in meat, dairy, eggs, or any animal product, many people are eating less fiber than they should. When you initially increase your intake of plant foods—and thus fiber—you may experience some discomfort. However, once your body adjusts, it's not really a problem for most people. In the beginning, if you feel you need to take in fewer high-fiber foods, you can still do so without adding animal products back into your diet. There are lower-fiber plant foods you can try, such as white rice instead of brown, bagels, pastas, crackers, tofu, nondairy yogurt, tomato sauce, pizza, fruit juices (with no pulp), apple sauce, and bananas. As you get more comfortable—and you will—you can continue adding more higher-fiber plant foods into your diet.

Creating a Movement

Unlike the soluble fiber that helps to reduce cholesterol and stabilize blood sugar, insoluble fiber is the plant roughage that stays intact and helps push everything through and out of our bodies, manifesting in more trips to the bathroom. Some people get nervous about this, but I assure you it's not only normal, it's optimal. The average nonvegan has sub-optimal fiber intakes, which contributes to less-frequent bowel movements and constipation, marked by hard, dry, difficult-to-pass stool. So, even though you may be surprised by the new sensations in your colon, or by the change in your stool from hard pellets to a softer final product, you can celebrate the fact that this is quite literally contributing to reduced risk of colon disease and cancer.

Discomforting Beans

It's the sugar molecules—called oligosaccharides—in beans that people have a hard time digesting, resulting in gas, cramping, or bloating. Rather than avoiding eating these incredibly healthful legumes, there are a few things you can do if beans are giving you trouble.

- *Gradually* increase your intake of beans. Counterintuitive though it may seem, the more your body adjusts to these oligosaccharides, the easier it is for it to digest them. Throw a few on a salad or into a soup, and slowly begin to eat more concentrated bean dishes.

- Eat more canned beans than beans made from scratch. In canned beans, the sugars have been aggressively cooked out, and the beans have been thoroughly rinsed, lowering the oligosaccharides and thus reducing the problem.

- If you cook beans from scratch, DO NOT cook the beans in the same water you soaked them in (because the oligosaccharides are now in the water).

- People tend to do better with the smaller lentils than with the larger beans. Try them and see if it helps.

- Some species of a particular mold produce an anti-oligosaccharide enzyme, which facilitates digestion of oligosaccharides in the small intestine. This enzyme (Alpha-galactosidase enzyme) is sold as the brand *Beano*. By taking this enzyme at the same time you begin to eat the beans, there's a very good chance that you won't experience the gas and bloating. However, the only problem with Beano is that it uses gelatin, which is a slaughterhouse byproduct) to make its capsule. Fret not. A vegan version called *Bean-zyme* is available in health food stores, online vegan stores, and large natural grocery stores.

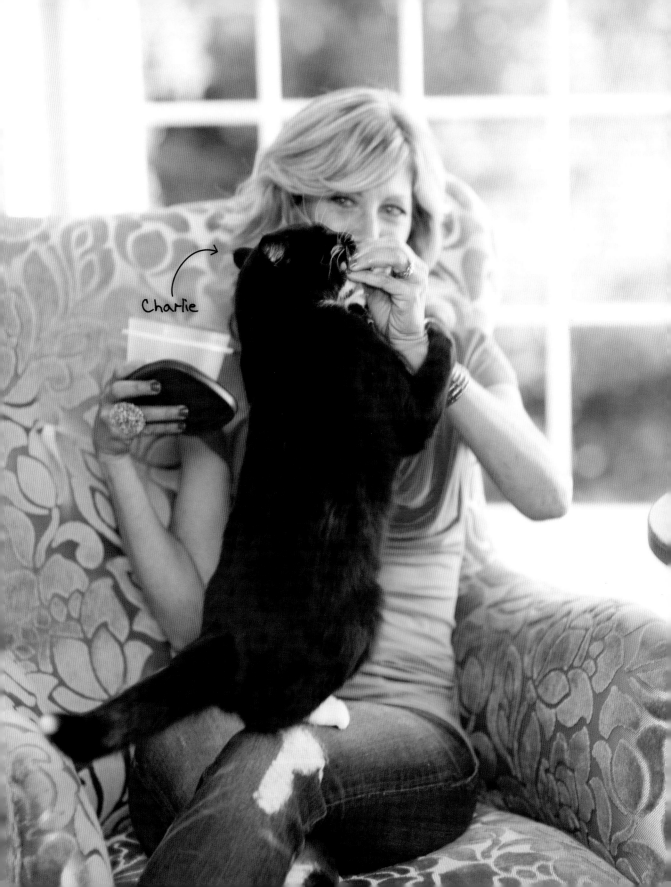

Charlie

Nutritional Needs for Specific Groups

Everyone taking The 30-Day Vegan Challenge will benefit from the changes they are making throughout; however, although we all have the same nutritional needs in terms of macronutrients, vitamins, and minerals, there are a few additional considerations if you belong to a particular group. This is true for vegans and nonvegans, but to increase your confidence even more, look at what the American Dietetic Association has to say:

> *Well-planned vegetarian diets are appropriate for individuals during all stages of the life cycle, including pregnancy, lactation, infancy, childhood, and adolescence, and for athletes.*

Even if you don't fall into any of these categories, my hope is that today's information will help you feel empowered and informed so you can respond confidently if you're ever asked questions about any of these groups—and certainly enable you to empower friends and family members who fall into these categories. Trust me—you *will* be asked questions about vegan pregnancy and vegan athletes—whether or not you're pregnant or athletic!

So let's look at what it means for the diets of these special groups of people to be "well-planned," as recommended by the ADA.

PREGNANT AND LACTATING WOMEN

Everyone already has a lot to say about how you should do things when you're pregnant, so it's no different when you're vegan during this process. Everyone will have their opinion on what you need to do and will no doubt express concern about the fact that you're not eating animal flesh and fluids while your baby grows.

Having said that, proper nutrition is critical during pregnancy, but that applies to vegan as well as non-vegan women. All the nutrients you consume support the growth and health of your baby, so being healthy and strong even before you get pregnant is key. Then, by the time you conceive, you will be drawing on nutrient reserves and healthful habits you have already established.

Several studies provide solid evidence that vegan pregnancies are perfectly healthy for momma and baby, particularly in looking at the weight gain of the pregnant woman and the birth weight of the infant, which are two important barometers for determining a healthful pregnancy. The findings of these studies show that the vegan women gained adequate weight during their pregnancies—sometimes more than nonvegan pregnant women did—and that the birth weight of their babies was totally normal—not affected at all.

The only studies that indicate lower birth weights in babies are those that saw pregnant vegan women on very *restricted* diets—either those who severely restricted calories or those following a strict low-fat (and thus also low-calorie) macrobiotic diet. So, it's important to be clear that that's not the fault of being *vegan*; it's because the diets were too low in fat and calories. Studies and experts looking at pregnant vegan women following a healthful, varied diet with all the calories and nutrients she needs to support her pregnancy indicate there is no reason to be concerned.

Calorie Increase: You don't have to "eat for two" by doubling the amount of calories you consume when you're pregnant, but pregnant women *are advised* to increase their daily calorie consumption by 10% to 15%, resulting in healthful, necessary weight gain. To be precise, additional calories aren't even necessary in the first trimester; in the second, you need about 340 extra calories per day; and in the third, you need about 450 extra calories per day. Depending on your current weight and frame, a recommended weight gain of between 25 and 45 pounds is to be expected. Here are a few simple ways to add nutrient-dense calories:

- ► Eating one cup of cooked oatmeal (~300 calories), plus 1 tablespoon of brown sugar or maple syrup (~50 calories) or whatever sweetener you like (they're all around the same calories), plus 1 apple chopped (~70 calories), a tablespoon of walnuts (~50 calories), and a tablespoon of ground flaxseeds (~50 calories).

- ► Making healthful fruit shakes with additional flax oil or ground flaxseeds.

- ► Increasing the consumption of nuts and seeds (and their butters), as well as avocados.

- ► Eating high-fiber, healthful baked goods, such as muffins, fruit crisps, and cookies.

Protein: The average-size woman needs 45 to 50 grams of protein per day; pregnant women would do well do take in about 70. Here are a few easy ways to add an extra 20 grams:

- ► ½ cup firm tofu (may vary according to brand and texture)

- ► 5 tablespoons peanut butter (make a PB&J)

- ► 3 ounces peanuts

- 1½ cups cooked beans such as: chickpeas, kidney beans, baked beans, pinto beans, refried beans, lentils or black beans

- Two to three 8-ounce glasses nondairy milk

- 3 ounces of seitan, which is wheat protein, provides about 17 grams of protein. Make a veggie stir-fry with seitan, and you're good to go!

Iron: Iron needs are 50% higher from 18 mg/day for menstruating women to 27 mg/day for pregnant women—all pregnant women, not just pregnant vegan women. These needs can be met by taking a supplement (see Resources for You for my recommended prenatal vitamin), though see Day 19: Strong Like Popeye: Increasing Your Iron Absorption for iron-rich foods as well as foods that increase iron's bioavailability. The experts, whose opinions I respect, don't think it's necessary for non-pregnant folks to take iron as a supplement (even in a multivitamin), but for pregnant women, it's usually recommended. So, a good prenatal supplement is what you want to look for.

Lactating women: It's recommended that lactating women take in 9 mg of iron/day; when you're breastfeeding, you're not menstruating, thus you're not losing iron. And, remember from our day on iron: it's recommended that nobody—not men, women, children, pregnant women, nonvegans—should exceed more than 45 mg a day.

Zinc: The recommended intake for zinc during pregnancy and lactation is about 15 mg/day. (It's around 10 mg for adult men and non-pregnant women.) As for zinc-rich food sources: 100 grams of toasted wheat germ provides 17 milligrams of zinc; 100 grams of cashews yields 6 milligrams; 100 grams of tahini offers 4.6 milligrams; one cup of cooked chickpeas provides 2.8 milligrams.

Calcium and Vitamin D: Pregnant and lactating women should meet the daily value of 1,000 mg/day for calcium and the 15 mcg (600 IU) daily value for vitamin D. Review past days for more information on calcium and vitamin D in general.

Vitamin B$_{12}$: Be sure you take a daily Vitamin B$_{12}$ supplement whether you're pregnant, or not (see Day 21). The RDA is 2.6 mcg/day for pregnant women and 2.8 mcg per day for lactating women, though B$_{12}$ supplements, multivitamins, and prenatal supplements will have substantially more than that. And, re-member, vitamin B$_{12}$ is water-soluble, so it's okay to take more than the recommended daily allowance.

Folate/Folic Acid: As I explain in detail in *Color Me Vegan,* folate is a water-soluble B vitamin that occurs naturally in food. *Folic acid* is the synthetic form of folate that is found in supplements and added to fortified foods,[63] such as rice, breads, pastas, and commercial cereals. Folate is prevalent in green leafy vegetables.

Although more research needs to be done, some studies have shown that too much of the synthetic supplement—folic acid— may raise the risk of bowel and prostate cancer. Therefore, some experts are concerned that people are getting too much folic acid because it's in multivitamins as well as in fortified foods. The RDA for anyone over 13 is 400 mcg; the RDA is 600 mcg for pregnant women and 500 mcg for lactating women, and though nutrient-rich vegan diets provide plenty of folate, some experts believe that a prenatal multivitamin/multimineral that contains folic acid is prudent during pregnancy. Some disagree. Consult with your physician.

Here are some folate-rich foods to demonstrate how easy it is to meet the folate recommendations with food:

- ► 1 cup cooked lentils gives you over 350 mcg of folate
- ► 1 cup cooked pinto beans—almost 300 mcg
- ► 2 cups romaine lettuce totals 150 mcg
- ► 4 spears of cooked asparagus have 85 mcg
- ► 1 cup orange juice has 74 mcg
- ► ½ cup cooked green peas equals 50 mcg

The Daily Value for folate is

- ► 150 micrograms (mcg) for children aged 1 to 3
- ► 200 micrograms (mcg) for children 4 to 8
- ► 300 micrograms (mcg) for children 9 to 13
- ► 400 micrograms (mcg) for anyone over 13 years of age
- ► 600 micrograms (mcg) for pregnant women and 500 micrograms for lactating women

Essential Fatty Acids: Experts recommend that pregnant and lactating vegans take a direct source of DHA, aiming for 300 mg/day. These recommendations are based on evidence that DHA intake during pregnancy and breast-feeding improves by brain function and vision in the infant.

INFANTS AND CHILDREN

Of course, all babies are vegan for the first four to six months, meaning they don't need anything other than the milk created just for them: human milk. The more nutrient-rich the mother's diet is, the healthier the baby will be.

Many experts recommend breastfeeding for a minimum of one year—preferably two years or more. Breastfeeding provides immune protection, reduces the chances that your baby will develop allergies, it decreases the risk of illnesses, including those related to the respiratory and gastrointestinal systems, and of course, it's economical!

Continuing to take B_{12} supplements and getting sufficient vitamin D and essential fatty acids (as well as all the other nutrients) is the best formula for success.

In addition, it's recommended that breast-fed infants should receive a vitamin B_{12} supplement of at least 0.3 mcg per day from the second week of life until at least two years of age. As for vitamin D—since breast milk is not a reliable source of this vitamin, it's recommended that breast-fed infants and children—starting at one week—should be given a vitamin D supplement of 5 to 10 mcg a day. At age 1, they can go up to the Daily Value of 600 IU/15 mcg a day, which most multivitamins contain.

In terms of protein needs:

- Healthy 1-to-3-year-old children need 0.5 grams of protein per pound of body weight per day.

- 4-to-13-year-olds should have 0.43 grams of protein per pound of body weight per day.

- 0.39 grams per pound of body weight is recommended 14-to-18-year-olds.

Research continues to support that our early eating habits determine our health in our later years. Instilling healthful habits in children can begin with this 30-Day Vegan Challenge. While breaking old habits requires patience, rest assured that the more variety they are offered, the less persnickety they will be. Anecdotal though it is, *every* vegan child I know eats a more varied diet than most nonvegan adults do.

MEN AND WOMEN OVER 50

The wisdom you have gained over your lifetime is clearly reflected in your commitment to The 30-Day Vegan Challenge. As we get older, our nutritional requirements need to be bumped up a bit. Here is a summary of the nutritional recommendations for seniors gleaned from their respective chapters:

Protein: As muscle tissue decreases, meeting protein requirements for your weight is essential. Although the RDA for protein doesn't change for seniors, some experts recommend increasing it just a bit. Instead of 0.36 gram of protein per pound of body weight, perhaps 0.45 would be the way to go.

Calcium: Because our ability to absorb this essential mineral decreases as we age, experts recommend bumping up the suggested 1,000 mg/day to 1,200 mg/day for women over 50 and men over 70.

Vitamin D: Although 600 IU (15 mcg) per day is sufficient for children and adults up to 70 years of age, vitamin D needs increase to 800 IU (20 mcg) per day if you are over 70. Because it is hard to achieve this through diet (or safe sun exposure) alone, supplementation is recommended. If you are limiting unprotected sun exposure, a vitamin D supplement of 1,000 IU is recommended.

Vitamin B_{12}: As I said when we discussed vitamin B_{12}, "because people over fifty tend to lack proper B_{12} absorption, the Food and Nutrition Board recommends that *everyone* (not just vegans) over age 50 should meet their RDA mainly by consuming foods fortified with B_{12} or a B_{12}-containing supplement."

Essential Fatty Acids: To ensure optimal absorption and conversion of the EFAs into DHA, experts recommend people over 65 take DHA directly in addition to making one tablespoon of ground flaxseeds (or one teaspoon of flax oil) a part of your daily diet. Between the healthful EFAs you're taking in through food and through the DHA supplement, you'll be lowering your risk of dementia, improving your memory, and helping to prevent arthritis.

And of course, consuming high amounts of healthful plant foods means taking in all the protective antioxidants to reduce your risk of cataracts, macular degeneration, heart disease, and even wrinkles. Aging need not mean illness.

Iron: Women in post-menopause have lower iron requirements since they no longer lose iron through menstruation on a monthly basis. A daily intake of 8 mg for post-menopausal women is recommended.

COMPETITIVE ATHLETES

Whole books are written on proper nutrition for athletes—including vegan athletes. If you are doing this challenge as a high-performance athlete, you're on your way to improving your performance. Many medal-winning, world-class athletes are vegan—and were so during their peaks, including ultramarathoner Scott Jurek; tennis champions Billie Jean King and Martina Navratilova; Olympian Carl Lewis; and baseball player Tony Gonzalez.

Because energy output (calorie expenditure) is so much greater, energy intake (calorie consumption) needs also increase, depending on the performance goals, body size, and composition of the athlete. Nutrient needs will be met because of the increased calories; if you're lacking energy, the first solution would be to eat more (increase energy intake).

Complex carbohydrates are the preferred fuel for athletes. The American Dietetic Association position paper on nutrition for physical fitness and athletic performance states:

"In general (i.e. for most athletes), it is recommended that 60-65% of total energy should come from carbohydrate. Athletes who train exhaustively on successive days or who compete in prolonged endurance events should consume a diet that provides 65-70% of energy from carbohydrate."

Complex carbohydrates are abundant in whole grains, vegetables, fruits, legumes, nuts, and seeds. The recommendations for protein for competitive athletes are higher—between 0.6 to 0.9 grams per pound of body weight—versus 0.4 to 0.5 for noncompetitive athletes. Fat recommendations for athletes are generally no more than 30% to 35% of total calories.

Although protein bars and shakes are unnecessary for your average Joe (or Joanne) to get *sufficient* protein, they are useful for those endurance and bodybuilding athletes who want *additional* protein. They're also just convenient when you're on the road. They tend to be made from soy, rice, hemp, or pea protein. (See Resources for You in the back of this book.)

Although individual athletes may hone their own diet to increase their own performance, in terms of vitamin and mineral requirements, all the same recommendations throughout this book apply to athletes.

DIABETICS

I'm including this group here, because there is a serious misconception that diabetics have to limit their intake of carbohydrates and thus would have a difficult time being vegan. Let's be clear: the 18 million Americans who now have diabetes did not get it from eating vegetables—including potatoes, perhaps the most disparaged of all the vegetables. There is a difference between simple and complex carbohydrates, and the latter are healthful and necessary. Diabetes is a symptom of subsisting on a poor animal-based diet. Not only has a whole foods vegan diet proven to prevent and treat the diabetes itself—particularly Type 2—it also addresses the diabetes-related consequences and causes, including obesity, cardiovascular disease, kidney disease, high blood pressure, and nervous system disease.[64] Type 1 diabetics are able to reduce their insulin when on a whole foods vegan diet.[65]

THE ALLERGY-PRONE

Whether you're just sensitive to a particular food or deathly allergic to a certain allergen, I think you'll find during these 30 days that you will still find abundant choices on a vegan diet.

Soy

Despite the stereotype, not all vegans eat foods made from soybeans. There are plenty of soy-free plant-based milks and creamers, ice creams, and vegan meats (such as Field Roast made from wheat). As noted on Day 18, there are plenty of protein-rich foods (legumes, nuts, seeds) in a soy-free diet. Whether you're vegan or not, if you have a soy allergy, any soy that appears in processed foods such as chocolate bars (as soy lecithin) or in energy bars (as isolated soy protein) is an issue for you. (However, soy-free energy bars are definitely available, and I've been hearing more about soy-lecithin-free chocolate.) But, for those who aren't sensitive, soybeans and the foods made from them are healthful and delicious additions to any diet.

Wheat/Gluten

People tend to be *sensitive* to wheat but *allergic* to gluten in that their bodies just aren't able to digest this protein. There is an entire spectrum, but in short, symptoms of wheat sensitivities tend to include lethargy and headaches, while gluten intolerance includes constipation, diarrhea, gas, bloating, and cramps. The process of learning to live wheat- or gluten-free is really the same as learning to live vegan. Once you know what to look for, you form new habits, and it becomes second nature. Today, many commercial wheat- and gluten-free vegan products are available, and although gluten-free baking is definitely a challenge, it can certainly be done. On the flip side, most savory recipes—such as my own—are naturally gluten-free when they're based on whole plant foods.

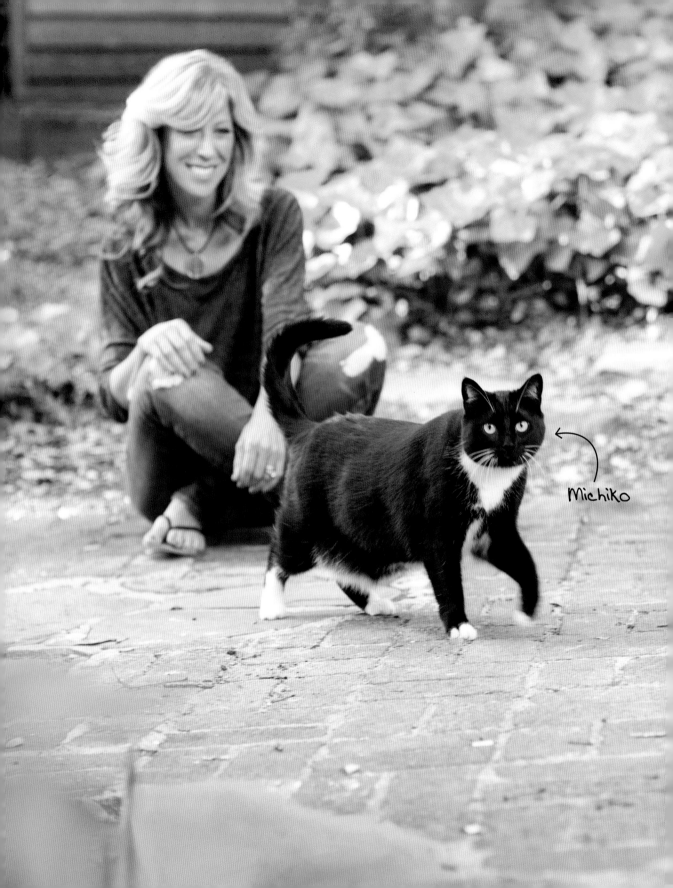

Michiko

CATS AND DOGS

One of the most common questions I'm asked is "What do you feed your cats?" And, since this is indeed a particular group we need to consider, it is important to include it here.

With their own diets reflecting compassion and optimal nutrition, many people are naturally reluctant to support the slaughter industry by feeding animal-based meat to their dogs and cats. It's a dilemma for many of us who want to do the right thing.

In short, dogs—as natural omnivores—are equipped to thrive on a plant-based diet; cats—as obligate carnivores—are not. Now, some dogs may have issues with allergens such as corn, soy, wheat, and gluten that are in commercial dog foods, so that's just a matter of finding the right food if that issue arises. Whenever you're making food changes in your dog's diet, you'll want to transition him or her slowly, incorporating the new food into his or her regular food little by little. See Resources for You in the back of the book for recommended brands of vegan dog food.

While there are many anecdotal tales of cats thriving on vegetarian and vegan diets, let's just say I'm not convinced—based on my own research and experience. Cats are physiologically built as carnivores and have very high protein requirements. They do not *require* plant products in their diet, though they do tend to consume some when they eat the stomach contents of their prey. Offering them some veggie food is fine, but the foundation of their diet—at least 75%—should be animal-based. Making their diet 25% vegan is one way to compromise a little—it enables you to give your cats what they need to be healthy, while allowing you to cut down somewhat on the amount of meat you're buying.

One of the potential problems in vegan cats is the risk of Feline Urologic Syndrome or feline urinary tract disease, which occurs when crystals form in the bladder and are unable to pass through the urethra. It's more common in males because their urethras are narrower than that of females, and it's fatal when not caught. A 100% vegan diet—even using the commercial cat food that's supplemented with taurine and other essential amino acids—often means that their urine is more alkaline than acidic, which can lead to the formation of crystals.

I feed my cats only canned food of aquatic animals (salmon, tuna, shrimp), and my main criterion is that the food not contain byproducts or grains. Many of the cheaper, lower-grade brands rely on byproducts (such as U.S. Department of Agriculture grade 4-D meat, which stands for dead, dying, disabled, and diseased animals) as well as filler in the form of corn that is difficult for many cats to ingest.

So, I think that just about covers special considerations for various groups. I hope that helps you feel empowered if you're in one of these groups or just more informed for when you're asked about any of these groups. And you *will* be asked.

Are Supplements Harmful or Helpful?

By this stage in the Challenge, you should feel empowered enough to understand that a plant-based diet based on whole foods is rich in the nutrients you need to thrive and that B_{12} is really the only vitamin that doesn't have a reliable food source. But, you may also be wondering if there are any other instances when supplements are necessary. You may also be asking if there are ever any risks to taking supplements, if they're just a waste of money, or if it's wise to take a daily multivitamin?

In our quick-fix, just-take-this-pill-and-all-will-be-well society, we have been conditioned to believe that the beneficial properties of whole foods can be contained in a single pill. However much we want to believe that we can live unhealthy lives and escape the consequences by compensating with a few pills each day, I'm here to tell you that's not how it works. Nature is a complex machine, and the nutrients found in plants—the fiber, phytonutrients, vitamins, minerals—all work together as part of a perfect package.

I go into this in great length in *Color Me Vegan*, but in short, recent studies indicate that the effects of antioxidant supplements—particularly vitamins A, E, and C, beta carotene, selenium, and zinc—may be nil at best and harmful at worst.[66] The researchers made it clear that they are talking about *synthetic* supplements—*not whole fruits and vegetables that naturally contain these antioxidants*. This is a very important distinction to make.

But, having said that, the effects of living in our modern age and in industrialized societies aren't all bad. Although we traded the diseases of deficiency—scurvy, rickets, kwashiorkor—for the "diseases of affluence," "diseases of civilization," or "diseases of excess" (cancer, atherosclerosis, and diabetes), how wonderful that with some lifestyle changes (comprehensively outlined in this book) and with access to all the nutrients we need, we have the potential to be the healthiest versions of our species that have ever lived—with no deficiencies. In other words, though the best place to get our vitamins, minerals, and antioxidants is from whole foods (and the sun), many experts still advocate taking a daily multivitamin—if only for insurance. After all, some days we might eat better than others, some days we might be sick and not eat at all, some days we may not absorb certain nutrients as well as others.

But, what are conscious consumers to do if they are not taking single supplements but are taking a multivitamin that contains vitamin E and vitamin A and/or beta-carotene? Before you panic, look at the label on your multivitamin bottle. Most likely, the amounts of these antioxidants fall just under or at the recommended daily value. You can determine that by looking at the column that reads "% Daily Value." For instance, the daily value for vitamin A is 5,000 IUs, and your multivitamin probably contains that many, so the percentage will read 100%.

Once you're ready to switch to a new multivitamin, look for one that doesn't include vitamin A. (See Resources for You on page 310 for brands.) Outside of the amount in your diet (which, I *repeat*, is safe coming from whole foods), the main concern is taking these *single* antioxidants *over and above* that which you get in your multivitamin. Unless you're in treatment for a specific deficiency and under the care of your doctor, there is no need to take them as isolated supplements.

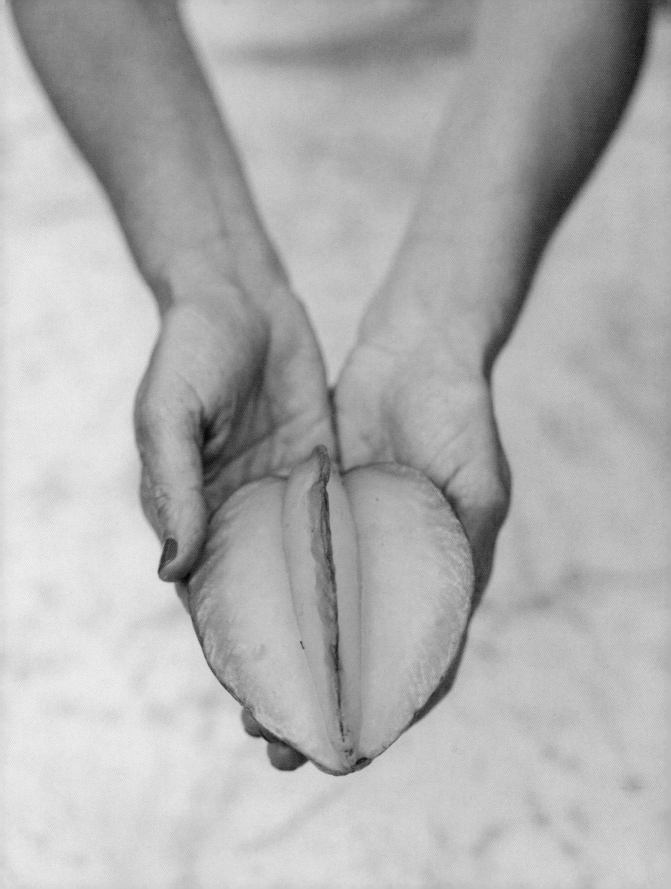

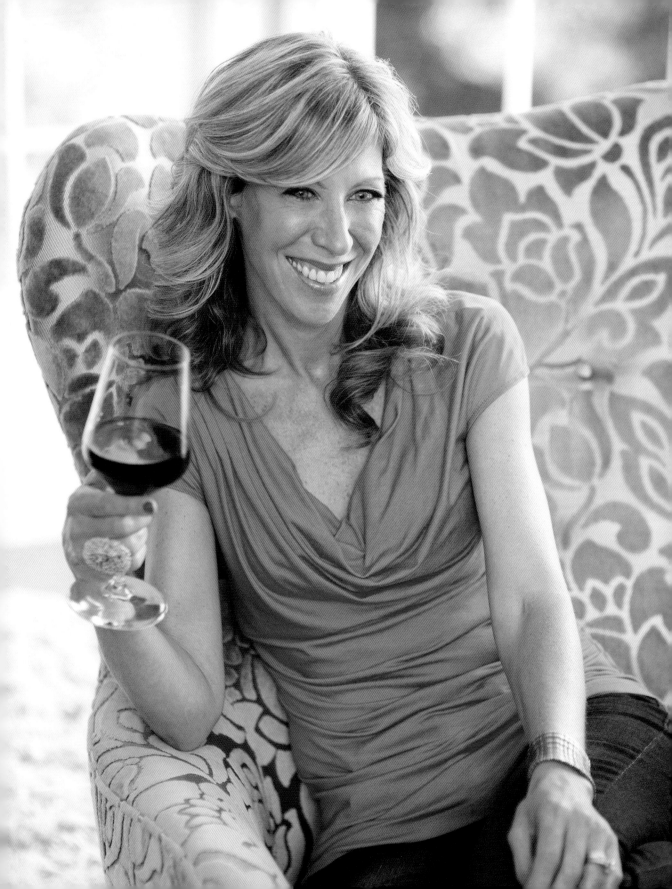

Eating Confidently and Joyfully in Social Situations

Since you're now in your last week of The 30-Day Vegan Challenge, no doubt you're learning what every vegan knows: that making your own diet changes can make other people uncomfortable. I often say that the food is the easy part of this lifestyle change—you learn some new recipes, you re-stock your kitchen, you read labels as though it were second nature.

Then, you're in a social situation and you're asked to defend your new way of eating. You're asked the same questions over and over —about protein, about how to replace cheese, about what the Bible says about eating animals. Next, someone begins pointing out all the areas in your life where you're not perfect, calling you a hypocrite for not solving world hunger or human rights abuses around the world.

You tell someone you're vegan, and you're expected to have multiple graduate degrees in philosophy, nutrition, ethics, ecology, history, religion, animal husbandry, anthropology, and the culinary arts. You tell someone you're vegan, and they take it personally, becoming defensive about their own eating habits.

To be honest, I think this pressure takes its toll on new vegans—especially if they are naturally shy or reticent about their opinions—and I believe it's why many people just give up and revert back to eating meat, dairy, and eggs. I think it's why many wind up feeling isolated and shy away from coming out of the "vegan closet," if you will. I think it's why many people resist becoming vegan in the first place.

And, although we can't change how people are going to react to us, we *can* change how we represent our "vegan-ness."

When you state, "I am vegan," you aren't simply saying, "I eat vegetables." You are a physical representation of someone who is living a conscious life with an awakened mind and heart. You're authentically manifesting what it means to truly eat healthfully and compassionately. And people know this. They feel it, and it rocks their world because *you're* doing what they say they want to do but haven't followed through on. For this reason, they would rather you just keep it to yourself and stop "making meat-eaters feel guilty," an accusation leveled at many vegans who often say nothing more than, "I'm vegan."

I call this the phenomenon "being the vegan in the room," which I think is a powerful and privileged position to be in. It can also be scary for those who don't want to look at their eating habits or consider changing them.

GIVING PEOPLE THE BENEFIT OF THE DOUBT

To avoid discomfort, many vegans figure it's a lot easier not to say anything at all, so they don't speak up for what they believe in, they don't reveal themselves as they truly are, or they "compromise" and eat an animal product just to make someone else happy. Although I understand that it is indeed easier to blend in and conform, the question we have to ask ourselves is "at what cost?" At the cost of our own health? At the cost of our own values? At the cost of our own integrity?

We often romanticize the idea of the independently minded individual, but I think we value this ideal less than we think. I don't think we feel comfortable around people who aren't part of the status quo; I think we appreciate people who conform more than we appreciate those who don't conform. Nonconformists are looked at with suspicion in our society. We all know this on an intuitive level, and so for fear of "being different," many people continue to eat animals and animal products because they're afraid of the attention they'll receive for not looking like everyone else.

This calls to mind an ancient Arabic folktale about a witch who visits a kingdom one night and taints the public water source with a poison that drives people mad. Everyone who drinks from this well indeed goes mad. The king, privy to what had transpired (but having his own water source) did not drink from the well. The next day, all of his subjects who had imbibed the poisoned water (and gone mad) arrived at the king's palace and accused *him* of being mad. The king had a decision to make. He could drink from the well, lose his sanity, conform to everyone else in his kingdom—but remain king. Or, he could *not* drink, remain sane, but be deposed from his throne and denied his power by those who would see his very sanity as madness.

For ordinary folk like you and me, the stakes may not be as high as those in this story, but I think they *feel* that way to many people. Though they may not have a kingdom to lose, I think people are afraid to lose relationships or their own comfort level, and all of these things may be valued as high to an ordinary citizen as a kingdom is to a king.

Most of us want to make a difference in this world. We want to leave our mark, do something meaningful, help others, effect change, and contribute something important. And, I do believe people when they say this, but I wonder sometimes if this all means as much to them as *not appearing different*.

Although we may want to make a difference, I think we need to remember that in order to make a difference, we may have to do something *different*. It's only people who are willing to assert their individuality and personal beliefs who actually make a difference. It's easy to go along with the status quo, but the question we have to ask ourselves is it what we really want at the cost of our own values?

But, let's be clear. Reflecting your values—whether they are motivated by health or ethics—in your behavior doesn't mean you have to constantly rock the boat. It's really just as simple as being authentically *you*. I don't have to apologize for my principles, and they certainly don't fluctuate depending to whom I'm talking. My values don't depend on someone else's comfort level, and they don't change even if they make people uneasy.

It's very possible that who I am and what I believe *will* make someone uncomfortable, but that's very different than *setting out* to make someone uncomfortable. If someone is offended or threatened by my beliefs or ethics, that's not my burden to carry. My regard for the life and autonomy of nonhuman animals is not something I'm ashamed of, and I certainly didn't come to my beliefs with the hope or intention of making others uncomfortable.

In other words, I've learned the boundary of where I end and another person begins.

And if you think about it, there's an element of self-centeredness—not self-effacement—in being afraid of telling people we don't consume or wear animals because it might make them uncomfortable. Truly, how can I possibly guess how someone else will react to my telling them I'm vegan? Time and again, when I tell someone I'm vegan, I'm met with mostly positive responses because *I'm* very positive about being vegan. Often, they start telling me about their own experiences with or feelings about animals. Or, they begin asking me questions about the nutritional benefits of being vegan. Or, they offer to make a meal for me so they can test out some new vegan recipes they just discovered.

To be honest, I think we're all guilty of underestimating the people in our lives—whether they are family or friends, strangers or co-workers. Although past experiences may lead us to conclude how we think someone will react, sometimes we'd be better off giving people the benefit of the doubt. People can surprise us all the time. And besides, in trying to avoid what we think will be uncomfortable, we're also potentially denying someone else the opportunity to stretch their own comfort zones, to learn something new, and to explore other options they may not have considered before. Because the truth is, how else are these things possible except through authentic communication with one another?

By speaking our truth and living our truth, we give others permission to speak and live theirs. When we raise the bar, others rise to meet it. When we speak to the highest in people, they rise to the highest that's in them. I know this is true. I see this every single day. And, if I understand the situation correctly, when we're talking about friends and family, these are presumably the people who care about us. Although

> **CHALLENGE YOUR THINKING:**
> We need to speak up for what we believe in without being attached to how our beliefs will affect someone else.

they might have their own adjustment period to the changes in our lives, the assumption is that the people in our lives want us to be happy.

If someone reacts with hostility to our changes or is resistant to who we are, to what we believe, and to us *speaking up* for ourselves, then perhaps that's a bigger issue in the relationship that needs to be examined. But, I think it's safe to say that our friends and family members love us and want us to be happy. If that's our perception, that will be our experience.

ASKING FOR WHAT YOU WANT

I highly recommend re-visiting the tips for Eating Out and Speaking Up on a previous day and taking a close look at the communication strategies I recommend. Being a joyful vegan in a nonvegan world is walking the line between being humble and speaking up for what you want, and the power of example is the most profound gift we can give. As I intimated above, if we are confident and joyful in our vegan-ness, others will respond in kind.

For example, my husband works for a company that provides breakfast for the employees every day. There are hot and cold options, consisting of a lot of animal flesh and fluids, but because of David's presence, there are more vegan options than before he told them he was vegan. Upon learning that David was vegan, the person in charge of the food made sure to serve nondairy yogurts, nondairy milks, and nondairy cream cheese for the bagels, along with vegan sausages and tofu scrambles. Of course, nonvegans (as well as other vegans in the office) eat the "vegan" breakfast items as well, so even their options increased. What's more: when David asked, his company agreed to make Mondays completely meatless.

Speak up and everyone benefits!

The same rules apply for any situation you're going to be in: going to a friend's home for dinner, the boss' house for brunch, a wedding, a summer BBQ, an office outing, etc. Simply letting the host know in advance, offering to help with the food, offering to bring food are all simple ways to make the situation pleasant and comfortable. It's a matter of speaking up with truth, graciousness, and integrity.

Truth be told, unlike the king in our story, we don't have to choose between reflecting our values and having a social life. We can have both, but we need to grant ourselves permission to ask for what we want. We need to express our values without being attached to how they might affect someone else.

After all, if we're afraid to stand up for who we are and what we believe in, what's the point of having any opinions at all? What's the point of having values if we don't reflect them in our behavior?

Vegan Kids in Social Situations

Family gatherings, children's birthday parties, and school events tend to revolve around food, and vegan parents naturally want to make sure their children aren't left out. With a little forethought and preparation, this need not be a problem at all.

Preparing for Parties

Depending on the event, you can always prepare something special for your child, or just ask the host if you can bring something to share with everyone. If your kids had a food allergy, you'd have no problem doing this, so why should it be any different when it comes to your family's ethical- or health-driven food choices?

My vegan friends who have kids teach them that it's okay for them not to have what everyone else is having all the time. Even though it won't always be "equal" for them in terms of food options, my friends teach their children that the person whose birthday they're celebrating is more important than a chocolate cupcake with sprinkles.

Vegan Kids in the Classroom

I know some brilliant vegan parents who prepare at the beginning of the school year, first by making sure the teacher knows their children are vegan, and next by packing a bag of nonperishable treats that are kept in the classroom, replenishing the supply as needed. Whenever another student brings in nonvegan cupcakes or treats, the teacher gifts my friends' children with their own special treats from their vegan goodie bag. These kids do not feel awkward or left out at school celebrations.

Teachers are hearing from parents all the time about special diets, allergies, and foods children don't eat for one reason or another. This situation is no different, so give the teacher the benefit of the doubt, and relax a little.

The other option—depending on how much time you want to invest—is to whip up a batch of vegan cupcakes to have your child bring to the school when you know there is a birthday being celebrated.

Though it may seem daunting at first, I assure you that in time it gets easier. Family and friends ultimately want to make sure your children are included in celebrations and will often make sure there is something vegan for them to eat. Just give them time to come around, while being clear and consistent about your family's dietary choices.

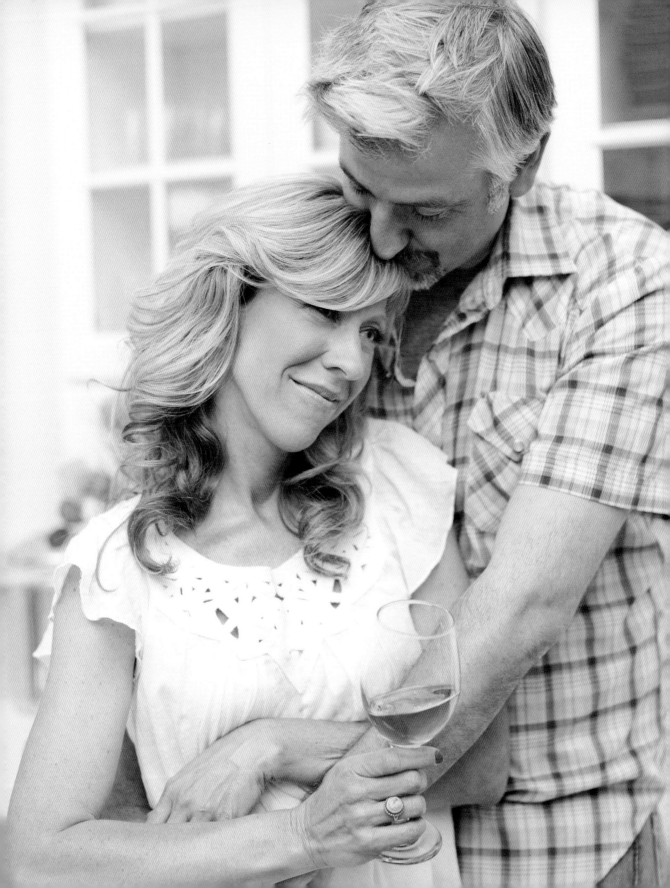

Finding Harmony While Living in a Mixed Household

In an earlier chapter preparing you for The 30-Day Vegan Challenge, I encouraged you to ask the people you live with to take the Challenge with you. Even if they didn't join you, you may find that they are supportive of your changes, making the process a lot less challenging for you.

However, not everyone has this experience, and new vegans are often surprised by how their own changes cause ripples in otherwise calm waters. Some nonvegan family members may be critical, resistant, or even hostile to your new way of eating. Understanding the reasons for their reaction will do wonders for your peace of mind and the ease of your journey.

YOUR JOURNEY MAY NOT BE THEIR JOURNEY

You may have come to this Challenge because you had health issues you heard could be helped by a plant-based diet, you may have decided you didn't want to contribute to violence against animals, or you may have become inspired by the desire to use fewer of the Earth's resources. By the time you arrived here, you most likely read, processed, and internalized a lot of information. By the time you picked up this book, you may have already created some new habits. With conviction and zeal, you declared this to your family members and were disappointed by their less-than-stellar reaction.

We have to remember that even though we may have become awakened to our own compassion or had a revelation about our health, it doesn't mean everyone around us has had the same experience. Even though our own perceptions and habits have completely changed, we have to consider how these changes might affect our loved ones. If we want them to be considerate and understanding of us, we have to show them the same consideration and understanding.

They may not have gone through the same process as you, read the same books, or watched the same videos. In fact, they *may not be willing to.* But, demanding that they understand the transformation you've experienced or calling them close-minded for not being supportive is ineffective and unfair. Just as you've taken the time to adjust to your new way of seeing the world, you have to honor the transition of the people with whom you share your life. That doesn't mean you should squelch your newfound enthusiasm; it just means you need to understand that not everyone around you may share it—at least not right now.

Navigating these tricky waters requires a little patience, a dash of psychology, and a lot of really good food, no matter how old you are or what your living situation is.

VEGAN TWEENS AND TEENS LIVING WITH NONVEGAN PARENTS

Part of becoming an adult means trying to understand someone else's perspective, and I always encourage new teen vegans to put themselves in their parents' shoes to understand why they may react with panic when they learn their child wants to be vegan.

Frankly, no matter what your age, parents need time to adjust to your new lifestyle. Like all of us, they are creatures of habit and have most likely been cooking the same meals for you day after day, year after year. They've gone through your picky-eating phases, they've made sandwiches just the way you like them, they've prepared special meals to accommodate your preferences. And now, you tell them that everything is different—and you wonder why they react emotionally. What I'm saying is, *let them have their reaction, and remember that it has nothing to do with you.*

On one hand, they're probably genuinely concerned because they don't know what to feed you. If they've been making your favorite meals for years, they're not exactly going to be enthusiastic about changing the repertoire.

CHALLENGE YOUR THINKING: Though we may have become awakened to our own compassion or had a revelation about our health, it doesn't mean everyone around us has had the same experience.

CHANGE YOUR BEHAVIOR: If we want our loved ones to be considerate and understanding of us, we have to show them the same consideration and understanding.

On a much deeper level, though, I believe that one of the reasons parents take our new way of living (or our newfound veganism) personally is because they've used food from the day we came into this world as a way to nourish us—literally and emotionally—and as a means of showing their love for us. When we turn down the food they've chosen to feed us, it may feel like we're rejecting *them* and their affections. They may defensively ask, "What's wrong with how we raised you? You always loved the food I made for you!" "How can you do this to me?" as if our being vegan is a judgment of their parenting skills.

Tell them you understand how different this must be for them; thank them for teaching you to be an open, compassionate, thoughtful person—all of the qualities that led you to make these new choices. Tell them how much you appreciate all the years they've spent feeding you and buying your favorite foods. Tell them this is not just another temporary fad; tell them why this means so much to you. Show them that you're serious. Be consistent. Tell them you need their support and that you're willing to help make it easier.

And then... help make it easier.

It would be utterly unfair to expect Mom or Dad—or whomever does the cooking—to change instantly. You absolutely need to take responsibility for your decision and help cook. This will not only take the burden off them and begin to hone your own cooking skills, but it will also show them how delicious and nutritious your new lifestyle is. I've never seen it fail. Even parents who were the most resistant in the beginning eventually come around and wind up being inspired and influenced, many becoming vegan themselves. I'm not saying that this should be your expectation, but I've seen many parents change because their teenager changed first. Whatever the outcome, I can assure you they will respond differently given some time.

To help with the process:

- ▶ Sit down with your parents, and write down all of the dishes you all eat on a regular basis. Show them how you can veganize the family favorites.

- ▶ Look through cookbooks together and pick out recipes you'd like to try.

- ▶ Shop with them. Participate.

Beyond food, your parents are probably genuinely concerned that you're not going to get all the nutrients a growing person needs. Help alleviate their fears. Show them the chapters in this book on protein, calcium, iron, omega-3 fatty acids, and vitamin B_{12}. Read them the American Dietetic Association's Position Paper on Vegetarianism. Show them—*by eating your vegetables*—that you're not a junk-food vegan. You can't expect them to support you if all you eat is potato chips. Vegan? Yes. Healthful? No.

The goal is to find solutions together and not let your being vegan become a power struggle between vegan teenager and nonvegan parent.

VEGAN PARENTS OF NONVEGAN CHILDREN

Teenagers aren't the only family members who bring veganism home. Often, one or both parents make dietary changes that inevitably affect the entire family. Your children and teens may already be joining you in this Challenge, but they also might be resisting. The difference may have to do with how old they are.

There's no doubt that it's more difficult to change the food habits *you* instilled in your children, but that's not to say it can't be done. Communication, consistency, and confidence are essential ingredients.

I say "confidence" because I've often heard people criticize parents for raising their children vegan, accusing them of "imposing their values on their children." Balderdash! Parents impose their values on their children all the time. It's called being a parent. So, if transitioning your children from an animal-based to a plant-based diet is what you feel is best for yourself and your family, be confident in your decision. There's nothing wrong with raising your children in such a way that reflects your values and the values you've most likely taught them already: compassion, kindness, empathy, and wellness.

I believe we come into this world fully compassionate, and the best gift we can give our children is to honor the empathy they have for animals by encouraging them to make choices that are aligned with these values. After all, we try and keep images of animal cruelty and suffering *from* children for a reason, so why would we go behind their backs and support the very thing they would (and we *do)* find anathema? Why should we pay other people to do things to animals what we could never do ourselves, things that children (and adults) are traumatized by when they witness?

Don't underestimate the compassion in your children. When they begin to understand that their new way of eating means animals will be helped, *they get it*. The actual transition process may be bumpy at first as they learn how to navigate in this new world, but as they internalize the lessons you're teaching them, it will become easier, and those values will become their own.

In terms of health, I think the most compelling research coming out about what we eat and how well we live is that which tells us that the food habits instilled in us as children dictate how we eat as adults; that the food choices we make as children are strong predictors of disease later in life. In other words, what children eat during their formative years has a profound impact on their future health, and since American children eat so few whole plant sources, there is *much* room for improvement.

As you discuss with your children the benefits of eating their veggies—for everyone involved—you can start changing their meals, and this is where vegan versions of their familiar foods will be helpful.

- ▶ Instead of animal-based hot dogs and hamburgers, give them veggie dogs and veggie burgers.

- ▶ If they're accustomed to cow's milk in their cereal, gradually reduce it by a quarter, then half, until you're using 100% plant-based milk. Do the same if they eat yogurt, ice cream, sour cream, or cream cheese.

- ▶ Make or buy other vegan versions of their favorite foods, but don't make a big commotion about the new food. They may turn their nose up at it just because it's new. Over time, you can casually tell them they're eating the cruelty-free versions.

VEGAN, LIVING WITH A DIE-HARD MEAT-EATER

I've heard from many vegan women over the years who lament that their husbands, riddled with health issues that could very well be improved or solved by eating a plant-based diet, fight tooth-and-nail when it comes to making any changes. Understandably, this causes friction—the wife pleading with her husband to change, the husband insisting that he's just fine. Nobody wins, and everyone is miserable.

Keep in mind that some people may not want information about eating differently *simply because it comes from you.* I think family members can be the hardest to reach because of all the other underlying dynamics that are already built in. Sometimes it's much easier to receive information from strangers.

Certainly there's nothing wrong with directing them to resources (such as *The 30-Day Vegan Challenge*!), but it's important to do so and then remain unattached to the outcome. Note the difference between, "You need to/should read this" and, "I just read a really compelling book I think you would really appreciate. I'll leave it here in case you want to take a look." Then leave it there and let them read it. Don't ask them if they have. Don't ask them why they haven't. Don't criticize them or take it personally if they never do.

> **CHALLENGE YOUR THINKING:**
> Sometimes family members may not want information about veganism *because* it comes from you. Sometimes it's easier for them to receive information from strangers.
>
> **CHANGE YOUR BEHAVIOR:**
> Guide loved ones to resources, but try to remain detached to the outcome. Know that you have planted seeds, whose germination is not your business.

Also, when you're concerned about someone's health, communicate openly from your heart. Telling your husband (or wife) that you're genuinely concerned, that you love him and are scared to lose him, will go much farther than prodding him about how unhealthful his diet is. Be sure to tell him that you cannot condone what you perceive as harmful behavior but that you won't hassle him about it anymore. And then be true to your word.

Planting seeds is a much more effective way of inspiring people than knocking them over the head.

I also hear from a lot of newly vegan women—who are still the primary cooks in most families—who feel obligated to continue cooking for their husbands all of the animal products he insists on eating. Add fussy kids or teens to the mix, and she winds up making three two or three different meals every night for dinner. When did home kitchens become restaurants?

I absolutely do not advocate people making more than one meal for their meat-, dairy-, and egg-eating family members. If you're the cook in the family, and the expectation has always been that the rest of the family eats what you create, then that applies in this situation, too. If your family members feel they need to eat meat at every meal, then they can cook it themselves. If they eat outside the home for lunch, then they can get whatever they want at that time. But at dinner, if you're in charge of the meals, then *you* decide what's on the menu. I'm not suggesting you do this in a dictatorial way, because of course deciding what's on the menu also means making vegan variations of their favorite meals. Some of their favorite meals may already be vegan by default. The point is to not become a short-order cook in your own kitchen.

After all, the surest way to inspire people to *eat* delicious plant-based food is to *make* delicious plant-based food. "If it tastes good, they will eat it" is my motto. If people eat food they find satisfying, filling, familiar, and tasty, they won't care if it has no animals in it.

ACCOMMODATIONS AND COMPROMISES

I realize that it's easier when you live with someone who shares the same perspective about keeping a vegan home, but how do you navigate the issue when you want to keep a vegan home and your partner does not? I think the answer lies in compromise and communication, which are what relationships are all about.

I suggest that we express ourselves openly, honestly, and vulnerably with our loved one, which might look something like, "This is *my* home and *your* home, but we have a problem here. It's difficult for me to have animal products in the house, because when I look at them, all I see are images of sorrow and pain. I know this is your house, too, and I appreciate that you are open to my sharing this with you. This is not a judgment of you at all; it's just a reflection of the sensitivity and I awareness I have around this issue." Whatever words you use, communicate your thoughts as clearly as possible, without judgment, attachment, or expectation.

However, because this issue is not simply about sharing how you feel but about finding a solution to a problem, you have to be very clear about asking for what you want. You're not asking your partner to "be vegan for you," and I think you need to make that very clear. You're asking for some decision to be made about what is brought into the home you both share. He or she may agree to keep a vegan home, but if not, I know people who have met each other halfway:

- He or she might be willing to forgo having any animal flesh in the house, including that of aquatic animals, but still wants to have animal-based cheese or eggs, and you—the vegan— might realize that it's not perfect, but it's better than nothing at all, and it's something you could live with. It's called compromise.

- He or she might not be willing to stop bringing meat, dairy, or eggs into the house, and so you can keep a separate small refrigerator for animal products. It's better than nothing, and it's something you could live with. It's called compromise.

- I know couples who might not keep a vegan home, but the nonvegan agrees that they won't *cook* animal meat in the house. They might still have things like lunchmeats (maybe in that separate fridge!), or they use a grill to cook animal-based meat outside so the smell doesn't permeate the house. It might not be perfect, but it's called compromise.

KEEPING A VEGAN HOME

I talk a lot about the importance of speaking your truth, and I emphasize the power of inspiring people rather than trying to "convert" them, as some say. I teach—as well as live by—the belief that the most effective way to advocate for what we believe in is to plant seeds, then step back and remain unattached to how those seeds will germinate. I'm very proud of the fact that I've heard from thousands of people over the years that have heeded this advice and have found themselves much happier, their message coming across much clearer, and their friends and family members much more receptive because of it.

Learning where we end and another person begins isn't always easy, but I've seen countless people draw the boundaries necessary to become compassionate, effective voices for this kind and healthy way of living. Yet, somehow—interestingly and ironically—people have a harder time keeping these boundaries in their own homes. They may have learned to ask for what they want in restaurants or politely laugh at a silly joke about veganism, but afraid of being considered controlling, extreme, or militant, they are reluctant to draw the line at their front door lest they "insult" or "offend" someone who visits. Things get even more complicated when you live with nonvegans who might not share your desire to draw that line.

In the least complicated scenario, both you and the people with whom you live (partners, spouses, and children) all agree that animal products have no place in the home—and all is well. In fact, I find often that one family member tends to go vegan first, which then dictates this house rule. That was certainly the case with me and my husband. When I became vegan, it was just a succinct way of saying that I became awakened to the compassion that had always been inside of me—it was viscerally painful to imagine having anything that came from the slaughter industry in my home. Bombarded as we are with images and stories of violence against animals, I wanted my home to be a refuge, a sanctuary, a place of peace. My husband, who wasn't vegan (yet) agreed on the spot. He was more concerned with my happiness than with the need to keep cow's milk in our fridge or fish's bodies in our freezer.

So, from that day in 1999 until today, the various homes we've lived in have been—for all intents and purposes—vegan. I am qualifying that statement, because the only exception is the fish-based commercial cat food we feed to our cats. But in every other way, our home is vegan, and that includes our furniture and décor. Nothing we buy—to our knowledge—is made with leather, silk, feathers, down, or anything else belonging to animal. (I discuss textiles on Day 28: Compassionate Fashion.)

The next scenario, however, is about that same couple or family who keep a vegan home but struggles with how to communicate this to friends and family. How do we tell neighbors not to bring nonvegan food into our home? How do we draw this line? How do we deal with contractors or house sitters who may be in our home temporarily? What about when we have parties and potlucks? What do we do when someone unwittingly *does* bring animal products in?

The short answer is:

- communicate clearly and compassionately

- be patient and sensitive

- keep things in perspective

- do the best you can

I share this with you as an invitation to learn from my mistakes. When I first became vegan, some friends arrived at our apartment with milkshakes in their hands—milkshakes made with cow's milk. Still emotionally raw from my newfound awakening about the violence inherent in the dairy industry, I remember standing in front of them poised to make a very important announcement while they sat on the couch drinking their shakes. I told them how it was just too upsetting to have animal products in the house knowing what I now knew. Not knowing anything about my transformation to veganism prior to this moment, of course they felt horrible sitting there with milkshakes in hand, apologizing, and offering to throw them out.

Making our friends feel guilty was never my intention, but I'm sure that's what I accomplished. The more gracious thing would have been to tell them in a neutral situation—when they were not eating animal products—and in a neutral location—when they were not in our home. I could have also done it in a more casual way, but I still would have done it. I have no qualms with setting this boundary to not have animal products in my home; I have qualms only with how I went about it in this situation, and I wouldn't recommend it. Lesson learned.

About six months after I became vegan, David joined me, and it became clear to our existing friends and family that we didn't allow animal products in the house, because we talked about having a vegan home as if it were the most natural thing in the world—because for us, it was; for us, it is. As more time passed, we also made more friends who were already vegetarian and vegan, and it just became a given that we keep a vegan home. One of the easiest and most direct ways we communicate this is when we have potlucks or casual parties. On the invitation (or when we speak to guests directly), we ask folks to bring a dish and say "vegan, of course." Right away, they understand. It's called setting boundaries, and people tend to respect them. Those who don't, well, that's a different story.

When we host a party or dinner for which I make all the food, and friends ask what they can bring, I thank them and say, "Nothing at all—just your fantastic self." If they persist, I invite them to bring wine. If they really want to bring a dessert, I ask if they would like any recipes for baking or any resources for buying vegan desserts. If he or she is a new friend, usually they know quickly in our relationship that we're vegan, so we don't have a problem saying, "You're so sweet to offer. Anything vegan would be great." Usually *they're* the ones who say, "What can I bring? Of course I'll make it vegan."

> **CHALLENGE YOUR THINKING:**
> Why should we value the customs dictated by religion but not those dictated by principles?

This goes for holidays, as well. Whenever we host Thanksgiving dinners with nonvegan friends, because we established the "house rules" in casual conversations, they are always gracious about contributing vegan-only dishes. As a result, our gastronomic gatherings are always filled with the most delicious food made by all of our friends. It has never been a problem.

Are there people who resent that we ask them to bring only plant foods into our home? Are there people who think we are rude? Are there people who don't come to our house because of it? I have no idea, but as far as I'm aware: no. I suppose it's certainly a possibility, but I just don't have the sense that this has ever been an issue. I have no idea what people say when we're not around, but from everything I have experienced in the last couple decades, everyone has always been—and continues to be—nothing but gracious.

If they *do* have a problem with it, frankly, that's too bad. It's our home! It's the one place in the world we can control. With the sights and smells of animal products everywhere around us in the world, our home is our refuge, and that feels really good.

Are there times when someone has brought in animal products unknowingly? Absolutely. Did we freak out? Absolutely not. We just made it clearer for the next time they were coming over. It's never been an issue (and our nonvegan friends and neighbors haven't stopped coming)!

I wonder if the folks who think it's rude to draw boundaries feel the same way when it's done for religious or health reasons rather than for ethics. Can you imagine someone saying, "Well I understand they keep a Kosher home when *they're* in it, but when guests come over, they should bend the rules. How rude to keep *me* from eating pork when I come to their house for dinner. How dare they impose their religion on me!" I can't imagine someone saying such a thing. Why should we value the customs dictated by religion but not those dictated by principles? Personally, I don't see a difference.

Maya Angelou, the late great American author, activist, and poet, believed that negative words are powerful enough to seep into our consciousness. I remember reading that because of this conviction, she didn't allow anyone to curse in her home. She didn't tolerate negative words, judgments, or profanity and forbade them to cross the threshold of her house because she didn't want to bring negativity into her own space. Was that unreasonable, rude, and ungracious of Maya Angelou? I don't think so. It was *her* home. Many people—including my husband and me—ask our guests to take off their shoes before entering their home. We supply slippers so their feet aren't cold. Is that rude? I don't think so. It's *our* home.

Inside and outside of my house, when I'm able, when it's possible, and when it's practical, I do my best to not contribute to violence against anyone, and there's a lot I can't control. But, if I can't draw that line at my front door, then where can I draw it?

The bottom line is that if you act like you're doing something wrong or that you're *depriving* your family members and friends of eating animals and animal products in your home, then that's how they're going to take it. This goes back to what I said in the very beginning—that the decision you make about the rules in your home have to stem from the overall confidence you feel being vegan. If you think you're being a pain in the *derrière* to those around you or are putting people out or are being a rude or ungracious host, then that's how people will perceive it.

For me, being vegan is a reflection of—and extension of—my compassion. Because that's how I perceive it, that's how I present it to the world, and that's how it's received. The joy you feel making compassionate, healthful choices will quite literally be a magnet to those around you. Your enthusiasm will be contagious and will arouse curiosity and interest, and the amazing food you serve will seal the deal.

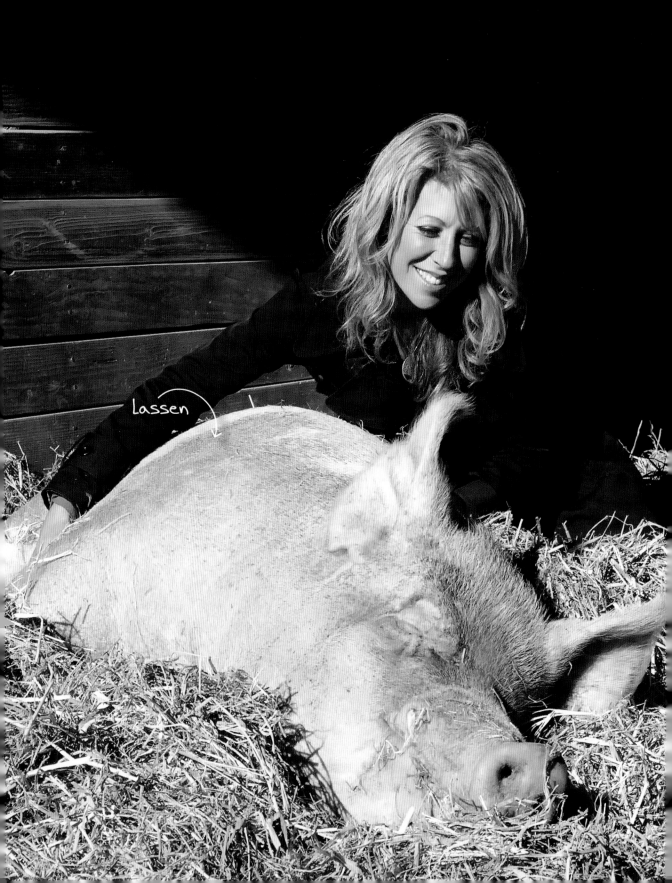

Celebrating the Holidays and Honoring Your Values

Whether you're vegan or not, holidays can be stressful. Self- and family-imposed expectations, unexpected expenses, and cross-country travel can take its toll on even the most balanced individual. Add food to the equation, and it can be a recipe for disaster. Though food exists in our lives for mere utilitarian reasons—to provide the sustenance we need to survive—it plays a complicated and emotional role for many of us.

Within the familial microcosm, most likely, everyone has been cooking the same favorites year after year, making a ritual of carving the "holiday bird," and passing down recipes from years past. For the larger society, by not eating turkeys, lambs, eggs, "corned beef," "ham," dairy, and any other number of animal flesh and fluids on the various holidays throughout the year, vegans are perceived as upsetting the natural order of things.

Those who defend the consumption of animals on the basis of culture and tradition seem to imply that we're entitled to do whatever we want simply because it brings us pleasure—or comfort. Not only does this presume there is no pleasure to be found in rejecting such products, it also presumes there is no victim—or that if there is one, considerations for him or her are secondary to fulfilling our own desires.

CHALLENGE YOUR THINKING: Just because we are capable of doing something doesn't mean we should do it. Just because we've always done something doesn't mean we have to keep doing it. Once we know better, we do better.

CHALLENGE YOUR THINKING: Ethics and traditions need not be mutually exclusive. We can care about both at the same time.

CHANGE YOUR BEHAVIOR: Demonstrate to your loved ones that our food choices aren't about rejecting *their* traditions but rather about manifesting our own values.

When pressed, I think most people would agree that tradition is no excuse for violence. Just because we are capable of doing something doesn't mean we should do it. Just because we've always done something doesn't mean we have to keep doing it. One of the ways we progress as a society is by deciding that once-acceptable behaviors are no longer acceptable, particularly when they harm someone else. Present laws are windows into a past littered with cruel customs and offensive practices. Once we know better, we do better.

Moreover, ethics and traditions need not be mutually exclusive. We can care about, reflect, and celebrate both at the same time. Holiday meals can be the perfect time to show family members that in becoming vegan, we are manifesting *our* own values—not rejecting *their* traditions. Communicating this distinction to them can work wonders in alleviating tension.

AUTUMN HOLIDAYS: THANKSGIVING AND HALLOWEEN

Thanksgiving can be a tough time for vegans—not because delicious autumnal food isn't abundant this time of year, but because the cultural rhetoric is dominated by talk of baked turkeys, roasted turkeys, leftover turkeys, and—just when you thought it couldn't get worse—turkducken, an increasingly popular dish where a chicken is stuffed into a duck, who is then stuffed into a turkey (and sometimes wrapped in bacon). I don't think anyone has the corner on what this holiday is "supposed" to be about, but I have a feeling that most would agree that it should be about more than gluttony and wasted lives.

Romanticized notions rather than historical facts are what inform our consciousness about Thanksgiving. This is especially true when you look at what is considered "traditional Thanksgiving food," how it came to be such, and the stories we have created about what we consider the "First Thanksgiving."

Although we cannot be 100% certain, it is most likely that the animals eaten when 90 Wampanoag Indians gathered for a three-day feast with 52 colonists were deer, geese, ducks, and different species of fish. If cranberries were on the table, it would have been for their red color—not cooked with sugar as we eat them today. Potatoes hadn't even arrived in the colonies yet, so nobody was enjoying mashed, baked, sweet, or whipped potatoes; and apples—not native to North America—were not even in New England at the time. And, even if they had an oven in which to bake them, pies, tarts, and cakes were unlikely on the menu given the unavailability of flour and the difficulty in acquiring butter.

Oh, and we do know that forks would not have been used. They weren't customary yet.

Even though vegans (and vegetarians) are often accused of "breaking tradition" for not eating turkeys at Thanksgiving, if historical accuracy is the standard for being true to "tradition," then *anyone* who eats bread stuffing, mashed potatoes slathered in dairy-based butter, cranberries boiled with sugar, candied sweet potatoes, apple cobbler, pumpkin pie, buttermilk biscuits, or other foods *not* on the menu of the First Thanksgiving, is breaking tradition. To further the point, we are also breaking tradition when we eat with forks.

Of course, it's an absurd notion that any of us are so tied to tradition that we try to mimic exactly what was done in the past. At many times throughout our lives, we selectively choose which customs and traditions we want to uphold depending on how convenient, healthful, or ethical they are. We take what we want from the past to create our myths, customs, and traditions, and we leave behind what doesn't suit us anymore. Although staged reenactments of historic events can momentarily bring the past back to life, we tend to regard them as quaint reproductions rather than as a model for everyday living.

In other words, we turn to traditions because they act as touchstones for us. Our desire to feel connected to something is greater than any desire to perfectly replicate the original source of our tradition. We bend the rules all of the time, and so in the end, it doesn't *matter* that people choose not to consume turkeys on Thanksgiving. They're creating *new* traditions based on their ideals or tastes, which is exactly how we came to associate turkeys with Thanksgiving: someone arbitrarily chose to highlight that animal because it was familiar to *her*. That someone was a very real person with a very specific agenda.

The menu we associate with Thanksgiving was conceived by a woman named Sarah Josepha Hale (1788-1879), who appealed to various U.S. presidents over the course of several decades to make Thanksgiving an official American holiday. As the editor of a popular and influential women's magazine (she was also the author of "Mary Had a Little Lamb"), she had the perfect medium for furthering her cause. To appeal to her readership, she fictionalized and romanticized the events and the menu of that first Thanksgiving. She shared recipes and illustrations for roasted turkeys, pumpkin pies, mashed potatoes, and biscuits—none of which would have been served in 1621 in Plymouth, Massachusetts. Her advocacy paid off, and in 1863, President Lincoln signed legislation to accept Thanksgiving as a national holiday. The menu that Hale contrived for this fall holiday continues to permeate our culture's consciousness.

Fast forward almost 100 years, when out of a USDA-funded breeding program came the "Beltsville white" turkey breed, which replaced the darker feathers—and thus darker flesh—of wild turkeys. (White feathers means white flesh.) Sadly, the marketing muscle of the turkey industry has so successfully increased the demand for turkey meat that, in 2012, according to the Department of Agriculture's National Agricultural Statistics, an estimated 254 million turkeys were brought into this world only to be killed.[67] (These birds must be artificially inseminated since they've been bred to have obscenely large breasts and thus cannot naturally copulate).

For the English colonists and Wampanoag Indians, that first gathering was a celebration of food and feasting, and for praising God and the Three Sisters (corn, beans, and squash), respectively. Before Hale's mythologizing of that First Thanksgiving, it was considered a simple regional holiday that was celebrated solemnly through fasting and quiet reflection: quite a bit different from the gluttonous and commercial celebrations of today.

CHANGE YOUR BEHAVIOR: Create new traditions that stem from your own values, and embrace them with pride and joy.

Creating a beautiful Thanksgiving menu that draws from all the riches of the autumn's harvest is easy and not very different from what most of us grew up with. Make a few tweaks by using nondairy butter, nondairy milk, and vegetable stock instead of animal-based versions, and the side dishes remain the same. As for the main dish, I believe that what people are attached to is a beautiful *centerpiece* on the table and a focal point on the plate. Most of us were raised conditioned to believe that the centerpiece and focal point had to be animal-based meat, but really I think most people would agree that vegetables are so much more conducive to being stuffed than a bird is. I'll say no more about *that*, but please revisit the suggestions for creating a beautiful focal point outlined in Day 2: Trying New Foods.

Options for side dishes abound:

- ► Mashed potatoes and gravy
- ► Green beans sautéed in garlic and tossed with almond slices
- ► Traditional bread stuffing using vegetable broth and nondairy butter
- ► Cranberry relish
- ► Fresh or frozen corn
- ► Mashed rutabagas
- ► Roasted brussels sprouts or root vegetables
- ► Cornbread
- ► Biscuits or sliced bread
- ► Green salad

And of course, dessert options are never lacking, ranging from pies, cakes, and cobblers, to crisps, cookies, and breads.

These are just some of the dishes my husband and I enjoy at the annual Thanksgiving meal we host in our home. All of our friends pick a different dish to bring, and it's a veritable feast! When we go back east to celebrate the holidays with our families, they've always been so happy to host a vegan-only feast. We cook alongside our family, and everyone enjoys delicious, seasonal, plant-based fare.

Don't underestimate how your family will respond. Give them the benefit of the doubt, and don't forget: if you agree to cook, it means they don't have to, and who can resist someone else cooking the holiday meal?

HALLOWEEN

Another holiday connected to autumn and the harvest is an ancient Celtic holiday called Samhain (pronounced SAH-win). Its roots can be found in our modern-day Halloween and in the Catholic holiday, All Soul's Day. ("Halloween" means "hallowed evening"; "hallowed" means *holy*). Many European cultural traditions hold that Halloween is one of the times of the year when spirits can make contact with the physical world, and this is also seen in the Mexican holiday, *Día de los Muertos* (Day of the Dead), whose emphasis is on honoring the lives of those who died and celebrating the continuation of life.

Many of our modern customs related to this holiday have been borrowed from those in Celtic-speaking countries such as Scotland, Wales, and Ireland, where traditionally, adults and children disguised themselves and went from door to door singing or reciting verse in exchange for food or coins. This ritual is also called *mumming* or *guising* and is still found in the "Mummers plays" in the British Isles and parts of the United States.

All Hallows' Eve as a Christian observance is a time to honor the saints and pray for departed souls of loved ones. One of the early requirements during what was originally a 3-day vigil was to abstain from the consumption of animal flesh, and though this is no longer enforced, the tradition of eating certain plant foods persists, hence the popularity of apples, apple cider, colcannon (mashed potatoes mixed with greens), potato pancakes, and soul cakes. A "soul cake" is a cross between a scone and a cookie—small, round, and often filled with fruit and spices. The cakes themselves were called "souls" and were handed out to "soulers" (often the poor) who would go around from house to house on "All Hallow's Eve" reciting and singing prayers for the dead—a precursor to our modern-day custom of "Trick-or-Treating."

Like Thanksgiving, Halloween is a food-centered holiday, though in this case it's mostly *junk food;* i.e. candy. Apples and soul cakes aside, the primary way this holiday tends to be celebrated is by purchasing large amounts of commercial candy to give away to Trick-or-Treaters (who may as well be called Treaters at this point, because no one ever says, "Forget the treat! Let me show you a trick!").

Many newly vegan parents worry about how their children will fit into this popular ritual. Fear not. It turns out that a lot of candy given out during Halloween is vegan. It's *junk*, but it's vegan junk. So, don't worry. Your kid can be a normal kid—just like everyone else and get to eat *junk*, including:

Skittles, Mary Janes, Lemonheads, Smarties, Redhots, Blow Pops, Oreos, Dum Dums, Airheads, Atomic Fireballs, Cracker Jacks, Dots, Dubble Bubble and Hubba Bubba bubblegum, Big League Chew, Jolly Ranchers, Sour Patch Kids, Sweet Tarts, Red Vines, Twizzlers, Jujubes, Jujyfruits, Pez, Now and Later, Junior Mints, and Swedish Fish, plus nonsugary treats, such as potato chips, tortilla chips, pretzels, crackers, and nuts.

> **CHALLENGE YOUR THINKING:**
> We are social creatures indeed, but that doesn't mean that we need to teach our children that they always have to do what everyone else does. *Different* doesn't mean *inferior.*

I can't emphasize enough that if you're raising your children consistent with your values—compassion, kindness, and wellness—then this is just one more extension of that, and children will understand. Just as you do with other principles you are instilling in them, talk to them about why your family doesn't eat animal flesh and fluids—using age-appropriate language, tools, and resources, of course. We are social creatures indeed, but that doesn't mean that we need to teach our children that they always have to do what everyone else does. Different doesn't mean inferior. Individuality need not mean isolation. Living according to principles you believe in doesn't necessarily mean deprivation.

> **CHALLENGE YOUR THINKING:**
> Individuality need not mean isolation. Living by something you believe in doesn't necessarily mean deprivation.

And truly, these days with everyone allergic or sensitive to one thing or another, it's not odd at all for someone to have particular food preferences. Your child will not be ostracized because they don't eat Milk Duds, especially if you help give them a voice with which to express the reasons for your family's choices. Kids can develop a sense of strength and confidence when they don't have a fear of being different but are instead proud to make compassionate choices. When they show this confidence to their peers, they are often respected and happily accommodated by their friends. Of course, as adults, we need to model this confidence for our children.

So, on one hand, talk to your children about why your family doesn't eat animal products—sometimes found in processed foods and candies—but also try to put less of an emphasis on the candy during this holiday. Really, what kids enjoy so much about Halloween is the independence they feel running up to a stranger's front door (while you watch from the curb), the excitement of not knowing who will answer or what they will offer, the intrigue of dressing up, and the social aspect of parties and Trick-or-Treating. Emphasize these aspects more than the candy.

When it comes to the actual Trick-or-Treating, there are also a few practical things you can do:

- ▶ Let your kids know that the rule is they cannot eat any candy until they arrive home. This was what my parents insisted on when I was a child—not because we were vegan but because they wanted to instill self-restraint. Different motivation; same effect.

- ▶ Let your children help pick through the nonvegan treats they receive. Make a game of separating the vegan from nonvegan candy and use it as an opportunity to talk about such animal products as gelatin or cow's milk and why your family doesn't eat such things.

- ▶ Keep a stash of vegan treats for them at home, so they can trade the nonvegan candy for their favorite vegan candy you set aside for them.

SPRING HOLIDAYS: EASTER/PASSOVER

Easter is a Christian holiday that marks the end of Lent—a 40-day period of fasting, penance, and prayer—and celebrates the resurrection of Jesus Christ. I grew up Catholic and loved this time of year. There was a profound mix of sorrow and joy, darkness and light, solemnity and jubilation.

I also loved the rabbit-shaped chocolates and baskets of candy that were hidden for me to find. During Lent, you choose something to "give up," so the memory that is equally vivid for me is the awareness that the intention during this time of the year was to stop, reflect, and temporarily relinquish something you loved to eat, drink, say, or do. As I grew older, I would use it as a time to practice self-discipline and not swear, gossip, watch my favorite television shows, or smoke (yes, it's true, and it's a habit I have long-since dropped). From a secular perspective, I saw Lent as an opportunity for self-improvement and learned that—with a little conviction—we are capable of doing whatever it is we set our minds to.

During the Middle Ages, the consumption of meat, dairy, and eggs was forbidden during Lent. Then, over time, "dispensations" (exceptions) were allowed for dairy and so that, too, became acceptable to eat during this "fasting time." Eventually, eggs were allowed, and so they, too, became part of the "fast." Although the original doctrine was to not eat animal products at all during the 40 days between Ash Wednesday and Good Friday, by the time I was growing up, we had to abstain only on Fridays. And fish was acceptable. Whereas the original idea was for Catholics to abstain from consuming animal flesh *every Friday* throughout the year, these days, if a special holiday or occasion, such as a wedding, falls on a Friday, you're exempt; you can eat meat. In fact, here is what AmericanCatholic.org has to say about the rules for "abstinence" during Lent:

> *Abstinence does not include meat juices and liquid foods made from meat. Thus, such foods as chicken broth, consommé, soups cooked or flavored with meat, meat gravies or sauces, as well as seasonings or condiments made from animal fat are not forbidden. So it is permissible to use margarine and lard. Even bacon drippings which contain little bits of meat may be poured over lettuce as seasoning.* [68]

Although some Orthodox Christians still follow the earlier teachings to abstain from animal products altogether, clearly the bar is kept pretty low in terms of what is required of people. I'm certain that there are folks holding this book right now who decided to try The 30-Day Vegan Challenge during the Lenten season or who became vegan on their own volition during Lent and decided to stick with it.

My discussion of Lent is here to illustrate what I said previously in this chapter about picking and choosing the traditions we want to uphold. We justify the consumption of turkeys on Thanksgiving, eggs at Easter, and meat during Lent on the grounds of "tradition" even though it doesn't really hold up. To authentically honor the traditions of this Christian holiday would mean to abstain from meat, dairy, and eggs entirely during Lent, but rules have been relaxed to suit people's modern tastes and desires.

As I write in *The Vegan Table*, the bottom line is that "our holiday foods and rituals are often symbols for something much deeper. In being attached to the form (turkeys at Thanksgiving, eggs at Passover, 'ham' at Easter), we risk losing the true meaning of whatever it is we are celebrating or honoring. If we uncover the meanings of these symbols, we will find that a plant-based menu better reflects the values and significance of these holidays." [69]

For instance, the Easter eggs we boiled and colored as children *represented* something much deeper. Eggs are the perfect embodiment of the *hope* that after death comes life, that after winter comes spring, and that after despair comes hope itself. That's the point: the egg is the *symbol* of these ideas, but we have come to put more weight on the symbol rather than on its meaning. And for the hens whose reproductive cycles are exploited for this symbol, there is no life. There is no hope.

Individual Americans consume about 250 chicken eggs each year, and to keep this consumption steady, the egg industry currently confines over 290 million hens. With ad campaigns romantically touting the nutritional benefits of what the egg industry calls "nature's perfect food," egg consumption is on the rise.

Labels such as "organic, "cage-free," or "free-range" are effective marketing terms, but they mean very little to the birds themselves. Like all females (including humans), the reproductive cycles of hens slow down over time and eventually hens stop producing eggs. No longer "valuable" to the egg industry, all "unproductive" hens are sold to the meat industry and are killed to be used for "lower-grade" products such as canned soup or frozen pot pies. Most birds in operations labeled "humane" are still confined and crowded indoors, many are debeaked, and most come from the same hatcheries that kill over 250 million newly hatched male chicks each year in ways that make horror movies seem like Romantic Comedies.

Males are killed upon birth because they don't have eggs; it doesn't make economic sense to feed animals who will not produce anything in return. They're not kept and raised for "meat" because through selective breeding, egg-laying breeds are created for the purpose of high egg production—not fast flesh growth that is valued in the meat industry. Male chicks are ground up and used as fertilizer, as food for other "livestock," or as filler for dog and cat food.

This is all very different from what we envision this spring holiday to be about, but we can still experience the meaning of this holiday without compromising our values.

▶ We can still use the egg as a symbol for life, birth, and hope, but paint wooden, ceramic, or papier mâché eggs that can be cherished each year as decoration. Or, fill plastic eggs with treats for children and hide them at Easter Egg hunts; the plastic eggs can be re-used each year. No waste. No suffering.

▶ When I reflect on the Easter Egg Hunts I loved as a child, it wasn't the eggs themselves (or the dairy-based chocolate candy) as much as the fact that it was a community event with friends and family—and all the children were tasked with a quest to *find* what was hidden just for us. That excitement isn't lessened because animal products aren't used.

▶ A more consistent—and compassionate—symbol for spring would be a flower bulb or vegetable seeds or a tree. In fact, they are more than just a symbol in that they really do hold (and deliver!) the promise of a flower or vegetables or leaves and fruit. What better way for our children to understand the processes of nature—that with tenderness, attention, and water—there is a beautiful (and even edible) outcome.

Celebrate the foods of the season and create your menu around arugula, asparagus, basil, broccoli, cabbage, carrots, cauliflower, corn, fava beans, grapefruit, green onions, leeks, lemons, lettuce, limes, mint, nettles, new potatoes, parsnips, pea greens, peppers, radicchio, spinach, spring greens, and watercress.

▶ Many vegan chocolatiers sell chocolate bunnies, chocolate eggs, and other candy we associate with Easter baskets this time of year, including AllisonsGourmet.com (which also features the most delicious brownies, fudge, cookies, and confections throughout the year).

EASTER/SPRING EQUINOX—RECIPES TO CELEBRATE RENEWAL

PASSOVER

Of course, Easter and Lent are not the only religious observances that fall in the beginning of spring. Passover (*Pesach*) is a Jewish festival that commemorates the exodus of Jews out of Egypt and thus from slavery to freedom. The central ritual of Passover is a special dinner called a Seder, the etymology of which is derived from the Hebrew word for "order," referring to the specific order of the ritual meal itself.

Each food and beverage chosen for the meal represents an element of the narrative told in Exodus in the Bible and represents the very significant journey to freedom. For instance, leavened foods are not eaten because when fleeing Egypt, the Jews wouldn't have had time to allow their dough to rise, so the only acceptable bread is made from matzo and is used to make everything from cakes and cookies (matzo flour), breadcrumbs (matzo meal), and bread itself (in the form of full-sized matzos).

The six symbolic foods on the Seder Plate play an important role, since they're used to recount the story of the exodus, but like Easter eggs *representing* renewal and rebirth, these Seder foods stand for something else. They convey the elements of the powerful message of Passover: that freedom is possible, that slavery can end, and that the future can be better than the past or the present. Although many plant foods are traditionally part of the dinner, a few animal products are also used as symbols, though plant foods can be used in those cases as well:

▶ Fruit (both dried and fresh), along with nuts and sweet spices are soaked in wine resulting in a flavorful dish called Charoset (or Haroset), representing the mortar that Jews worked with when they were enslaved by the Egyptians.

▶ Bitter herbs represent the harshness of slavery. Ashkenazi Jews tend to use horseradish or the bitter-tasting heart of romaine lettuce; Sephardic Jews often use celery leaves, green onion, or parsley.

▶ A vegetable, other than bitter herbs, is dipped in salt water to signify the slaves' tears.

▶ A boiled egg—a symbol of fertility and new life—is replaced at vegan Seders with roasted nuts, a flower, or a small white egg-sized eggplant. Same symbolic meaning. No suffering for anyone.

► The only meat on the Seder plate is the "shankbone" of a lamb or goat (or the neck or wing of a chicken) and is meant to represent the lamb that was offered for sacrifice. Jewish vegans use roasted beets, expressly allowed by the Talmud, or a sweet potato.

What better way to celebrate the freedom from slavery than to use symbols that do not merely convey compassion, freedom, and liberation but that actually *are* products of compassion, freedom, and liberation; i.e. plants? Certainly, the animals themselves—the victims of our appetites—would have us include *them* in our circle of compassion. Like us, they want to live. If they have wings, they want to fly. If they have legs, they want to walk. If they have voices, they want to communicate. If they have offspring, they want to nurture them.

To center our holiday meals on foods that give life rather than take life is in keeping with the values we hold and the ideals we are celebrating.

Understanding Weight Loss: Calorie Reduction and Calorie Expenditure

You may have chosen to take the Challenge out of a desire to lose weight, and you wouldn't be alone, but I want to clarify something up front: I'm not a fan of so-called "experts" who promise that if you go vegan, you are *guaranteed* to lose weight (assuming you need to). I don't think it's accurate or fair to make such an overgeneralization. For one thing, I don't think that's a good enough reason to become vegan; rather, I think (potential) weight loss and all the health benefits are byproducts of living a conscious, compassionate life filled with nutrient-rich plant-based foods.

Second, I don't see veganism as a *diet*.

Third, I think it is irresponsible to promise someone that his or her weight will drop immediately upon becoming vegan, because if it doesn't, that person winds up feeling like a failure. To boot, they think "being vegan" isn't what they hoped it would be—and they give up. That's not good at all. Not good for them, not good for me, and not good for the animals.

Having said that, it's accurate to say that *some* people *do* lose weight upon eliminating animal products from their diet. Although there are always exceptions, studies do indicate that people who eat a plant-based diet have a lower body mass index,[70] have less body fat, are less likely to be overweight or obese than people who eat animals.[71] And, that translates to being at lower risk for certain disease such as diabetes and atherosclerosis (which leads to heart attacks and strokes).

But, weight loss is not a *guarantee* of becoming vegan—and, of course, many people don't want to and don't need to lose weight. Some people may actually want or need to *gain* weight—and that can be done on a vegan "diet," as well, because—after all—there are a million ways to "be vegan."

Regarding weight loss and veganism, I think it's far more appropriate—and accurate—to say, "People who switch from an animal-based diet to a plant-based diet *tend* to healthfully lose unnecessary pounds because plants are much less calorie-dense than animal flesh and fluids."

The main reason for this is fat. Remember the basics behind macronutrients and calories? There are:

4 calories in 1 gram of protein,

4 calories in 1 gram of carbohydrates, and

9 calories in 1 gram of fat.

Most nonvegan's fat consumption comes from animal products: meat, cheese, and eggs, and though there is indeed fat in plant foods, there is generally much less than there is in animal products. As a result, on a plant-based diet, you tend to consume fewer calories without much effort. And, everyone knows that eating fewer calories leads to weight loss.

When you burn more calories than you consume, you experience weight loss, so if you want to lose weight, you need to do one of two things: take in fewer calories or burn more calories. (Or do both at the same time.) If weight loss is your goal, it is a simple numbers game. Weight loss is all about *decreasing* your energy (calorie) intake and increasing your calorie (energy) output so that you end up with a *calorie deficit* at the end of the day.

Here's how it works:

3,500 calories represents one pound of body fat. Let's say your aim is to lose 20 pounds. Here's what I mean when I say it's a numbers game. 20 pounds is the equivalent of 70,000 calories. (To get that number, I multiplied 3,500 by 20.) So, to lose 20 pounds, you must *burn* 70,000 more calories than you *consume.* That's just basic math. The question is: over what time period should this happen? Most experts agree that losing no more than 2 pounds a week is the safest and most sustainable rate for healthy weight loss. So, let's break this down: if you aim to lose 2 pounds a week, it would take you 10 weeks to lose 20 pounds. (10 weeks is the equivalent of 70 days.)

So, sticking with our numbers game, then, you want to aim for a daily deficit of 1,000 calories (70,000 calories divided by our 70 days). You can do that either by eating 1,000 fewer calories a day or by burning 1,000 additional calories a day for 10 weeks. Or you can do it by eating 500 fewer calories and burning 500 more calories. I'm using this example because these numbers are just easy, but you can create your own calculation. You can lose the same amount—20 pounds—but lose

> **CHALLENGE YOUR THINKING:**
> On a plant-based diet, you tend to consume fewer calories without much effort, and eating fewer calories leads to weight loss.

> **CHALLENGE YOUR THINKING:**
> Weight loss is a numbers game. When you burn more calories than you consume, you experience weight loss.
>
> **CHANGE YOUR BEHAVIOR:**
> To lose weight, either take in fewer calories or burn more calories.

one pound a week, which means you lose it slower and just have a daily deficit of 500 calories. The point is you can create the calculation yourself based on your own goals.

You can have a lot of fun just deciding how you want to achieve this deficit. (Yes, I just said weight loss can be fun.)

CALORIE REDUCTION

Let's talk first about reducing the number of calories taken in. As I said, this may happen very naturally for you within these 30 days, but what I hope you realize is that *eating fewer calories does not necessarily mean eating less food.* We are not talking about a *diet* here but rather a mathematical principle. Essentially, you can eat more and weigh less because a plant-based diet enables you to eat *more* food in terms of volume and still take in fewer calories.

It's true that there are fewer calories in plant foods because there is less fat in plant foods, but if you're aiming to lose weight, you'll want to have a smaller ratio of high-fat plant foods such as avocados, nuts, and seeds. You'll also want to limit or eliminate deep-fried foods and empty-calorie snack foods, which is a good thing, because instead you'll be filling your body with high-nutrient plant foods.

The Cost of Calories

In fact, what if we reduced the calories we ate and experienced weight loss in a joyful, empowering way? Think of it this way. There are inherent costs associated with what we eat: monetary costs, environmental costs, health costs, costs to our values, costs to the animals, etc. There is also the *cost* of calories. Each time we eat, we make either an investment in or a withdrawal from our health and well-being account.

The idea is this: choose the number of calories you want to "spend" (i.e. *eat*) throughout each day, but choose to spend (*eat*) them as effectively as possible—spending (eating) calories that are nutrient-dense rather than empty. (Empty calories refer to foods that are calorie-rich but nutrient-poor.) The goal is to make sure that every calorie we spend (i.e. *take in*) goes towards giving us the best bang for our caloric buck. We want the calories we eat to give us the most amount of energy, provide us with a plethora of healthful nutrients, contribute to both short- and long-term health, and give us pleasure.

We *can* have all of that. It's not about experiencing deprivation. It's not about sacrifice; it's about creating a budget.

Just as when you do your financial budget you determine how much money you have and then figure out how you want to spend it, I suggest you do the same for your calorie budget. You can spend it however you

CHALLENGE YOUR THINKING:
Every time we eat, we make either an investment in or a withdrawal from our health and well-being.

CHANGE YOUR BEHAVIOR:
Choose the number of calories you want to spend throughout the day and spend them as effectively as possible: spending calories that are nutrient-dense rather than nutrient-poor.

like each day. You don't even have to deprive yourself of your favorite cookie or eggless mayonnaise on your sandwich. *You* can decide how to spend your calories, but—like all good budgeters, you learn to spend them wisely.

And just as *credit* really isn't the best way to make purchases with your dollars—because you're spending money you don't have—you also learn that if you *spend* (eat) calories, you have to *pay* for them! So, if you really want that piece of chocolate—let's say it's 200 calories—you just have to realize that you need to pay for it by burning those 200 calories (or spending 200 less elsewhere).

HOW MANY CALORIES TO SPEND EACH DAY?

Since in terms of healthful weight loss, it's a matter of having a calorie *deficit*, the number of calories you consume each day matters less than the fact that you consume fewer calories than you burn (or burn more calories than you take in). For example, if you're aiming to lose one pound a week, then you'll want to have a calorie deficit of 500 calories a day (or 3,500 calories a week—the equivalent of one pound). So, if you *take in* 2,000 calories in one day, and your goal is to have a *deficit* of 500 calories that day, then you need to burn *a total* of 2,500 calories, which you will do through normal activities as well as through *intentional* cardiovascular movement.

Your weight loss can be slow or fast depending on the deficit you choose, though most experts would recommend losing no more than 2 pounds a week.

Wisely Spending 500 Calories

Let's look at some ways to wisely "spend" (eat) 500 calories.

Breakfast

▶ One 6-ounce container of coconut milk yogurt is about 140 calories. (Soy milk yogurt tends to be between 160 and 170 calories, depending on the flavor). Add to that 2 tablespoons walnuts (100 calories), 1 tablespoon of ground flaxseeds (50 calories), and you've got plenty of calories to spend on fruit: 110 calories or so for a medium banana; about 40 calories for an entire half-cup of blueberries; 20 calories for a half-cup of whole strawberries.

▶ One-half cup of cooked oatmeal is about 150 calories. Add to that 1 tablespoon of brown sugar or maple syrup (~50 calories) or whatever sweetener you like (they're all around the same calories), plus 1 apple chopped (70 calories), a tablespoon of walnuts (50 calories), and a tablespoon of ground flaxseeds (50 calories). You still have calories to spare—add more fruit or oats.

Fruit smoothies can be calorie-dense or calorie-light, depending on your goal. Add one banana (110 calories), half-cup blueberries (40 calories), 1 tablespoon peanut butter (80 calories), 1 tablespoon ground flaxseeds (50 calories), and 1 cup of nondairy milk (90 calories) for about 370 calories. Make it less calorie-dense by using reduced calorie plant-based milk or halving the milk and adding cold filtered water. The options abound!

▶ If you want to spend 500 calories on a heartier breakfast, there are 150 calories in an average-size pancake. People usually have three or more, so that's about 450 calories. Adding one teaspoon of Earth Balance would add 33 calories, and two tablespoons of maple syrup would add 100 more. Instead of the nondairy butter and liquid sweeteners, however, just pile on the fruit!

▶ When choosing cold cereals, I recommend the ones that are the least processed, like Grape Nuts (200 calories for ½ cup) or Shredded Wheat (183 calories for 1 cup for bite-sized shredded wheat). Although they're a little more processed, All Bran (81 calories for ½ cup) and Bran Flakes (95 calories for ¾ cup) are also options. Add to your cereal bowl some nondairy milk (all of them average about 90 calories for 8 fluid ounces), and of course a banana (110 calories) and berries (40 calories), and you're good to go.

▶ You're not going to get a lot of bang for your calorie buck if you just have a bagel (about 350 calories) and peanut butter (190 calories for 2 tablespoons), but you can still choose that option, choosing whole grain versions.

The question to ask is, "Is that how I want to spend my precious calories?" The answer is up to you.

Lunch/Dinner

▶ Five Tofurky slices (100 calories) on two slices of whole-wheat bread (200 calories) or whole-wheat pita bread (170 calories), with one tablespoon of vegan mayonnaise (80 calories) or mustard (15 calories per tablespoon), allows you to pile on the lettuce, tomato, and alfalfa sprouts. Make a bunch of kale chips to go with that sandwich. One whole bunch of kale is only 50 calories, and only one teaspoon of oil (40 calories) is needed to make the whole bunch of chips. That still leaves room for two or three carrots cut up.

▶ Two Wildwood Southwest Tofu Burgers are 340 calories; two Dr. Praeger's California burgers are 220 calories; or two of Amy's California Veggie Burger are 140 calories. Add a whole grain bun (or not), a side of sautéed veggies or a salad, and you're under or around 500 calories.

▶ Green salads are the best way to spend your calories wisely. The greens (lettuce, arugula, kale, chard, etc.) needed for an entire salad add a mere 50 calories—but with loads of nutrients. Top with beans (a can of rinsed and drained beans averages 330 calories, so use half a can if you want to spend more calories on raw veggies) or 3 ounces of extra firm tofu (around 90 calories.) Pile on the veggies: 1 tomato is 15 calories; 1 medium raw carrot is 35 calories; 1 cup of cauliflower is 25 calories. There are many low-calorie dressings, though my favorite is just seasoned rice vinegar mixed with minced garlic and miso.

Snacks

▶ The best way to spend calories for weight loss and nutrition is on raw veggies and fruit. Cut them up so you can savor each bite, and choose them according to what's in season. Raw carrots, bell peppers, cauliflower florets are wonderful snacks. Dip them in a little hummus or peanut butter.

▶ One cup of air-popped popcorn is 30 calories (though I never eat just a cup!). Toss it with a few mists of spray-on olive oil, nutritional yeast, and salt. (My favorite is truffle salt!) See recipe on page 185 for my Truffle Popcorn.

▶ Vegan ice creams vary, but a cup of ice cream is anywhere from between 250 and 400 calories, depending on the brand and flavor. My favorite "ice cream" is just frozen bananas thrown in the blender, along with some almond milk, vanilla extract, and cinnamon. Try varying the flavor by adding in some frozen strawberries, mango, pineapple or other favorite frozen fruit. Add a few walnuts and a little maple syrup and vanilla for a "maple walnut ice cream"!

Beverages

Beverages can be a part of your total calories for the day, but they can really add many calories very quickly. If that's where you want to spend, that's up to you, but consider:

▶ A 4-ounce glass of red table wine is about 100 calories; a dry white is between 80 and 100.

▶ A 12-ounce bottle of beer is typically 150 calories.

▶ 8 ounces of nondairy milk is about 90 calories.

▶ 8 ounces of orange juice is 110 calories.

▶ Exotic coffee drinks vary, but you may be surprised at how calorically high some of them are, including fruit shakes and smoothies. Try not to spend all of your calories on drinks!

When you realize *you* have the power to spend calories the way you want to—and pay for it with a little calorie expenditure, then you can allow yourself to have more indulgent food for a special occasion or dinner at a special restaurant. Just as when you buy a new pair of fabulous leather-free shoes, you have to cough up the dough, so, too, with food. You can have the birthday cake or special treat, but just know that you'll have pay in the form of extra calories. There are no free rides.

A FEW TIPS FOR LOSING WEIGHT

▶ **Set a goal.** Studies indicate that setting goals really do help people more successfully lose weight. The goals might be pounds lost, inches lost, muscle gained, body fat lost—or whatever works for you—but set a goal, and make it realistic. And, remember, experts recommend losing no more than two pounds per week.

- ► **Keep temptations out of the house.** A big part of being tempted by the high-calorie foods we love is figuring out how they are put in front of us in the first place. If they are not in our homes, we will be less tempted by them. If you want to do yourself the biggest favor, keep the stuff that tempts you out of the house! When I was writing *The Joy of Vegan Baking*, I tested 150 desserts! That's a lot of baked goods in my home in a short period. So, to resist the temptation of having so many treats in the house, I would bake, take a bite or two to confirm taste and texture, and then give the rest to my husband to take to his co-workers. It's not that I don't have self-control; it's that it just that it doesn't make any sense to make it any harder on me than I had to. With treats like that in the house, it's too easy to eat them.

- ► **Know what your temptations are.** For some, it's baked goods; for some it's bread; for some it's pretzels; for others, it's chips or ice cream. Only you know, so be honest with yourself and keep those things out of your cupboards if it helps.

- ► **Write down your calorie intake for the first 30 days when you're trying to lose weight,** after which time you'll have a better idea of the calorie content of your favorite foods.

- ► **Find a buddy.** It should be enough that we're accountable to ourselves, but sometimes it's helpful to have to be accountable to someone else, too. Find someone you trust and either create a commitment to each other—or just find someone that you can confide in and tell what your goals are so someone else knows you are striving toward something.

CALORIE BURN/EXPENDITURE

We are beings made to *move*—not lead sedentary lives. We need to move—and we need to give our bones a reason to live.

In terms of intentional calorie burn, we have a million options. When I say "intentional calorie burn," I mean that which is in the form of cardiovascular exercise versus the calories we burn just breathing and being alive. The best form of exercise for you is that which makes you most excited and gets you most motivated.

Personally, I'm not a gym person—I prefer to run, walk, and hike outside—those are my preferred forms of "intentional exercise," and I love them. Being excited about what forms you choose makes it so much more enjoyable!

- ► **Running:** The number of calories you burn during any cardiovascular exercise depends on your weight. On average, women burn approximately 105 calories and men burn approximately 124 calories on a 1-mile (1.6 km) run. So, we're talking about 300 calories for a 3-mile run. That's pretty good! If you're going for a 500-calorie deficit each day, bump it to five miles. That kind of math will help you set your goals and stick to them.

- ▶ **Walking:** If you're not a runner, that's fine. Perhaps you like walking. It's a low-impact exercise that can be done anywhere—just remember that it takes more time to burn more calories when you're walking versus doing something more intense. In terms of calorie burn, women burn about 75 calories and men burn about 87 calories for a 1-mile (1.6 km) walk. A 160-pound person walking briskly could burn about 275 calories in one hour; if you increase your pace to a 5-mph jog, you can burn almost twice that amount in the same time.

- ▶ **Hiking:** As someone who has to be outside as much as possible, when I'm not running or walking, I'm hiking, which is really just walking in the woods but perhaps with more hills. By choosing a trail with hills, you expend some extra calories, and if you run a little bit (or at least walk briskly), you burn more, too.

- ▶ **Cycling:** Cycling is another way to take in the outdoors, and it's also an option at your fitness club. If your gym offers spinning classes, it's an effective workout in a short period. In terms of calorie burn: a 160-pound person cycling at a leisurely 10 miles per hour will burn almost 300 calories in an hour; a 200-pound person would burn about 365 in an hour. You definitely burn more calories on a mobile bicycle than when you're on a stationary bike, but a stationary bike is better than nothing.

- ▶ **Swimming:** Although appropriate for anyone, water exercise is an especially good option for people who cannot tolerate impact. Swimming, water jogging, and water aerobics are easier on the joints and back than running or jumping rope. One hour of swimming consistent laps burns a little over 500 calories for a 160-pound person.

There are so many additional ways to get moving. Take your pick: join a gym, jump rope, dance, lift weights, join a sports team, practice yoga, play tennis, bowl, skate, rollerblade, ski, golf, take an aerobics class, or buy a workout video. Though they all vary in terms of calories burned, the point is to get moving.

Setting goals for something like a race proves to be very helpful, because you're working toward a goal, and you tend to push yourself a little more. If you don't want to do a formal race and you have a lot of self-discipline, then at least create goals for yourself that involve increasing your pace, increasing your distance, or increasing the number of times you exercise. Creating goals really makes a difference for people.

You might be asking how to calculate calories burned throughout the day to better keep track of your weight loss. You have a couple options.

1. **Estimate.** Once you have an idea of how many calories you burn in a cardio interval (let's say 500 for a run), that's a start. I know many machines in gyms have read-outs telling you how many calories you burned, but they're not *that* accurate. Frankly, I'd subtract 100 calories from whatever it tells you, especially if you are using a machine that doesn't ask you to enter your weight and other information. There are a number of calculators online, such as healthstatus.com, that enable you to calculate various activities.

2. **Use a monitor.** There are a number of monitors available to track your calorie-burn throughout the day. The best and most heavily studied devices are the BodyMedia arm band (featured on The Biggest Loser TV show) and Fitbit (fitbit.com).

STRENGTH TRAINING

Many people who are exercising solely to lose weight may not spend much (or any) time on strength training exercises under the belief that only cardiovascular exercises will help them burn calories and lose weight. Although cardiovascular exercises will burn more calories per workout, strength-training workouts play a very important role in burning calories. Strength training improves muscle mass, which helps the body burn calories more efficiently. Strength training helps the body burn more calories during other types of exercises.

And, since muscle holds less water and takes up less room than the equivalent weight of fat, by shedding fat and gaining muscle, you can lose inches and sizes without losing actual pounds on the scale. And, measuring inches lost and clothing sizes is another measuring stick besides just looking at pounds.

But, keep in mind that the time spent doing resistance exercise burns fewer calories than if the same time were spent on aerobic activities. So, in terms of the most effective use of your time in relation to calorie burn—you're going to get that with cardio. If you want both, though—calorie burn and toned muscles— then make both part of your routine. It's worth saying, though, that strength training has benefits beyond being part of a weight loss regiment.

- By stressing your bones, you increase bone density and reduce the risk of osteoporosis, which is a good thing.

- Building muscle protects your joints from injury. It also helps you maintain flexibility and balance.

- Strength training can boost your self-confidence, improve your body image, and reduce the risk of depression.

- Strength training can reduce the signs and symptoms of many chronic conditions, including arthritis, back pain, depression, diabetes, obesity, and osteoporosis.

So, get moving—even if weight loss isn't your goal. *Lack* of physical activity is associated with many diseases, including cardiovascular disease, high blood pressure, diabetes, osteoporosis, and depression, and it's a leading cause of obesity.

On the positive side, cardiovascular exercise has a number of positive psychological, emotional, and physiological affects. It even has social benefits, such as when we combine exercise with social activities, such as spending time with friends, neighbors, or family.

And remember: if we don't have time to be sick, we have to make time to be healthy.

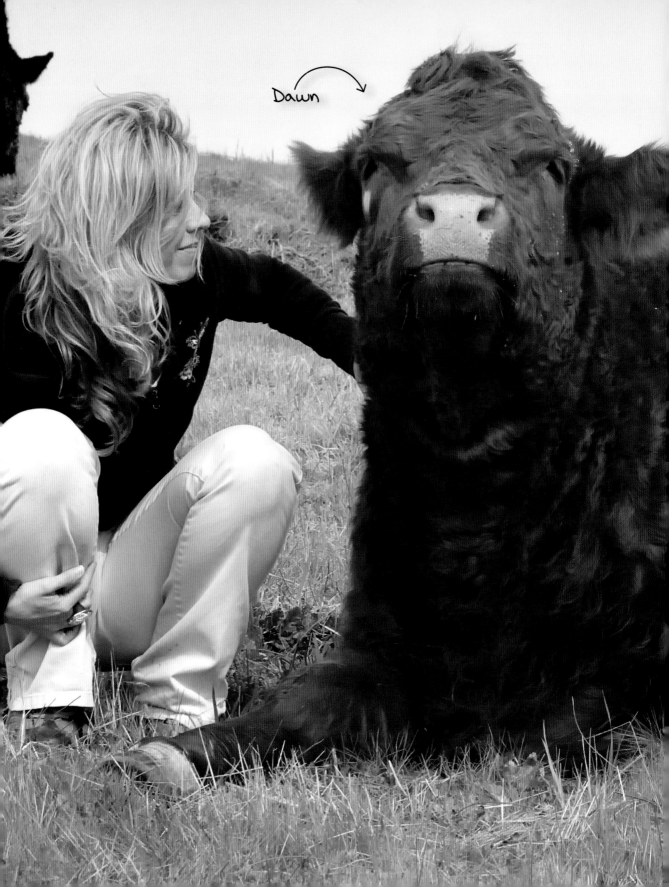

Dawn

Compassionate Fashion: It's Cool to Be Kind

As you wrap up your 30 days, reaping the many benefits of a compassionate, plant-fueled diet, you may be more keenly aware not only of the animals you once put in your mouth but also of the animals you may be wearing on your body in the form of leather shoes, leather purse, wool suits and dresses, silk ties, Pashmina scarves, and cashmere sweaters. You may suddenly realize there's goose down in your winter coat, duck feathers in your pillows and comforter, and fur lining in your gloves.

As our awareness expands, so does our desire to be consistent in our values, which is why many people extend their compassionate ethics beyond their diet to their wardrobe and home goods. But just as we have been conditioned to believe that meat, dairy, and eggs are healthful, so, too, has animal skin, fur, and hair been touted as "natural," "humane," and even "eco-friendly," leading many compassionate people to unknowingly support practices they really are opposed to. Below is a brief overview of leather, wool, feathers/down, silk, and fur with many recommendations for choosing compassionate versions.

LEATHER

When I was about 17 years old, there was a leather store in the mall near where I lived, which sold everything from coats, belts, and jackets to purses, wallets, and shoes—all made out of leather. I was obsessed with a particular black leather skirt they carried, and I saved up my money to buy it. Around the same time, I had a brown leather bomber jacket that I wore with affection, as well as a pair of brown leather cowboy boots. I absolutely loved all of these things, and I had no idea what I was contributing to. I was already someone who cared about animals, and yet I had successfully compartmentalized my compassion and my understanding—blissfully ignorant of the impact I was having. In fact, I continued to wear leather shoes even after I had stopped eating land animals. I simply did not make the connection.

Denial is deep and vast, and it tends to manifest itself in the excuses we tell ourselves to justify our behavior—not only to feel *better* about what we're doing but also to feel *good* about it. When it comes to leather, we often declare that it is just a byproduct of the meat industry, and say we feel good knowing they're at least doing something with the leftover parts of the animals instead of having them go to waste. As much as we like to believe the leather industry is motivated by waste-conscious altruism, it is not the case. The U.S. leather industry is a $1.5 billion business tanning over 100 million animal skins every year; worldwide, it's even bigger, representing $46 billion, ranking among the most important internationally traded commodities.

CHALLENGE YOUR THINKING:
One of the reasons meat is so cheap (aside from the government subsidies the meat industry receives) is because slaughterhouse byproducts are so profitable. The leather industry subsidizes the meat industry.

What most people don't understand is that the meat industry is *not* sustainable on its own. It *relies* on skin sales to remain profitable. Let me put this another way: One of the reasons meat is so cheap (aside from the subsidies it receives from the government) is because they can sell so much of the animal's other body parts, such as the skin and fat, for a profit. According to the U.S. Department of Agriculture, the skin represents the most economically important byproduct of the meat-packing industry.[72]

Most leather is from cattle—bulls, steers, cows, and calves—though not all. Buckskin comes from deer; suede is made from lambs, goats, pigs, calves, and deer; pigskin is from pigs and often used to make riding saddles; horses' skin tends to be used for baseballs; and a "shearling" garment is created from the skin of young lambs, which is tanned with the wool still on. And, even though the slaughter industry relies on the leather industry to be profitable, that doesn't mean wild animals are safe. Some animals in the U.S., such as deer, sharks and alligators are killed only for their skins, and animals killed outside the U.S. include zebras, bison, water buffaloes, kangaroos, elephants, eels, dolphins, seals, walruses, frogs, crocodiles and lizards. Australia exports approximately three million kangaroo skins every year, and though you won't see "Kangaroo" on the label, but you will see "K leather" or "RKT."

Much of the leather sold in the U.S. comes from overseas, especially from India. That may surprise people who thought cattle were considered "sacred" in this country. Not everyone in India follows Hindu principles, and the law dictates that cattle can be killed in certain provinces. In fact, they can be raised in one province but killed in another, which often means the cattle are forced to travel hundreds of miles on foot, in the hot sun, with their noses tied together. China is also another of the world's leading exporters of leather. In addition to using cattle and sheep, an estimated two million cats and dogs in China are killed for their hides each year.

From an environmental and health perspective, the tanning process is incredibly energy-intensive and pollution producing. In fact, tanneries are listed as top polluters on the Environmental Protection Agency's Superfund list, which identifies the most critical industrial sites in need of environmental cleanup. Because of their high toxic levels, many old tannery sites can't even be used for agriculture, built on, or even sold. Tanning is bad for the workers, bad for people who live near these tanneries, bad for the rivers that ultimately collect these toxins (formaldehyde, coal tar derivatives, oils, dyes, and cyanide-based compounds), and bad for the animals and eco-systems affected by these toxins in the environment.

ALTERNATIVES TO LEATHER

What's a compassionate fashionista to do? Well, once you've decided not to contribute to the leather and meat industry, you have plenty of options, and they're everywhere you look!

The main thing to look for on the label when you're buying synthetic leather is "manmade materials." (Note that you might see "manmade materials" for the main part of the shoe but "leather uppers," so look carefully at the label.) You can find synthetic shoes in virtually every store from Macy's and Saks Fifth Avenue to Birkenstock and Payless. Even higher-end lines, including Stella McCartney, Steve Madden, Chinese Laundry, Kenneth Cole, Nine West, and Kate Spade all feature stylish, affordable synthetic footwear and accessories.

As a runner, I have to make sure I have the best running sneakers in terms of comfort and safety, and I never have a problem finding what I need. New Balance is my go-to brand for running sneakers—though there many are other brands, as well—and Merrell makes great walking and hiking shoes. Whenever I visit a shoe store, I just ask them to tell me which ones are leather-free, and they're always happy to assist, or I just search on their websites for "synthetic" or "vegan."

There are also many online and brick-and-mortar stores dedicated to only to vegan shoes, and the options continue to expand. MooShoes (mooshoes.com) has a beautiful shoe store in New York City as well as their entire inventory online. No Harm (noharm.com) is a UK-based online shoe store featuring professional men's shoes. Coral 8 (coral8.com) is an online shoe store featuring trendy women's shoes, including flats, pumps, and boots. These purveyors are conscious not only of carrying animal-free wares, but they extend those ethics to every aspect of the manufacturing process. For instance, you'll find that they only use suppliers who adhere to fair labor practices, ensuring that workers get fair pay and safe working conditions. These vegan companies—and the ones listed below—go to great lengths to make sure their products are high-quality, ethical, and sustainable—as well as fashionable.

Alternative Outfitters (alternativeoutfitters.com) is another fabulous fashion-conscious vegan-owned store, and they carry super cute shoes, bags, wallets, and accessories. They also carry the vegan ethic to all aspects of their business and ensure that the products made outside of the U.S. and Canada are made under fair trade conditions and are not manufactured with child labor or under sweatshop conditions.

Outside of the U.S., there are the pioneers: Vegetarian Shoes and Bags (vegetarian-shoes.co.uk). A vegan-owned shoe store based in England, they have been around since 1990. They're also concerned with human rights as well as animal rights and work to make sure they are buying from companies that don't exploit the humans. There are so many other online retailers, including zappos.com (search for "vegan"), overstock.com (search for "faux"), veganchic.com, veganessentials.com, and veganstore.com.

Many of these companies also carry non-leather wallets, guitar straps, briefcases, gloves, purses, and belts for men and women, including those from Truth Belts (vegetarianbelts.com), and Matt and Nat (mattandnat.com). Of course, there are also other wonderful alternatives to leather, such as "microsuede," "microfiber," cotton, linen, rubber, ramie, canvas, bamboo, and a whole range of synthetics.

FEATHERS AND DOWN

During the second half of the nineteenth century, plumaged headwear was incredibly popular in the United States, and I'm not talking about just a few feathers in a hat! Veritable birds' nests complete with stuffed birds, perched atop a woman's head. Early animal advocacy pioneers campaigned against these hats and won a huge legislative, cultural, and ethical victory. Sadly, it didn't end the practice of killing birds for their feathers or down, and we see them used today in everything from comforters to winter coats.

Sometimes our attachment to certain comfort items can be so tenacious that we genuinely believe that no one is harmed in their production; what's more is that we give more credence to the people selling the goods than we give to our own consciences, economic realities, and basic common sense. Ask people how they think feathers and down are acquired, and many will insist they just fall off the birds and are collected by opportunists. Some even think the feathers are massaged off, while the birds live a pampered life. Unfortunately, this is not the case.

Geese and ducks are the primary victims of the feather and down industries (chickens and turkeys don't produce down), but ostriches are also exploited for their beautiful plumes. A very lucrative multimillion-dollar industry, most of it is situated in China, Hungary, and Poland, though more than 25 countries are involved in the production of feathers and down, taken either from live geese (referred to as "live plucking" or "ripping") or dead. Feathers from live animals are considered better quality and thus have a higher value. The geese are plucked three to four times a year before they're killed. Many are force-fed to produce foie gras before they meet their end.

ALTERNATIVES TO FEATHER AND DOWN

Feather- and down-free blankets, coats, and sleeping bags are widely available. Many bedding stores, such as The Company Store (thecompanystore.com) and West Elm (westelm.com), sell down-free comforters, duvets, and pillows in various colors and sizes. Look for "down alternatives" or "Primaloft" on their website. Many other companies market their own down-free versions, "hypo-allergenic down alternatives" called MICROMAX™, Nature's Touch™, Sensuelle, and Thinsulate.

Consider another advantage of synthetic down: when wet, the thermal properties of animal-based down are virtually eliminated, making it a much worse insulator than equally wet synthetic fills. To make up for this, sleeping bags insulated with down also require the use of a sleeping pad to provide insulation from warmth that would otherwise be conducted into the ground. So, essentially, the down is useless. And, that applies to coats. Coats made with down are not waterproof, whereas if you get a down-free jacket with a waterproof material like Gore Tex, you have the advantage of good insulation.

In fact, many outdoor clothing stores and brands (REI, Patagonia, North Face) carry puffy, warm, down-free jackets and vests, using synthetic Primaloft and recycled Thermogreen materials. Many options abound, and they're less expensive than the animal versions. Just visit sporting goods stores and ask the sales people for down-free coats, or search for "synthetic down" on their websites.

WOOL

Wool is like the leather industry in that you can't support the wool industry without supporting the meat industry, and all sheep raised for their wool are eventually killed for their flesh. Australia and China dominate the wool industry, with Iran, New Zealand, and Turkey following closely behind.

The dominant breed used in the wool industry is the Merino sheep, bred specifically to have wrinkled skin to increase the amount of wool they carry. Besides causing many sheep to die of heat exhaustion from carrying so much bulk and weight, the wrinkled skin gets moisture trapped building up an odor that attracts flies and maggots, whose bites cause the sheep tremendous discomfort and pain. The industry calls this "fly-strike" or "blow-strike." To remedy this and smooth out the skin, the sheep farmers cut off chunks of the sheep's skin around the tail without anesthesia, a process called mulesing.

Sheep are sheared at an incredible pace (shearers who are hired are paid by volume, not by the hour), a rough process that stresses out these already sensitive prey animals and often results in cuts and wounds that are left untreated. Just as with dairy cows, when sheep are no longer considered economically viable to provide shelter and food for, they are culled from the herd usually at 4 or 5 years old (their life expectancy is 15 to 20 years) and sold to slaughter. With so many "excess animals," the live animal export industry materialized. Livestock ships can carry up to 100,000 animals for voyages that last up to three weeks, painful, arduous journeys during which many sheep die. Once the sheep arrive at their destination, unloading them at the ports takes its own toll, and the sheep are sent straight to backyard butchers or dirty slaughterhouses where anti-cruelty laws are nonexistent. I'll spare you the gruesome details, though you can view undercover footage online.

In addition to being used for their milk and meat, goats are also bred and killed for their hair, which goes by several names: mohair, fleece, goat wool, angora, cashmere, or Pashmina, depending on the breed being used for the desired purpose. (Angora goats produce the fiber known as mohair.) Their end is the same as all other animals used only for what we can extract from them.

ALTERNATIVES TO WOOL

Wool-free materials have been around forever, mostly because so many people are allergic to wool clothing and blankets. Check labels for cotton, cotton flannel, polyester fleece, synthetic shearling, and other cruelty-free fibers such as Tencel—breathable, durable, and biodegradable—and Polartec Wind Pro—made primarily from recycled plastic soda bottles. Olefin—also known as polypropylene, polyethylene, or polyolefin—is a synthetic fiber used to make clothing, but also rugs, upholstery, wallpaper, and car interiors.

When shopping during the winter months, it's true that many stores tout their wool and cashmere clothing lines, but many—less expensive—brands make beautiful sweaters, pants, suits, and coats using acrylic, nylon, and polyester. And, for those of you who are avid knitters, wool-free yarn is even available; look for it at big-box retailers like Jo-Ann's or search for it online.

Aside from countless mainstream retailers selling clothing made from synthetic fibers, there is a growing number of fashion designers dedicated to creating vegan and often eco-friendly clothing, shoes, and accessories, especially Leanne Mai-ly Hilgart of Vaute Couture (vautecouture.com), Stella McCartney (stellamccartney.com), and Steve Madden (stevemadden.com). Non-wool tuxedos can be found at etuxedo.com and cheaptux.com. For area rugs, many options are available and are less expensive than those made with animal hair. Check out rugsusa.com or your favorite home goods store and look for synthetic versions.

There are also a number of online bloggers dedicated to vegan fashion for both men and women, but the two go-to experts I recommend are Chloe Jo Davis of Girlie Girl Army (girliegirlarmy.com) and Joshua Katcher of The Discerning Brute (thediscerningbrute.com), who is also the brains behind Brave Gentle Man (bravegentleman.com), which is the "premiere resource for principled attire."

SILK

Many people may have a hard time including worms in their circle of compassion, but if our intention is to foster kindness rather than harm, it's a no-brainer, especially once you know that silk is obtained from silkworms by submerging them in boiling water just before the adult moths emerge.

ALTERNATIVES TO SILK

Artificial silk, namely rayon, has the same beautiful sheen and texture as that made by worms, and nylon has been used as an alternative to silk since the 1930s. Many clothing items for both men and women, including scarves, blouses, and dresses, are made from these materials. For men's suits and neckties, bowties, and ascots, check out Jaan J. (jaanj.com) or places like Men's Warehouse.

FUR

Despite losing popularity in the 1990s due to successful anti-fur campaigns by animal activists, fur has returned on runways across the globe, in large part due to efforts of the fur industry to reach out to designers. Worldwide, more than 30 million animals are killed annually on fur farms. In the U.S. alone, three million animals die on farms and another four million are trapped. Half of the fur sold in the United States is from China, where domestic dogs and cats are brutally killed for their fur. Whether they are raised in confinement or trapped in the wild, the gruesomeness of this industry is something we would all rather put out of our minds.

ALTERNATIVES TO FUR

Fur can be found as trim on parkas, sweaters, boots, and gloves or as the basis for an entire coat, and though synthetic fur is most definitely available, investigations revealed that because of a loophole in the labeling law, real fur was often mislabeled as faux fur. Because of the dedication of the Humane Society of the United States, a bill was recently signed into law that has closed this loophole. If you're unsure that a faux fur garment is indeed synthetic, you can check yourself by spreading apart the hairs to reveal the material at their base. If you see threadwork stitching from which the "hairs" emerge, it's synthetic. If you're still not certain, perhaps pass on the item.

All of Fabulous Furs (fabulousfurs.com) items are made of faux fur, and other designers and manufacturers are specializing in faux furs as well, including Charly Calder, Faux, Purrfect Fur, and Sweet Herb. Wearing faux fur is one of those tricky decisions that each person has to make on their own. On one hand, it's great for the public to see that they can be compassionate as well as trendy, but if people just assume you're wearing authentic animal fur, then you might be inadvertently promoting the fur industry.

If you have old furs you want to get rid of, check out Coats for Cubs (coatsforcubs.com), an organization which collects fur and fur-trimmed garments for donation to wildlife rehabilitators, who use the furs to provide warmth and comfort for the injured or orphaned animals under their care. Animal shelters for dogs, cats, and rabbits also accept furs to use to line the shelter cages.

The reality is we live at a time when more and more compassionate options are available to us. Convenient, affordable, and fashionable, they eliminate every excuse to purchase anything but.

Keeping it in Perspective: Intention, Not Perfection

Perhaps in these last 30 days, you've received questions from people all around you—strangers, friends, co-workers, family members—and, unfortunately, some of them may have been antagonistic. Some may have tried to undermine your decision, some may have challenged the entire concept of being vegan, some may have tried to find fault with your choices. Because many people mistakenly believe that being vegan is about being perfect, they often accuse vegans of being hypocrites and sometimes don't hesitate to point out all the areas where they are indeed imperfect.

This pressure might not even come from others; it might come from *you*. Perhaps over these last few weeks, while striving to do your best, you've accidentally eaten something that wasn't vegan and still feel bad for doing so.

Because you are looking at the world through a new lens, you may notice animal products in things you've never even thought of before. You feel guilty, you feel overwhelmed, and you feel judged by everyone around you for "not doing it right" or for "not being perfect." You just wait for the vegan police to come knocking on your door to take away your vegan status.

Let me assuage your fears: there is no such thing as a licensed, certified vegan, and if perfection and purity is what you're trying to attain in a world that is by its nature imperfect, then I'm afraid you'll be gravely disappointed. As I said in the very first chapter, being vegan is not an end in itself; it's a *means* to an end, and if we forget this, then we're missing the entire point of what it means to be vegan, whether we're doing it from a health or ethical perspective.

Unfortunately, I think this expectation of perfection is what stops many people from even trying veganism. They're afraid they're going to be expected to change everything in one fell swoop, and their fear is justified when they proudly declare to someone that they're vegan, and they're met with a smug reminder that the shoes they're wearing are made of are leather. "Ha!" they seem to say, deriving pleasure in catching you at not being perfect after all.

Whenever I've been in the situation where it seems someone's trying to *catch* me, I'm aware of what a great privilege and responsibility it is to help change the perception of what it means to be vegan. Unabashedly, I admit that I'm far from perfect and that I'm doing my very best to make a difference where I'm able.

I remind them that to not do anything because we can't do everything makes absolutely no sense. *Don't do nothing because you can't do everything. Do something. Anything.*

Some new vegans simply can't stand the thought of wearing any of the animal products that once gave them so much pleasure, and so they slowly replace them with the array of beautiful skin-free products available. Most people can't afford to do this all at once, and so they do it over time. That's *fine*. You do what you can as you're able, and you feel confident that you're doing the best you can.

> **CHALLENGE YOUR THINKING:**
> There is no such thing as a certified vegan. If perfection and purity is what you're trying to attain in this imperfect world, then you will be gravely disappointed. Being vegan is a means to an end—not an end in itself.

Whenever you're faced with this dilemma, the question to ask is, "How does keeping this leather couch, for instance, contribute to animal cruelty?" Or flip it around, "How does getting rid of it *help* animals?" As it becomes difficult to even have the couch in your home, then sell it and save for a new one. Or sell it, and donate the money to an animal organization.

The most counterproductive response is to beat yourself up for once having purchased these things. Being vegan is not about being perfect. It's about doing the best we can with the information we have at the time.

> **CHALLENGE YOUR THINKING:**
> Being vegan is about reflecting our compassion and desire for health in our actions. It doesn't mean we're going to succeed all the time, but just having the intention means we will manifest these values more often than not.
>
> **CHANGE YOUR BEHAVIOR:**
> Don't do nothing because you can't do everything. Do something. Anything.

ACCIDENTS HAPPEN

Although vegans do their best to avoid using or buying anything that came out of or off of an animal, it's neither practical nor possible to avoid animal products completely. Unfortunately, because so many billions of animals are bred, kept, and killed for our pleasure, their body parts and fluids are sold cheaply to be used as filler, fertilizer, and frills. But there is so much we *can* do to live a compassionate and healthful life.

Keeping in mind your goals—whether you're trying to avoid contributing to violence towards animals, to eat only life-enhancing rather than life-taking foods, or to reduce the use of the Earth's resource or all of these things—will help keep things in perspective when you accidentally eat something that has gelatin or eggs. Here's how I handle that situation: I write it off as an accident, and I move on. Every vegan I know has bitten into a sandwich that contained some nonvegan ingredient. Even in vegan-friendly restaurants, I've witnessed vegan friends chew on what they thought was tofu but turned out to be a piece of a chicken. I, myself, have eaten what I realized was pork after I swallowed—in both a Mexican and an Asian restaurant.

Although it's not pleasant, and it can be emotionally upsetting, accidents happen. I certainly recommend talking to the server and telling them of the mistake, and competent management will rectify the situation, but in terms of dwelling on it, there's no point. Take whatever lessons can be gleaned from the experience and utilize them for the future.

DRAWING THE LINE

Living with integrity in a world that seems to value convenience and pleasure over ethics can be challenging at best, and since we can't be perfect, we do have to draw the line somewhere. After all, the rubber in my car tires have the remnants of animals in them; I kill insects every time I walk on the ground or drive my car; many municipal water systems use animal bones as filtering agents; and white sugar and wine is sometimes refined through activated charcoal, some of which comes from animal bones. Clearly, we have to find a line to draw, or we'll drive ourselves crazy.

Some people draw that line at white sugar (choosing unrefined cane sugar or "raw" sugar/turbinado, beet sugar, sucanat, or white sugar clearly labeled "vegan," as in Whole Foods' brand). Some people draw it at honey. In fact, a great debate rages over whether honey is "vegan" or not, and I confess, it's clear to me that it's not.

I believe that one of the reasons we're in such a sorry state in terms of our relationship with and treatment of animals is because we view them as here for *us* to do with as we please. We see their flesh, skin, reproductive outputs (milk and eggs), fur, hair, bodies as here for *us* to use and consume. Of course there are natural cycles we all benefit from (bees pollinating trees enabling us to eat nuts and fruit, for instance), but that need not include taking everything animals produce and making commodities out of them.

Some people feel that honey is the deal-breaker—that many who would try to be vegan would just change their minds upon realizing they'd have to "give up honey, too." Honestly, I don't think that's what keeps people from becoming vegan. If it weren't honey, it would be something else. I just don't believe that people are *this* close to being vegan but then say, "Oh—it means I couldn't eat honey either? Well, just forget the whole thing."

I think the other aspect of the honey issue is that there is still debate as to whether keeping bees constitutes cruelty or whether bees really are harmed when their food is taken. As a result, some people argue that including honey in the fold of products that vegans avoid makes veganism seem difficult, unreasonable, rigid, or impossible. I just don't agree. If someone is already resistant to being vegan, then they will make that same argument about other animal products, too.

To me, the bottom line is that honey is not made for me, and so it's not something I eat.

Besides, honey fills no nutritional need; it's just one of many liquid sweeteners. The people who *sell* honey and its by-product "royal jelly" (secreted from the heads of bees to feed their new queen) will tell you it's a "wonder" food, which is ridiculous. We have no more need to consume the regurgitated food of bees than we do to consume the colostrum of cows, which is also sold in health food stores with promises of optimal health.

Agave nectar is a delicious plant-based liquid sweetener that has the viscosity and flavor of honey. It comes from a cactus-like plant, and if you've ever had tequila, you've had agave. For baking, you can use it for such desserts as baklava, or use it to sweeten tea. Of course, other liquid sweeteners include maple syrup, rice syrup, molasses, sorghum syrup, and barley malt, but we don't have any nutritional need for any of them either. Although many of them are touted as health food, just keep in mind that they're all sweeteners. But, when we want them as a treat, we have many choices in the plant kingdom and can live without the *one* in the animal kingdom.

KEEPING IT IN PERSPECTIVE

I was once asked by someone if I'm a "hardcore" vegan. I asked her what she meant. She said, "Do you ever cheat? Do you ever sneak a piece of cheese, or are you hardcore?" I told her that if by "hardcore" she meant, "Am I consistent?" then, by that definition, yes, I suppose I'm hardcore. Honestly, I don't think living consistently according to your values is "hardcore," but I don't think people are accustomed to meeting people who walk the walk. We tend to be surprised by someone who actually lives by their principles and convictions.

I think the other reason people tend to ask the question about "cheating" is because "veganism" has been marketed as a diet, which is associated with deprivation, restriction, temperance, cheating, abstaining, suppressing, portion controlling, losing, failing, and wagon-falling-offing. In this negative light, veganism carries the weight of being "difficult," "temporary," or "extreme."

For me, being vegan is about expansiveness and openness. Not restriction. Not limitation. Not rules. Not doctrine. I'm not *forbidden* to eat animals or their milk or their eggs. I don't *want* to eat animals or their milk or their eggs. And, there is freedom and serenity in that choice.

For me, being vegan is about living my life with intention, doing my best to avoid causing harm to another – where it's "possible and practical" to do so. Being vegan is about reflecting our compassion and desire for health in our actions. It doesn't mean we're going to succeed all the time, but just having the intention means that we will manifest these values more often than not.

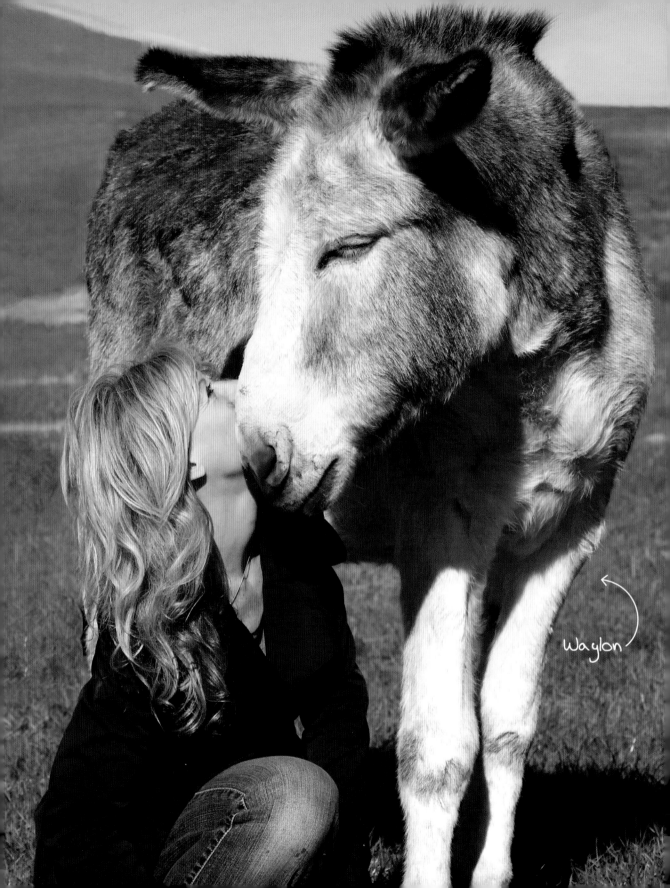

Waylon

Being a Joyful Vegan in a Non-Vegan World

My intention in writing *The 30-Day Vegan Challenge* was to provide you with the tools and resources you needed to do it for 30 days while I held your hand, answered your most pressing questions, debunked prevailing myths, and helped create a strong foundation on which to stand should you want to continue.

Giving you what you need, to eat delicious food and live as healthfully as possible is the easy part, and my hope is that this book will continue to serve as a resource and recipe guide for you long after you finish the 30 days. But, there is still much to say—about the social, ethical, and spiritual aspects of living in a world that seeks to encourage empathy, kindness, and compassion in children but seems suspicious of these same values in adults. We live in a world where human privilege and the desire for convenience and pleasure drive the socially sanctioned violence against billions and billions of nonhuman animals. We live in a world where it's considered normal to have your chest cut open and your arteries rerouted. We live in a world where it's normal to support these things and unpopular to oppose them.

The excuses people come up with to justify tradition and habit can range from the absurd to the offensive, and new vegans are often caught off guard by the defensiveness that seems to be directed toward what to them is simply a healthful, kind way for them to live. Even when the reaction isn't hostile, vegans are often asked to defend how and why they eat the way they do. Although nonvegans are never asked to explain why they eat meat, dairy, and eggs, the most common question meat-eaters ask those who don't is, "Why are you vegan?"

This can be difficult for some people to reconcile; not everyone wants to have to explain why they're vegan every time they sit down for a meal. And, I understand; just because you're vegan doesn't mean you're necessarily an activist. But, the truth is when we're the vegan someone meets, we represent *all vegans*. It's just the way it is. I realize that puts a lot of pressure on vegans, but with so many myths perpetuated about and against veganism, if we brush off people's questions or if we answer without patience and understanding, then we may be squandering an opportunity to show how positive and healthful this way of living really is.

We certainly don't have to become experts in all fields, but I do believe we have an obligation to speak our truth when someone asks us why we're vegan—not only for ourselves (and for the animals, if that's part of your story) but also for the benefit of the person asking. When someone asks me why vegan, I simply tell *my* reason for being vegan. *Your* reason may be different than mine; your *story* certainly will be, because it's your own. I understand that you may want to talk about the statistics and studies that support the health benefits of a plant-based diet, and there are many. If that's part of your story, your truth, your motivation, then express it. The power of authentically speaking from the heart is that nobody can argue with you or say "that's not true." You don't have to provide evidence or worry that you got the citation wrong. You just have to speak your truth.

I think people are often reluctant to talk about why they're vegan—especially if they're passionate about it—lest they be accused of proselytizing. But, as in other situations I described throughout this book, we have to understand where we end and another person begins. We have to be comfortable speaking up for our principles without being so afraid that someone will be upset by what we say. They may be upset by something we say, but that doesn't mean we set out to upset them. There is a difference between sharing the truth and trying to "convert" someone. There is a difference between sharing information and evangelizing. The difference has everything to do with being clear about what our intention is.

When our intention or goal is simply to plant seeds and remain unattached to the outcome, then we can't *but* succeed in having a pleasant and effective dialogue with people who inquire about our lifestyle (and they will inquire). I believe we're here to be teachers for one another, and I'm grateful for my role as a conduit, but that's all any of us are.

Don't feel so much pressure to have all the answers or speak so eloquently on behalf of a vegan lifestyle that you wind up not speaking at all. In your truth lies your eloquence. In *your* story lies someone else's. But to tell your story, you first have to remember it.

REMEMBERING OUR STORIES

In an earlier chapter, I talk about the phenomenon of nonvegans feeling threatened in the presence of a vegan because a mirror is held up to them that forces them to look at their own behavior. I call this being the "vegan in the room." But just as nonvegans need to confront this reflection and choose to either accept or reject what comes up for them, so, too do vegans need to look in the mirror when we meet someone who is still eating animal flesh and fluids and look squarely at what comes up for what it is. Is it impatience? Judgment? Self-righteousness? Arrogance? All of the above?

These reactions are understandable. When you stop eating animals, you become keenly aware of how often people are eating them, and

> **CHANGE YOUR BEHAVIOR:**
> Remember your story, and connect with like-minded people. Ask them to tell their story.

it can be very upsetting. When you look at the world through this new lens, you tend to want to shake everyone and make them see what you see. But, I guarantee that if we're pushy, hostile, angry, passive-aggressive, self-righteous, or arrogant, we *will* turn people away, and that will help neither them nor you—nor the animals.

We absolutely have to remember that we once ate animal flesh and fluids and that we, too, may have made excuses for eating them. Perhaps we even made fun of "those crazy vegans." In forgetting our own stories and our own process, we lose both our humility and the ability to be effective, compassionate spokes-people for this wonderful lifestyle.

Remember your story, and tell your story. Connect with other vegans—either online or in person, and ask them to tell their story. Creating a community of like-minded people is vital to staying a joyful vegan, but finding common ground with people who aren't where you're at yet is also essential.

LOOKING FORWARD—NOT BACKWARDS

When animals were first herded and domesticated for human use and consumption about 10,000 years ago, they became the alternatives to the plant foods that were then the foundation of the human diet. While humans ate mostly small animals and little of them, plant foods played the larger role. Thousands of years later, entrenched in an archaic animal-based agricultural system controlled by those who benefit financially, the roles have reversed. Animal-based products are dominant in most people's diets, while plant foods are regarded as side dishes or garnish.

With a determination that belies an irrational attachment to animal flesh and fluids, I've seen otherwise sensible and sensitive people spend time and energy extolling the human history of eating and domesticating animals. Using lyrical and exalted language, they wax poetic about the virtues of animal husbandry and glorify the prehistoric hunter-gatherer, who anthropologists now assert was more likely a gatherer-hunter. Still, the argument goes something like this: since early humans ate animals, we're justified in continuing to eat them now.

Some contemporary food writers even charge vegetarians and vegans with turning their backs on their "evolutionary heritage," apparently perceiving Darwinian evolution as a moral system by which we should justify our actions. By eschewing meat, they say unabashedly, we're "sacrificing a part of our identity." It seems to me that we have the ability and responsibility to make moral and rational decisions—not abdicate our ethics to an amoral process. Surely, our identities are defined by more than our paleontological past. And yet, determined to dwell perpetually on this past, these same people even romanticize the life of "cavemen" to rationalize our contemporary consumption of animals. Certainly, there are lessons to learn from our human predecessors, but do we really want to use Neanderthals as the model for our ethics? Can't we do better than that?

We often say that we want to do better than we did a generation ago, two generations ago. I presume we want to do better than we did hundreds of thousands of years ago. That's the point of being human, isn't it? To learn from our past and make better, more healthful, more compassionate choices once we know better, especially once we have the ability and opportunity to do so?

TAKING THE LONG VIEW

Having coined the word "vegan," founded the first vegan organization, and dedicated his life to inspiring a compassionate world, Donald Watson was asked in an interview a few years before he died if he had any message for the millions of people who are now vegan.

His answer was this, "Take the broad view of what veganism stands for—something beyond finding a new alternative to scrambled eggs on toast or a new recipe for Christmas cake. Realize that you're on to something really big, something that hadn't been tried until sixty years ago, and something which is meeting every reasonable criticism that anyone can level against it. And, this doesn't involve weeks or months of studying diet charts or reading books by so-called experts; it means grasping a few simple facts and applying them."

"We don't know the spiritual advancements that long-term veganism—over generations—would have for human life. It would be certainly a different civilization, and the first one in the whole of our history that would truly deserve the title of being a civilization."

May you realize you are indeed onto something really big. It's up to each one of us to reflect our deepest values in our daily choices and in doing so create the healthful, compassionate world we all imagine. If not you, then who? If not now, then when?

Share Your Experience!

Your feedback is so valuable to me and to future readers of *The 30-Day Vegan Challenge*. Please visit:

www.30dayveganchallenge.com

Click on Survey to answer a few questions about your experience reading and taking *The 30-Day Vegan Challenge!* Thank you, and I look forward to hearing from you!

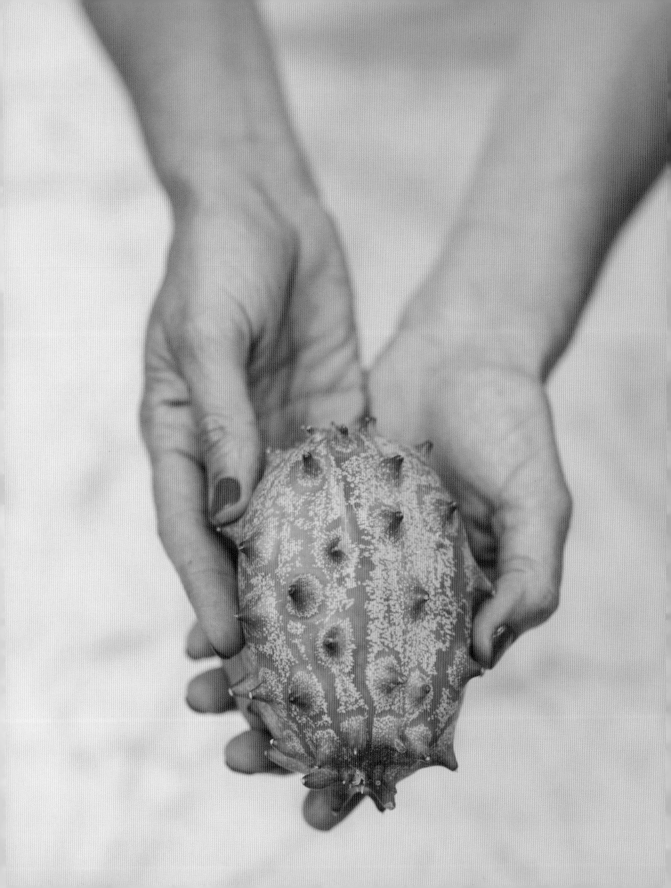

Resources for You

Here are a number of resources and recommendations for your edification and enjoyment.

VEGAN MEDICAL/NUTRITION EXPERTS

The experts below specialize in the fields of research and treatment of preventable diseases. Many of them have several or seminal books, which you can find on their websites. But I must recommend Brenda Davis, RD brendadavisrd.com first and foremost as my go-to resource. *Becoming Vegan* by Brenda Davis and Vesanto Melina is *the* bible of vegan nutrition, and their book *Becoming Raw* demystifies the questions around raw diets. Brenda vetted all of the nutrition information of this entire book, and I'm so grateful for her huge heart and brilliant mind.

Dr. T. Colin Campbell, nutritionstudies.org

Caldwell Esselstyn, MD, dresselstyn.com

Joel Fuhrman, MD, drfuhrman.com

Michael Greger, MD, drgreger.org

Michael Klaper, MD, doctorklaper.com

Vesanto Melina, RD, nutrispeak.com

John McDougall, MD, drmcdougall.com

Jack Norris, RD, veganhealth.org

Dr. Pam Popper, wellnessforum.com

Physicians Committee for Responsible Medicine, pcrm.org

STOCKING A VEGAN KITCHEN

Earth Balance butter, earthbalancenatural.com

Whole Soy & Co. yogurt, wholesoyco.com

Turtle Mountain So Delicious yogurt, ice cream, and coconut milk beverage, sodeliciousdairyfree.com

Almond Dream yogurt, tastethedream.com

Ricera yogurt, ricerafoods.com

Wildwood Organics eggless mayonnaise (aioli), yogurt, milk, tofu, tempeh, and tofu burgers, pulmuonewildwood.com

Follow Your Heart eggless mayonnaise (Vegenaise), cream cheese, salad dressings, and cheese, followyourheart.com

Nasoya tofu and eggless mayonnaise (Nayonaise), nasoya.com

Just Mayo eggless mayonnaise (Hampton Creek Foods), hamptoncreek.com

Tofurky deli slices, sausages, franks, pizza, tempeh bacon, jerky, tofurky roast, tofurky.com

Field Roast deli slices, sausages, burgers, cutlets, frankfurters, meat loaf, fieldroast.com

Gardein meatless meals and meats, gardein.com

Yves deli slices, franks, sausages, yvesveggie.com

Match Meat sausages, ground meatless meats, matchmeats.com

Rudi's Organic Bakery sliced breads, rudisbakery.com

Chicago Soydairy Temptations ice cream and Dandies vegan marshmallows, chicagosoydairy.com

Sweet and Sara vegan marshmallows sweetandsara.com

Visit peta.org/living/food/accidentally-vegan/ for more standard brands whose products happen to be vegan.

LIFE AFTER (NONDAIRY) CHEESE

Parma by Eat in the Raw, eatintheraw.com

Soymage Vegan Parmesan by Galaxy Nutritional Foods, goveggiefoods.com

Daiya, daiyafoods.com

Violife, violife.gr

Dr. Cow's aged Tree Nut Cheese, dr-cow.com

Sheese, by Bute Island Foods, buteisland.com

Teese by Chicago Vegan Foods, chicagoveganfoods.com

Better than Cream Cheese by Tofutti, tofutti.com

We Can't Say It's Cheese by WayFare, wayfarefoods.com

PLANT-BASED MILKS

There are almost too many brands to name, but here are a few.

Soy Milks: Wildwood (wildwoodfoods.com), Earth Balance (earthbalancenatural.com), Eden Soy (edenfoods.com), Soy Dream (imaginefoods.com), Vitasoy (vitasoy.com), Whole Foods 365 (wholefoods.com)

Almond Milks: Almond Breeze (almondbreeze.com), Pacific Foods (pacificfoods.com), Almond Dream (tastethedream.com), Whole Foods 365

Rice Milks: Rice Dream (imaginefoods.com), Pacific Foods

Coconut Milk (beverage and creamer): So Delicious by Turtle Mountain (sodeliciousdairyfree.com)

Hemp Milks: Tempt Living Harvest (livingharvest.com), Hemp Bliss by Manitoba Harvest (manitobaharvest.com), Pacific Foods

Coffee Creamers: Mimicreme (mimiccreme.com), Silk Creamers (silksoymilk.com), Wildwood, Trader Joe's

ATHLETES

Protein Powders: Nutiva hemp-based (nutiva.com), Nutribiotic rice-based (nutribiotic.com), Vega pea-protein (myvega.com)

Resources and community for vegan athletes: Organic Athlete (organicathlete.org), Brendan Brazier (brendanbrazier.com), Vegan Body Building (veganbodybuilding.com)

VEGAN DOG FOOD AND TREATS

V-Dog, v-dog.com

Evolution Diet, petfoodshop.com

Natural Life Pet Products, nlpp.com

Natural Balance, naturalbalanceinc.com

Nature's Recipe, naturesrecipe.com

Pet Guard, petguard.com

Boston Baked Bonz, bostonbakedbonz.com

SUPPLEMENTS

Dr. Fuhrman (drfuhrman.com) for multivitamin, vitamin D, DHA Purity, and other supplements for various stages of life. Also sold through joyfulvegan.com

O-Mega Zen3 and other supplements sold by NuTru (nutru.com)

DEVA Omega-3 DHA (devanutrition.com)

VegLife (nutraceutical.com) sold in various online stores

FINDING HARMONY IN A MIXED HOUSEHOLD

vegfamily.com

Teen's Vegetarian Cookbook by Judy Krizmanic

Help! My Child Has Stopped Eating Meat! by Carol Adams

BOOKS FOR VEGAN CHILDREN

A Turkey for Thanksgiving by Even Bunting

Herb the Vegetarian Dragon by Jules Bass and Debbie Harter

'Twas the Night Before Thanksgiving by Dav Pilkey

Victor's Picnic and *Victor, the Vegetarian* by Radha Vignola

Benji Bean Sprout Doesn't Eat Meat by Sarah Rudy

This is Why We Don't Eat Animals by Ruby Roth

Vegan is Love by Ruby Roth

Our Farm: By the Animals of Farm Sanctuary by Maya Gottfried

RECOMMENDED READING

Why We Love Dogs, Eat Pigs, and Wear Cows by Dr. Melanie Joy

Diet for a New America: How Your Food Choices Affect Your Health, Happiness and the Future of Life on Earth by John Robbins

An Unnatural Order: Roots of Our Destruction of Nature by Jim Mason

Animal Liberation by Peter Singer

Slaughterhouse: The Shocking Story of Greed, Neglect, and Inhumane Treatment Inside the U.S. Meat Industry by Gail Eisnitz

Mad Cowboy: Plain Truth from the Cattle Rancher who Won't Eat Meat by Howard Lyman

Dominion: The Power of Man, the Suffering of Animals, and the Call to Mercy by Matthew Scully

For the Prevention of Cruelty: The History and Legacy of Animal Rights Activism in the United States by Diane Beers

Food Politics: How the Food Industry Influences Nutrition and Health by Marion Nestle, chair of nutrition and food studies at NYU

World Peace Diet: Eating for Spiritual Health and Social Harmony by Will Tuttle

RECOMMENDED VIEWING

The people who work undercover to get footage of the plights of animals are unsung heroes, and the best way we can honor their work is to view what they have documented via video, audio, and still photos. Though these short videos contain footage I admit is difficult to watch, I think it is essential viewing for anyone who eats or has eaten meat, dairy, and eggs.

Many animal organizations have videos of undercover investigations available to view on their websites. Please visit humanesociety.org, farmsanctuary.org, animalplace.org, mercyforanimals.org, cok.net (Compassion Over Killing), and peta.org.

Earthlings, earthlings.com

Peaceable Kingdom, peaceablekingdomfilm.org

Vegucated, *getvegucated.com*

Cowspiracy, cowspiracy.com

Speciesism, *speciesismthemovie.com*

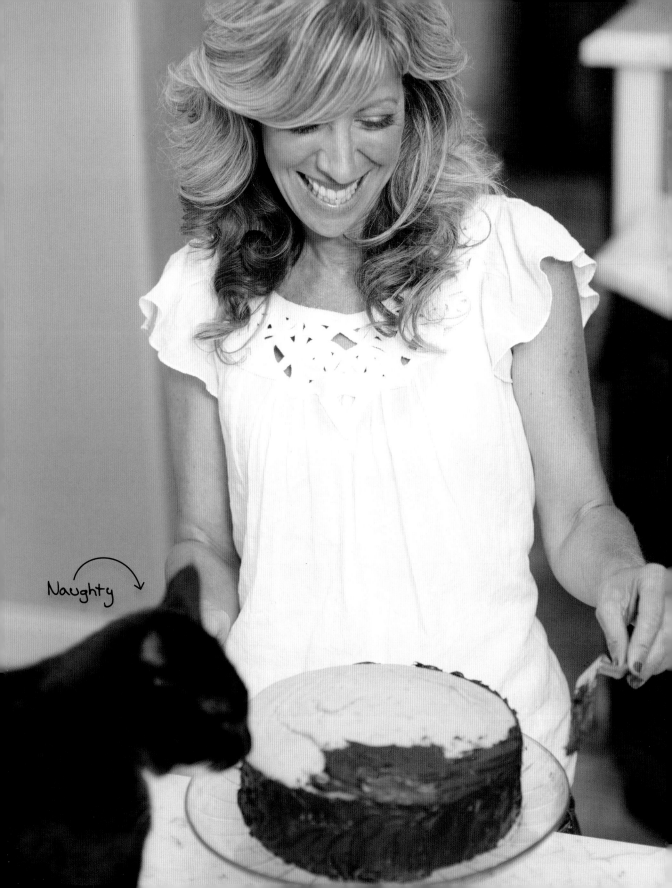

Naughty

ACKNOWLEDGMENTS

The making of a book starts with a seed that grows with the help of many hands, and I'm incredibly thankful for everyone who helped my idea for this book germinate, take root, blossom, and literally take shape. And I couldn't do any of it without the immense love and support of my beautiful husband, David Goudreau, my partner in life, love, laughter, and compassion! Each day with you is better than the one before.

Cliché as it sounds, the book you're holding in your hands would not have been published had it not been for the 1,000 individuals who funded it through our Indiegogo campaign. Contributions ranging from $1 to $2,500 poured in to put this book back on the shelves. (The original edition went out of print in 2011.) Thank you to each of you for seeing the value of this information and for enabling me to share it with the world in this form.

Thank you especially to generous contributors Tim Anderson and Dianne Waltner.

And thank you to those of you who spent hours helping me to shape, spread the word, and maintain the energy required for any crowdfunding campaign – Keegan Kuhn, Florian Radke, Kent Gustavson, Stephanie Gorchynski, and Erin Grayson.

My fairy godfathers, Alexander Gray and David Cabrera, celebrated the success of our campaign with a beautiful party in NYC at their gorgeous art gallery space, where dear friends and colleagues joyfully gathered together. I'm grateful to all who attended not only for contributing to the book's rebirth but also for their dedication to creating a compassionate world for all.

As for the making of the book itself, I'm blessed to be surrounded by so many incredibly talented, compassionate artists and advocates. The overall look and feel of the book started with Maria Villano's cover photo and the photographs of me, my hubby, and my kitties in my home. She perfectly captured what it looks like to be a joyful vegan and live a compassionate life.

Next came the food and recipe photographs of the amazing Marie Laforêt. I first connected with Marie in 2012 when she wrote to thank me for "changing her life." With information and inspiration she gleaned from my podcast, she became vegan, started a food blog, met the love of her life, and transformed her photography business to one that focuses on sustainable products, ethical businesses, and vegan living. When I looked at her photography, I knew right away that I wanted to work with her when I had the chance. As soon as I decided to publish the new edition of *The 30-Day Vegan Challenge*, I contacted Marie. All the way from France, she purchased, prepped, and shot all of the gorgeous food photographs throughout this book.

When I was looking for an intern to help me organize my own graphic-based content and photographs for my social media outlets, I didn't expect to stumble upon yet another talented (vegan) woman to join the creative team for the book. Sarah Cadwell is a Portland-based graphic designer, who has adeptly taken my written content and elevated it via a visual design that is captivating, bright, and joyful – like Sarah herself. My hope is that this book launches Sarah into the graphic design stratosphere – but only if I get to benefit from her greatness now and then.

Having found these three perfect women to graphically illustrate my content, my next task was to find an editor to proofread and perfect my text, and this superhero came in the form of a male – another vegan familiar with my work. Nat Denkin spent countless hours making sure my voice was clear and without error. I'm humbled and moved by his dedication, commitment, generosity, and skill.

When it comes to gathering the most accurate, up-to-date, unbiased nutrition information, it doesn't get better than Brenda Davis RD, who is tirelessly committed to empowering people to live compassionately and healthfully. The time, energy, generosity, and thoughtfulness Brenda brought to this book are beyond measure, as she scrupulously and expertly ensured that every nutrition-related fact lived up to the high standards we both seek to reflect in our work. I revere her as a colleague and adore her as a friend.

When it came to creating new recipes for this book, I wanted them to be completely different from my previous cookbooks but still reflect what I think characterizes all of my recipes: recognizable ingredients, ease of preparation, and familiar flavors and textures. Developing original recipes is not easy to do, and so I turned to the fabulously gifted vegan chef (and dear friend), Alicia Smiley, to create some recipes for me that I would make my own and pass onto you. After a few creative sessions discussing what my needs were, she created the White Bean Chowder, Strawberry Parfait, Homemade Almond Milk, Alfredo Sauce, Lentil Salad with Beets and Citrus Vinaigrette, Green Goddess Dressing, and the Everyday Vinaigrette. Now you will get to experience the deliciousness that is Alicia's food – even if you don't live in the San Francisco Bay Area where she tantalizes taste buds every day.

The list goes on. Julita Baker, who attended a few of my cooking classes in Oakland many years ago, was just finishing her PhD. in nutritional biology when she serendipitously re-appeared in my life as I was searching for an expert to compile the nutritional information for each recipe. She worked diligently and patiently to make sure everything was precise.

Speaking of precision, my amazing group of recipe testers helped me ensure that not only were the recipes delicious but that the directions were clear and easy to follow. I'm so grateful to them for their attention to detail, enthusiasm, and generosity: Jenn Bridge, Kathryn Bulver, Michelle Crisp, Michelle Donati-Grayman, Katharina Ikels, Erin Jeffries, Beth Morris, Danielle Puller, Kyleigh Rapanos, and Yvonne Vitt.

I'm so blessed to be surrounded by so many loving friends (you know who you are) and to have the love and support of mom Arlene, dad John, and parents-by-marriage, Mary Jane and Paul.

And what a blessing it is to live in the company of cats. Charlie and Michiko bring me immense joy every moment of every day. Courageous Simon, magical Schuster, and sweet Cassandra continue to live in my heart.

I am so incredibly thankful to have the honor and privilege of hearing from so many remarkable people whose eyes and hearts have been opened and who let me be part of their journey. Thank you to everyone who has ever listened to my podcast, read my books, used my recipes, watched my videos, or attended my talks. You are the reason I awaken with hope every day.

Thank you to each and every person who uses his or her voice to speak for those who have no voice. Whether you do it formally as part of a larger organization or on your own as a grassroots activist, every seed you plant contributes to the compassionate world we all envision.

My greatest inspirations are the nonhuman animals of the world. I dedicate my work to them, and I look forward to the day when online dictionaries don't try to replace my use of "he" and "she," and "who" to "it" and "that" when referring to these beautiful, sensitive, living, feeling beings.

For Your Inspiration

mariavillano.com

marielaforet.com

sarahcadwell.com

allwellfed.com (Alicia Smiley)

julitabaker.com

BIBLIOGRAPHY

[1] Serena Tonstad, Terry Butler, and Gary E. Fraser, "Type of vegetarian diet, body weight, and prevalence of type 2 diabetes," *Diabetes Care* 32 (2009): 791–796.

[2] Lap Tai Le and Joan Sabaté. "Beyond Meatless, the Health Effects of Vegan Diets: Findings from the Adventist Cohorts," *Nutrients* 6 (2014): 2135.

[3] Ibid.

[4] Isabel dos Santos Silva, Punam Mangtani, Valerie McCormack, Dee Bhakta, Leena Sevak andAnthony J. McMichael. "Lifelong vegetarianism and risk of breast cancer: a population-based case-control study among South Asian migrant women living in England," *International Journal of Cancer* 99 (2002): 238–244.

[5] Antonella Dewell, Gerdi Weidner, Michael D. Sumner, Christine S. Chi, Dean Ornish, "A very-low-fat vegan diet increases intake of protective dietary factors and decreases intake of pathogenic dietary factors." *Journal of the American Dietetic Association* 108 (2008): 347.

[6] Paul N Appleby, Naomi E Allen, and Timothy J Key, "Diet, vegetarianism, and cataract risk," *American Journal of Clinical Nutrition* 5 (2011): 1128–35.

[7] I. Hafström, B. Ringertz, A. Spångberg, L. von Zweigbergk, S. Brannemark, I. Nylander, J. Rönnelid, L. Laasonen, and L. Klareskog, "A vegan diet free of gluten improves the signs and symptoms of rheumatoid arthritis: the effects on arthritis correlate with a reduction in antibodies to food antigens." *Rheumatology* 40 (2001): 1175–9.

[8] Alexander Ströhle, Annika Waldmann, Maike Wolters, Andreas Hahn, "Vegetarian nutrition: preventive potential and possible risks. Part 1: plant foods," *Wiener Klinische Wochenschrift* 118 (2006): 580–93.

[9] Neal Barnard, "Seasonal Allergies," *Ask the Doc*, accessed August 13, 2014 http://www.vegetariantimes.com/article/ask-the-doc-seasonal-allergies/.

[10] N. D. Barnard, A. R. Scialli, D. Hurlock, and P. Bertron, "Diet and sex-hormone binding globulin, dysmenorrhea, and premenstrual symptoms," *Obstetrics and Gynecology* 95 (2000): 245–50.

[11] "Donald Watson: Vegan Society Founder & Patron, interview by George D. Rodger on 15 December 2002," *The Vegan*, Summer 2003, 17–18, accessed http://issuu.com/vegan_society/docs/the-vegan-summer-2003/1.

[12] Caldwell B. Esselstyn, Jr., *Prevent and Reverse heart Disease: The Revolutionary, Scientifically Proven, Nutrition-Based Cure*, (New York: Avery, 2007): 44.

[13] Metropolitan Life Insurance Company, "Ideal weights for men 1942." *Statistical Bulletin—Metropolitan Life Insurance Company* 23 (1942): 6–8.

Metropolitan Life Insurance Company, "Ideal weights for women 1943." *Statistical Bulletin—Metropolitan Life Insurance Company* 24 (1943): 6–8.[14] Mayo Clinic, "Apple and pear body shapes." *Diseases and Conditions*, accessed August 13, 2014, http://www.mayoclinic.org/diseases-conditions/metabolic-syndrome/multimedia/apple-and-pear-body-shapes/img-20006114.

[15] National Heart, Lung, and Blood Institute, "Clinical Guidelines on the Identification, Evaluation, and Treatment of Overweight and Obesity in Adults: The Evidence Report." (1998): xv, accessed July 7, 2014, http://www.nhlbi.nih.gov/guidelines/obesity/ob_gdlns.htm.

[16] The American Council on Exercise, "Percent Body Fat Calculator: Skinfold Method," accessed July 7, 2014, http://www.acefitness.org/acefit/healthy_living_tools_content.aspx?id=2.

[17] National Heart, Lung, and Blood Institute, *"Seventh Report of the Joint National Committee on Prevention, Detection, Evaluation, and Treatment of High Blood Pressure."* (2004): xiv, accessed July 7, 2014, http://www.ncbi.nlm.nih.gov/books/NBK9630/.

[18] Centers for Disease Control and Prevention, "National Diabetes Statistics Report, 2014" (2014): 1–3, accessed July 7, 2014, http://www.cdc.gov/diabetes/pubs/statsreport14/national-diabetes-report-web.pdf.

[19] U.S. National Library of Medicine and National Institutes of Health, "MedlinePlus: Glucose test – blood" accessed July 6, 2014, http://www.nlm.nih.gov/medlineplus/ency/article/003482.htm.

[20] Ibid.

[21] William P. Castelli, "Take this letter to your doctor," *Prevention* 48 (1996): 61–4.

[22] Centers for Disease Control and Prevention, "Cholesterol Facts," accessed July 7, 2014, http://www.cdc.gov/cholesterol/facts.htm.

[23] Caldwell B. Esselstyn, Jr., "Updating a 12-year experience with arrest and reversal therapy for coronary heart disease (an overdue requiem for palliative cardiology)," *American Journal of Cardiology* 84 (1999): 339–41, A8.

[24] Yuhua Sun, Yuejin Yang, Weidong Pei, Yongjian Wu, and Jinglin Zhao, "Is elevated high-density lipoprotein cholesterol always good for coronary heart disease?" *Clinical Cardiology* 30 (2007): 576–80.

[25] Mayo Clinic, "High cholesterol: Triglycerides: Why do they matter?" accessed July 6, 2014, http://www.mayoclinic.org/diseases-conditions/high-blood-cholesterol/in-depth/triglycerides/art-20048186

[26] Jack Norris, "Calcium and Vitamin D." *VeganHealth.org* last updated October 2013, accessed July 6, 2014, http://www.veganhealth.org/articles/bones#ideal+levels.

[27] United States Department of Agriculture, National Agricultural Statistics Service, "Poultry Slaughter 2013 Summary, February 2014," accessed July 7, 2014, http://www.nass.usda.gov/Publications/Todays_Reports/reports/pslaan14.pdf. The total number of animals killed includes those animals intended for slaughter, those killed while being processed, and bykill. Commercial fishing causes large numbers of fish and sea mammals to be killed en masse. Reports include the total tonnage for the desired catch is reported. The number fish killed each year is much greater than the number of land animals killed, and the number of shellfish killed is greater still.

[28] Morrisons, "Brits Stuck in a Repeat Meal Rut," (2013), accessed July 7, 2014, http://www.morrisons-corporate.com/media-centre/Consumer-news/Brits-Stuck-in-a-Repeat-Meal-Rut/.

[29] Colleen Patrick-Goudreau, *Vegan's Daily Companion: 365 Days of Inspiration for Cooking, Eating, and Living Compassionately* (Beverly, MA: Quarry Books, 2011), 175.

[30] U.S. Geological Survey, "NOAA: Gulf of Mexico 'Dead Zone' Predictions Feature Uncertainty," released June 21, 2012, accessed July 6, 2014, http://www.usgs.gov/newsroom/article.asp?ID=3252#.U7NSVPldXh4.

[31] Neal D. Barnard, Andrew Nicholson, and Jo Lil Howard, "The Medical Costs Attributable to Meat Consumption," *Preventive Medicine* 24 (1995): 646–655.

[32] Arman Kilic, Ashish S. Shah, John V. Conte, Kaushik Mandal, William A. Baumgartner, Duke E. Cameron, and Glenn J. R. Whitman,. "Understanding variability in hospital-specific costs of coronary artery bypass grafting represents an opportunity for standardizing care and improving resource use." *The Journal of Thoracic and Cardiovascular Surgery* 147 (2014): 109–116.

[33] Houston Northwest Medical Center, "Women and Heart Disease," accessed July 6, 2014, http://www.hnmc.com/en-us/ourservices/communityservices/pages/women%20and%20heart%20disease_v1.aspx

[34] Alan S. Go, Dariush Mozaffarian, Véronique L. Roger, Emelia J. Benjamin, Jarett D. Berry, Michael J. Blaha, Shifan Dai, Earl S. Ford, Caroline S. Fox, Sheila Franco, Heather J. Fullerton, Cathleen Gillespie, Susan M. Hailpern, John A. Heit, Virginia J. Howard, Mark D. Huffman, Suzanne E. Judd, Brett M. Kissela, Steven J. Kittner, Daniel T. Lackland, Judith H. Lichtman, Lynda D. Lisabeth, Rachel H. Mackey, David J. Magid, Gregory M. Marcus, Ariane Marelli, David B. Matchar, Darren K. McGuire, Emile R. Mohler III, Claudia S. Moy, Michael E. Mussolino, Robert W. Neumar, Graham Nichol, Dilip K. Pandey, Nina P. Paynter, Matthew J. Reeves, Paul D. Sorlie, Joel Stein, Amytis Towfighi, Tanya

N. Turan, Salim S. Virani, Nathan D. Wong, Daniel Woo and Melanie B. Turner on behalf of the American Heart Association Statistics Committee and Stroke Statistics Subcommittee, "Heart disease and stroke statistics—2014 update: a report from the American Heart Association," *Circulation*, 129 (2014): e30, published online December 18, 2013, accessed July 6, 2014, http://circ.ahajournals.org/content/129/3/e28.full.pdf+html.

[35] Ibid., e232.

[36] David J. A. Jenkins, Cyril W. C. Kendall, Augustine Marchie, Dorothea A. Faulkner, Julia M. W. Wong, Russell de Souza, Azadeh Emam, Tina L. Parker, Edward Vidgen, Karen G. Lapsley, Elke A. Trautwein, Robert G. Josse, Lawrence A. Leiter, and Philip W. Connelly, "Effects of a dietary portfolio of cholesterol-lowering foods vs lovastatin on serum lipids and C-reactive protein," *JAMA*, 290 (July 23, 2003): 502–10.

[37] United States Department of Agriculture, "Food Away from Home," updated November 22, 2013, accessed July 6, 2014. http://www.ers.usda.gov/topics/food-choices-health/food-consumption-demand/food-away-from-home.aspx#.U7RoJrHySrY.[38] Sean Poulter, "Fast food Britain: More than half our meals out are burgers or kebabs," *Mail Online*, January 17, 2012, accessed July 6, 2014, http://www.dailymail.co.uk/news/article-2087361/Fast-food-Britain-More-half-meals-burgers-kebabs.html.

[39] Environmental Working Group, "EWG's Shopper's Guide To Pesticides In Produce." April 29, 2014, accessed July 6, 2014, http://www.ewg.org/release/ewgs-2014-shoppers-guide-pesticides-produce.

[40] Ibid.

[41] T. Colin Campbell, "Protein—Meat and Dairy—Cause Cancer," (Lecture, VegSource Healthy Lifestyle Expo, 2005).

[42] Michael W. Robbins, *Whole Green Catalog: 1000 Best Things for You and the Earth* (New York: Rodale Books, 2009), 31.

[43] Colleen Patrick-Goudreau, *The Joy of Vegan Baking: The Compassionate Cooks' Traditional Treats and Sinful Secrets* (Beverly, MA: Fair Winds Press, 2007), 18.

[44] U.S. Food and Drug Administration, "Sodium in Your Diet: Using the Nutrition Facts Label to Reduce Your Intake," *Food Facts From the U.S. Food and Drug Administration*, July 2012, accessed July 6, 2014, http://www.fda.gov/food/ingredientspackaginglabeling/labelingnutrition/ucm315393.htm.

[45] Food and Nutrition Board, Institute of Medicine, National Academies, "Dietary Reference Intakes Essential Guide Nutrient Requirements," (2006): 529–542, accessed July 6, 2014, http://www.iom.edu/Reports/2006/Dietary-Reference-Intakes-Essential-Guide-Nutrient-Requirements.aspx. A PDF containing the summary tables is available at http://www.iom.edu/Activities/Nutrition/SummaryDRIs/~/media/Files/Activity%20Files/Nutrition/DRIs/5_Summary%20Table%20Tables%201-4.pdf

[46] Bethany A. Pribila, Steve R. Hertzler, Berdine R. Martin, Connie M. Weaver, and Dennis A. Savaiano, "Improved lactose digestion and intolerance among African-American adolescent girls fed a dairy-rich diet," *Journal of the American Dietetic Association* 100 (2000): 524–8, accessed July 7, 2014, http://www.ncbi.nlm.nih.gov/pubmed/10812376.

[47] Environmental Protection Agency, "Lifecycle Production Phases," updated June 27, 2012, accessed July 6, 3014, http://www.epa.gov/oecaagct/ag101/dairyphases.html.

[48] Marcy Lowe and Gary Gereffi, Center on Globalization, Governance & Competitiveness, Duke University, "A Value Chain Analysis of the U.S. Beef and Dairy Industries." (2009): 18, accessed July 6, 2014, http://www.cggc.duke.edu/environment/valuechainanalysis/CGGC_BeefDairyReport_2-16-09.pdf

[49] Brian Gould, Agricultural and Applied Economics, University of Wisconsin, Madison, "Dairy Cows on Farm/Dairy Cow Slaughter > Weekly Dairy Cattle Slaughtered." *Understanding Dairy Markets*, accessed July 6, 2014, http://future.aae.wisc.edu/data/weekly_values/by_area/2279.

[50] National Milk Producers Federation, "FDA Should Stop Imitation Products From Milking Dairy Terms, Says NMPF," released April 29, 2010, accessed August 13, 2014, http://nmpf.org/latest-news/press-releases/apr-2010/fda-should-stop-imitation-products-from-milking-dairy-terms-says.

[51] T. Colin Campbell, "Protein—Meat and Dairy—Cause Cancer."

[52] Physicians Committee for Responsible Medicine, "Analysis of Health Problems Associated with High-Protein, High-Fat, Carbohydrate-Restricted Diets Reported via an Online Registry," May 2004, accessed August 13, 2014, http://www.pcrm.org/health/reports/analysis-of-health-problems-associated-with-high.

[53] Robert M. Russell, and Carmen Castanada Sceppa, "How Much Protein Do You Need?" *The Doctor will see you now*. October 1, 1999, accessed July 7, 2014, http://www.thedoctorwillseeyounow.com/content/nutrition/art2059.html

[54] World Health Organization, "Micronutrient deficiencies: Iron deficiency anaemia," *Nutrition*, accessed August 13, 2014, http://www.who.int/nutrition/topics/ida/en/.

[55] National Institutes of Health Office of Dietary Supplements, "Iron Dietary Supplement Fact Sheet," April 8, 2014, accessed July 7, 2014, http://ods.od.nih.gov/factsheets/Iron-HealthProfessional/.

[56] Brenda Davis and Vesanto Melina, *Becoming Vegan*, (Summertown, TN: Book Publishing Company, 2000).

[57] Tomi-Pekka Tuomainen, Kristiina Nyyssönen, Riitita Salonen, Arja Tervahauta, Heikki Korpela, Timo Lakka, George A. Kaplan, and Jukka T. Salonen, "Body Iron Stores Are Associated With Serum Insulin and Blood Glucose Concentrations: Population study in 1,013 eastern Finnish men," *Diabetes Care* 20 (1997): 426–428, accessed July 7, 2014, http://care.diabetesjournals.org/content/20/3/426.

[58] Arch G. Mainous III, James M. Gill, Charles J. Everett, "Transferrin Saturation, Dietary Iron Intake, and Risk of Cancer," *Annals of Family Medicine* 3 (2005):131–137, accessed July 7, 2014, http://www.medscape.com/viewarticle/502752_4.

[59] Devra First, "Catch of the day?" *The Boston Globe*, July2, 2008, accessed July 24, 2014, http://www.boston.com/lifestyle/food/articles/2008/07/02/catch_of_the_day/?page=full.

[60] American Heart Association, "Homocysteine, Folic Acid and Cardiovascular Disease," updated March 18, 2014, accessed July 7, 2014, http://www.heart.org/HEARTORG/GettingHealthy/NutritionCenter/Homocysteine-Folic-

Acid-and-Cardiovascular-Disease_UCM_305997_Article.jsp.

[61] Steven Pratt, "Elaborate Study Of Rural Chinese Gives Big Points To The Health Value Of Their Plant-based Diets," *Chicago Tribune*, September 30, 1993, accessed July 24, 2014, http://articles.chicagotribune.com/1993-09-30/entertainment/9309300414_1_blood-cholesterol-china-study-cholesterol-levels.

[62] Margjie C.J.F. Jansen, H. Bas Bueno-de-Mesquita, Ratko Buzina, Flaminio Fidanza, Alessandro Menotti, Henry Blackburn, Aulikki M. Nissinen, Frans J. Kok, and Daan Kromhout, "Dietary Fiber and Plant Foods in Relation to Colorectal Cancer Mortality: The Seven Countries Study," International Journal of Cancer: 81 (1999): 174–179, accessed July 7, 2014, http://www.ncbi.nlm.nih.gov/pubmed/10188715.

[63] Colleen Patrick-Goudreau, *Color Me Vegan* (Beverly, MA: Fair Winds Press, 2010), 83.

[64] T. Colin Campbell and Thomas M. Campbell, II, *The China Study: The Most Comprehensive Study of Nutrition Ever Conducted And the Startling Implications for Diet, Weight Loss, And Long-term Health, (Dallas: BenBella Books, 2006), 145–156.*

[65] Alan Goldhamer, "Conservative Management of Diabetes," October 15, 2013, accessed August 13, 2014, http://nutritionstudies.org/conservative-management-diabetes/.

[66] Jaakko Mursu, Kim Robien, Lisa J. Harnack, Kyong Park, David R. Jacobs, "Dietary Supplements and Mortality Rate in Older Women, The Iowa Women's Health Study," *Archives of Internal Medicine*, 171 (2011): 1625–1633, accessed July 7, 2014, http://archinte.jamanetwork.com/article.aspx?articleid=1105975.

[67] United States Department of Agriculture, "2012 Census of Agriculture in Spotlight this Thanksgiving." Census of Agriculture, released November 14, 2012, accessed July 7, 2014, http://www.agcensus.usda.gov/Newsroom/2012/11_14_2012.php.

[68] American Catholic.org, "What is the Church's official position concerning penance and abstinence from meat during Lent?" accessed July 7, 2014, http://www.americancatholic.org/features/lent/lentrules.aspx.

[69] Colleen Patrick-Goudreau, *The Vegan Table: 200 Unforgettable Recipes for Entertaining Every Guest at Every Occasion* (Beverly, MA: Fair Winds Press, 2009), 198.

[70] E. A. Spencer, P. N. Appleby, G. K. Davey, T. J. Key, "Diet and body mass index in 38000 EPIC-Oxford meat-eaters, fish-eaters, vegetarians and vegans." *International Journal of Obesity and Related Metabolic Disorders.* 6 (2003): 728–34, accessed August 13, 2014, http://www.ncbi.nlm.nih.gov/pubmed/12833118.

[71] Mi Kyung Kim, Sang Woon Cho, and Yoo Kyoung Park, "Long-term vegetarians have low oxidative stress, body fat, and cholesterol levels," *Nutrition Research and Practice,* 6 (2012): 155–161, accessed August 13, 2014, http://www.ncbi.nlm.nih.gov/pmc/articles/PMC3349038/.

[72] Daniel L. Martl, Rachel J. Johnson, and Kenneth H. Mathews, Jr., "Where's the (Not) Meat? Byproducts From Beef and Pork Production," USDA report LDP-M-209-01, November 2011, accessed July7, 2014. http://www.ers.usda.gov/media/147867/ldpm20901.pdf.

RECIPE INDEX—ALPHABETICAL

RECIPE INDEX—BY TYPE

BEVERAGES

STARTERS

MAIN DISHES (BREAKFAST, LUNCH, OR DINNER)

SIDE DISHES

SOUPS

Herbed Lentil Soup	91
Smoky White Bean Chowder	89
Spicy Red Pepper Soup	102
Giambotta (Vegetable Stew)	96

SALADS / DRESSINGS / SAUCES

Broccoli Slaw	200
Coconut Peanut Sauce	146
Everyday Vinaigrette	101
Fish-Friendly Tuna Salad	141
Green Goddess Dressing	199
Lentil Salad with Beets and Citrus Vinaigrette	147
Panzanella (Bread Salad)	136
Southwestern Quinoa Pilaf	138
Spring Roll Salad	145
Waldorf Salad	51

TREATS / SNACKS / BAKED GOODS

Apple Breakfast Cake	114
Baked Oatmeal with Blueberries and Bananas	118
Chive and Black Pepper Cobbler Crust	100
Chipotle Roasted Chickpeas	139
Chocolate Gingersnaps	175
Coconut Bacon	113
Cowboy Cookies	176
Fresh Fruit Pops	179
Lemon Poppy Seed Muffins	121
Mexican Chocolate Cake	186
Strawberry Bruschetta	170
Strawberry Parfait with Vanilla Custard and Candied Almonds	180
Tiramisu	183
Truffle Popcorn	185

INDEX

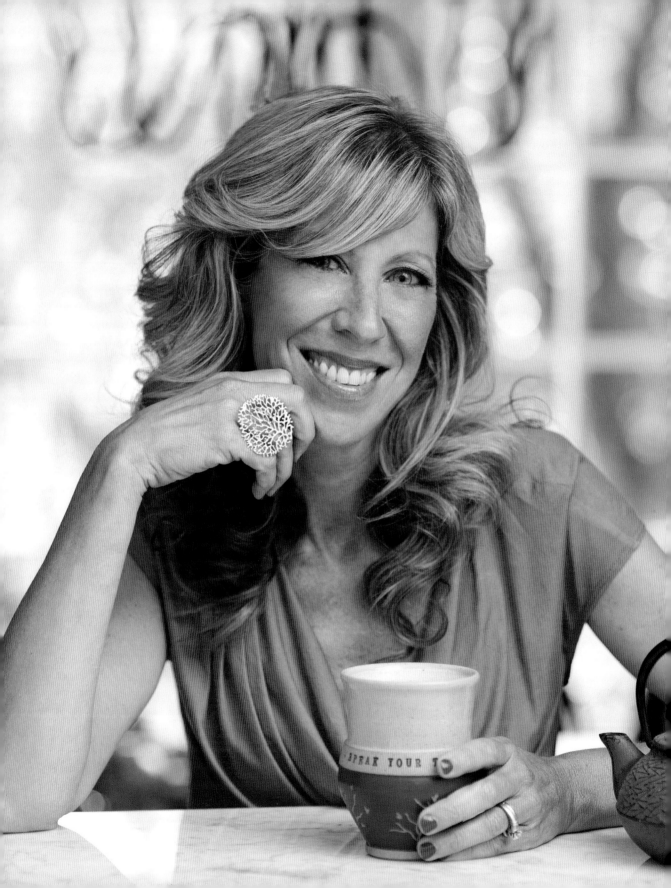

About the Author

Raised on a typical American diet of meat, dairy, and eggs, Colleen Patrick-Goudreau was moved to change when she read *Diet for a New America* at 19. No longer able to justify eating animals, Colleen began a journey of discovery that continues to this day.

For over 16 years, Colleen has guided people to becoming and staying vegan through bestselling books, inspiring lectures, engaging videos, and her immensely popular audio podcast, "Food for Thought." Using her unique blend of passion, humor, and common sense, she empowers and inspires people to live according to their own values of compassion and wellness.

With a master's degree in English literature and a command of traditional and new media, Colleen is an exhilarating speaker, a powerful writer, a talented chef, and a persuasive advocate, whose success can be measured by the thousands of people whose lives have been changed by her compassionate message that is propelling plant-based eating into the mainstream and forever changing how we regard animals.

The award-winning author of six books, including the bestselling *The Joy of Vegan Baking, The Vegan Table, On Being Vegan, Vegan's Daily Companion,* and *Color Me Vegan,* Colleen also contributes to National Public Radio and has appeared on The Food Network and PBS. She lives with her husband and feline babies in the San Francisco Bay area.

Colleen Patrick-Goudreau is available for select readings, book signings, and lectures. To inquire about a possible appearance, please visit:

joyfulvegan.com